T0276562

Current Developments in Endoscopic Surgery

Current Developments in Endoscopic Surgery

Edited by **Steven Notley**

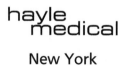

New York

Published by Hayle Medical,
30 West, 37th Street, Suite 612,
New York, NY 10018, USA
www.haylemedical.com

Current Developments in Endoscopic Surgery
Edited by Steven Notley

International Standard Book Number: 978-1-63241-101-3 (Hardback)

Printed in the United States of America.

Contents

Preface

This book has been an outcome of determined endeavour from a group of educationists in the field. The primary objective was to involve a broad spectrum of professionals from diverse cultural background involved in the field for developing new researches. The book not only targets students but also scholars pursuing higher research for further enhancement of the theoretical and practical applications of the subject.

Endoscopy has simplified medical diagnosis. Surgeons from varied domains have become extremely interested in endoscopy due to its low complication rates, high analytic yields and the opportunity to carry out a large diversity of therapeutic techniques. In the past few decades, the variety of surgical endoscopic methods has developed with many new techniques for both analysis and management, and these developments are presented in this book. It discusses the applications of endoscopic surgery in various areas such as the skull base, paranasal sinuses, the central nervous system and ophthalmology. Contributing to the expansion of endoscopic surgery around the world, this is a contemporary, informational, and interesting book.

It was an honour to edit such a profound book and also a challenging task to compile and examine all the relevant data for accuracy and originality. I wish to acknowledge the efforts of the contributors for submitting such brilliant and diverse chapters in the field and for endlessly working for the completion of the book. Last, but not the least; I thank my family for being a constant source of support in all my research endeavours.

Editor

Part 1

Endoscopy of the Paranasal Sinuses and the Skull Base

Endoscopic Endonasal Skull Base Surgery: Current State of the Art and Future Trends

Jouanneau Emmanuel, Messerer Mahmoud
and Berhouma Moncef
Department of Neurosurgery
Skull Base Surgery Unit Pierre Wertheimer
Neurological and Neurosurgical Hospital
Lyon
France

1. Introduction

Endoscopic endonasal skull base surgery (EESBS) is undergoing a remarkable evolution as in the last two decades it shifted from pituitary surgery to a myriad of approaches extending from the cribriform plate to C2 and laterally to the petrous apex and to the infratemporal fossa. The collaboration with ENT surgeons, technological advances in the field of instrumentation and endoscopic systems, a better comprehension of the skull base anatomy as seen from below and recent innovations in reconstruction techniques have led to obvious improvements in the management of cranial base lesions. EESBS is now becoming the gold-standard approach to the sellar, retrosellar and clival regions; however, its role in the management of anterior skull base tumors is still debated.

Through their experience of more than 400 endoscopic endonasal skull base procedures, the authors expose their modus operandi and discuss the current controversies as well as future trends.

2. A brief history of endoscopic procedures in neurosurgery

EESBS represents the recent meeting of endoscopic techniques, developed mainly by urologists, and pituitary transsphenoidal surgery.

2.1 First endoscopes

Endoscopic explorations of hollow organs appeared during the 19th century. A German physician, Philipp Bozzini (1773-1809), is considered as the inventor of the first endoscope which he named "*Lichtleiter*" (Figure 1, left). The latter was very difficult to handle and painful for the patients. Jean Desormeaux (1815-1894), a renowned French urologist, improved Bozzini's *Lichtleiter* using all the advances made during the second half of the 19th century in the fields of lighting (Castelnuovo et al., 2010a; Leger, 2004). The development of optic lenses led to the ergonomy optimization and the manoeuvrability improvement of endoscopes used mainly by urologists such as Max Nitze (1848-1906) (Herr, 2006; Litynski, 1999; Rathert, 1967). Paradoxically, the first ventricular neuroendoscopy with cauterization of choroid plexuses has been performed by an American urologist, Victor Darwin Lespinasse (1878-1946) (Grant JA, 1996), followed during the first half of the 20th century by Walter Dandy, one of the leading pioneers of neurosurgery (Dandy, 1926, 1932). Numerous improvements of optical systems made during the first half of the 20th century led to the modernization of endoscopic procedures. ENT surgeons like Messerklinger, Draf and Stammberger developed these endoscopic techniques in the management of paranasal sinuses diseases (Draf, 1973; Reuter, 2000; Wigand, 1981). After being used initially for cerebral third ventriculostomy, endoscopy changed dramatically the approach to the pituitary region at the end of the last century and initiated neurosurgeons to endoscopic endonasal skull base surgery.

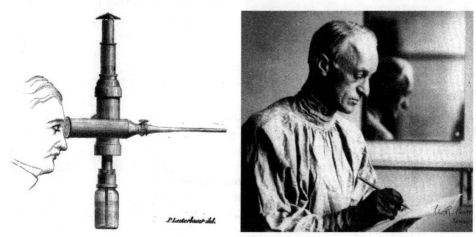

Fig. 1. Left: The "*Lichtleiter*", first endoscope designed by Philipp Bozzini (1773-1809)

Right: Harvey Cushing (1869-1939), the pioneer founder of the transsphenoidal pituitary surgery

2.2 Pituitary surgery
Modern pituitary surgery began with Harvey Cushing (Figure 1, right) during the early years of the 20th century, with the development of the sublabial transsphenoidal approach (Figure 2) and the use of a frontal light (Cushing, 1909). The initial poor results of this technique and the reduced visualization of the sella led to abandon the transsphenoidal route in favor of the transcranial approaches (Caton, 1893; Landolt, 2001; Lindholm, 2007; Pollock et al., 2003).

Gerard Guiot induced a rebirth of the trans-sphenoidal surgery in the middle of the last century with the introduction of the peroperative fluoroscopy and he first used an endoscope within the sella (Guiot et al., 1963a, 1963b). Later, Jules Hardy normalized the current pituitary surgery practice with the use of the operative microscope (Hardy, 2010; Liu et al., 2001). The application of endoscopic techniques in pituitary surgery and then in skull base surgery started progressively in the late 1980's before experiencing an exponential success during the last decade (Carrau et al., 2001).

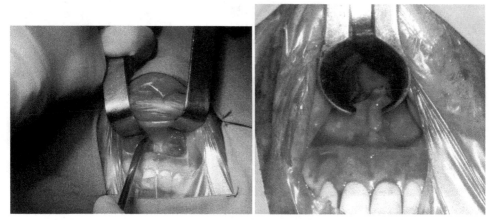

Fig. 2. Classical sublabial trans-sphenoidal microsurgical approach for pituitary adenomas.

3. Endoscopic endonasal anatomy of the skull base

The point of this section is to give the reader the main anatomical landmarks the surgeon has to deal with when using endonasal approach to the skull base (for more detailed and specific anatomical considerations, readers are invited to consult the references list at the end of this chapter).

3.1 Nasal fossa

The nasal cavity is marked medially by a rigid structure, the septum (S) (association of the perpendicular plate of the ethmoidal bone on the superior aspect, the vomer on the inferior aspect and anteriorly the quadrangular cartilage), and laterally by three longitudinal folds named the turbinates or conchae. Posteriorly both choanae (Ch) give access to the cavum. Placed immediately at the entry and below, the first seen turbinate is the inferior turbinate (IT) attached to the ethmoidal bone. Up, above and more posterior is the middle turbinate (MT), a part of the ethmoid (Figure 3, left).

The head of the middle turbinate is free and may be pneumatised (concha bullosa) and then narrows the surgical corridor (in such cases its complete or partial resection may be required). Septal deviation or spines can also complicate the surgical approach and have to be studied scrupulously on the preoperative imaging. During the nasal step, the middle turbinate has to be pushed gently aside laterally placing a spatula up to its posterior part (Figure 3, right). Caution will be taken when mobilizing those turbinates to avoid any skull base fracture and CFS leaks. Thereafter, the superior turbinate and medially the sphenoid ostium will appear (Figure 3). This key landmark is the entry point to the sphenoid sinus, placed about one and a half centimeter above the choanae (Ch). A branch of the sphenopalatine artery, the posterior nasal artery (dotted red arrow) passes just below to the sphenoid ostium to join the septum and may be cauterized to avoid postoperative nasal hemorrhages.

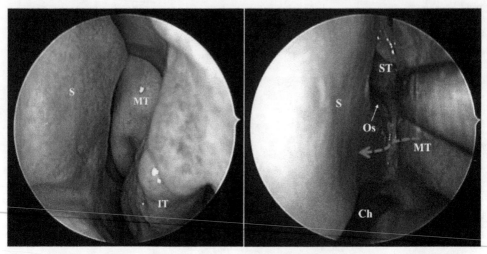

Fig. 3. Nasal step of a left endoscopic endonasal approach: Middle (MT) and inferior (IT) turbinates with the nasal septum (S) on the midline. Note the sphenoid ostium (Os) boarded by the posterior nasal branch of the sphenopalatine artery and superiorly the superior turbinate (ST)

3.2 Sphenoid sinus

The degrees of pneumatization of the sphenoid sinus and its septa have numerous variations which have to be studied on the preoperative MRI and/or CT-Scan. More often, the sphenoid sinus is largely pneumatized (sellar type). After removing the septa, the following landmarks are identified (Figure 4):
- Up and anteriorly the tuberculum of the sella (TS) and the planum (Planum)
- Centrally, the sella and the pituitary fossa.
- Laterally and up the optic nerve, paraclinoid carotid processes (C5) and the medial (OCR med) and lateral (OCR lat) opticocarotid recesses.
- Laterally, the anterior wall of the cavernous sinus and below the paraclival carotid processes (C3).
- Below the clivus corresponding posteriorly to the brainstem.

3.3 Perisellar anatomy
3.3.1 Parasellar compartment

Opening up laterally both sphenoid recesses gives access to the superior orbital fissure and straight below to the infratemporal fossa (Figure 5). After removing the bone, passing laterally and below to the cavernous sinus, the surgeon can get access to Meckel's cave with the V2 and V3 branches of the trigeminal nerve (Alfieri et al., 2001a, 2001b; Rivera-Serrano et al., 2010).

An important key for safer surgery of this area is to perfectly control the internal carotid artery (ICA). Within a sphenoid sinus of sellar type, the paraclival segment C3 is usually directly visible into the sinus just below and laterally to the sella as shown in figure 5. It is much more difficult to individualize the C2 segment of the ICA which can be retrieved following the vidian nerve in its canal (Figure 5, right) (Prevedello et al., 2010).

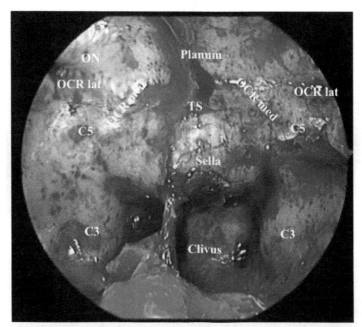

Fig. 4. Endoscopic operative view of the sphenoid sinus. Internal carotid arteries (paraclival segment C3, paraclinoid segment C5); right optic nerve: ON; Opticocarotid recesses medial (OCR med) and lateral (OCR lat).

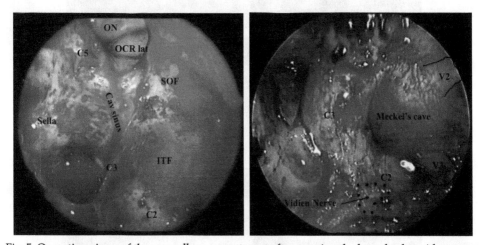

Fig. 5. Operative views of the parasellar compartment after opening the lateral sphenoid recesses.

Left (bone wall preserved): Optic nerve (ON); internal carotid artery (ICA) paraclinoid segment C5, paraclival segment C3, petrous segment C2; lateral opticocarotid recess (OCR lat); superior orbital fissure (SOF); infratemporal fossa (ITF); cavernous sinus (Cav sinus).
Right: the bone has been removed especially on the ITF exposing the Meckel's cave and the branches V2 and V3 of the trigeminal nerve.

3.3.2 Transplanum approach anatomy

Opening the sella with its tuberculum and the planum provides an access to the suprasellar cistern and the optic tract. The C6 segment of the ICA and the ON will be seen laterally as well as the pituitary stalk posteriorly. Above the optic chiasm are the anterior cerebral arteries and on the midline the anterior communicating artery (Figure 6).

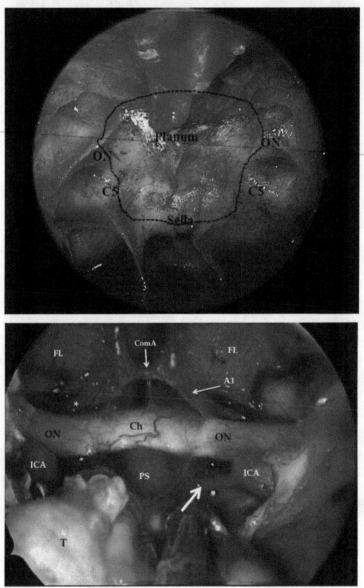

Fig. 6. Endoscopic endonasal resection of a tuberculum sellae meningioma through a transplanum transtubercular approach.

Up: Sphenoid sinus and bone aperture (dotted line). Internal carotid artery (ICA) C5; optic nerve (ON).

Down: Intradural dissection: meningioma (T); optic nerves (ON), the chiasm (Ch), the pituitary stalk (PS), the internal carotid arteries (ICA), the A1 artery (A1) and Heubner artery (*), the anterior communicating artery (ComA) and frontal lobes (FL). A useful mark to find the PS when removing a tumor is to follow the ICA and until after the superior hypophyseal arteries (SHA, white arrow) which always lead to the PS.

3.3.3 Transclival - transodontoid approach anatomy

Going through the choanae and below to the sphenoid sinus (white dotted arrow, figure 7 left) gives access to the cavum. An important landmark is the Eustachian tube as the ICA passes laterally very closely (Alfieri, 2002). The mucosa can be opened as a flap that can be placed in the cavum during the surgery. After removing the lower third of the clivus bone as well as the anterior arch of C1 and the odontoid process, an intradural and anterior access of the brainstem is easily obtained, making the removal of lesions located in this critical area possible (Cavallo et al., 2007).

Drawing a line from the nasal bone to the palatine one (Kassam's line, orange line, figure 7 left) gives the surgeon a good evaluation of how far he can go inferiorly by an endonasal approach (usually odontoid process and upper part of C2).

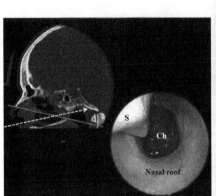
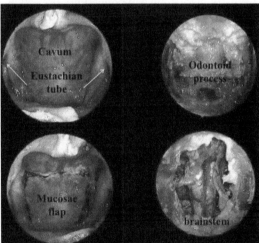

Fig. 7. Anatomic views of the endonasal approach to the clivus and cranio-cervical junction.

4. Operative characteristics, anesthetic considerations and instrumentation

4.1 Preoperative protocol

Preoperative craniofacial CT-Scan and MRI (Gardner et al., 2008) are systematically done as well as endocrinological assessment for sellar or perisellar tumors and ophthalmological examination. For cavernous sinus or Meckel's cave tumors, a cerebral angiography with occlusion tests is mandatory to avoid any unacceptable peroperative arterial occlusion in case of vascular injury during the surgery (vascular occlusion, clipping alone or associated with extra-intracranial anastomosis).

The preoperative protocol includes polyvidone shower and nasal disinfection with polyvidone cream, the day before surgery, and also on the morning of surgery. For extended approaches, vaccines against pneumococcus, meningococcus and haemophilus are usually used to prevent postoperative meningitis risk, whenever possible.

4.2 Anesthetic considerations

Specific considerations for anesthesia have to be tailored to endonasal endoscopic surgery, as well as to the extent of the approach (Ramachandran et al., 2011).

Under general anesthesia, an orotracheal intubation is used, with the tube placed on the left side. Invasive blood pressure monitoring is discussed with the surgeon, depending on the invasiveness of the approach and the vascularization of the tumor.

A bloodless surgical field is of paramount importance to the neurosurgeon. Many means help to achieve this goal: preoperative planning with rigorous study of the vasculature of the tumor, which may be embolized, total intravenous anesthesia (TIVA) with propofol and short-acting opioids, the use of sympathetic blockers as hypotensive agents, the use of diluted adrenalin-soaked pledgets before endoscope introduction.

In selected cases of extended endoscopic approaches, direct submucosal infiltration with diluted adrenalin (or other vasoconstrictor) may be useful to minimize peroperative bleeding especially if a nasoseptal flap is planned.

The use of peroperative hypopharyngeal packing should be systematic to avoid the pooling of blood and to minimize the risk of postoperative vomiting related to intragastric blood accumulation.

4.3 Dedicated instrumentation and operative room organization

Our endonasal endoscopic technique is derived from the one described by Jho (Jho & Carrau, 1997) and Cappabianca (Cappabianca et al. 1998).

Zero, 30° and more rarely 45°, 4 mm diameter rigid endoscopes are currently used during the surgery, the short one (18 cm) for the nasal step and the longer one (30 cm) during the tumor removal stage. For pediatric patients or for narrowed nostrils, small endoscopes (2.7 mm of diameter) have been designed.

The endoscope column is composed of a HD screen and camera, a Xenon light with an automated irrigation system to clean the endoscope during surgery without removing the endoscope.

Kassam, Cappabianca and Frank have designed dedicated sets of instrumentation (Storz®). High-speed bone drills and a mucosal automated shaver are useful. A microprobe Doppler is also used for extended approaches and for some specific pituitary surgery to localize accurately the nasoseptal flap pedicle or to individualize internal carotid arteries.

The neuronavigation system with CT-scan/MRI fusion is used for almost all our surgeries with a major role for recurrent tumors or when extended transbasal approaches have to be performed to remove intradural tumors.

The operative room organization is depicted in figure 8. The patient is in a supine position, the trunk slightly elevated (30°) with the head flexed up and turned to the right side to face the surgeon (figure 9). We prefer to raise both the trunk and the head so that the blood accumulates into the sphenoid sinus, falling down into the cavum during surgery to improve the visualization. This position also enables a better venous drainage from the head and less peroperative venous bleeding. A real supine position is preferred for anterior skull base tumors and a more flexed position when dealing with clival tumors.

Nevertheless, other teams work with a strict supine position whatever the type of surgery and strictly at the head of the patient. The lateral side of the right thigh is systematically draped in case of fascia lata and/or fat are needed for closure in specific cases of peroperative CSF leaks.

During the patient's positioning and after disinfection with polyvidone iodine, cotton pledgets soaked with diluted adrenalin and lidocain are placed on both nostrils. Those cottons, kept in place several minutes, allow retraction of the middle turbinate and minimize the bleeding during the nasal step.

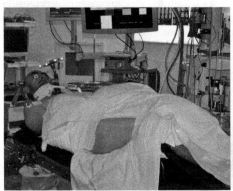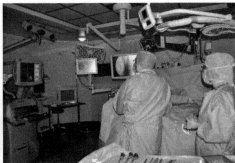

Fig. 8. Left: Patient's positioning. Right: Room organization with the neuronavigation system on the left surgeon's side and on the right the endoscopic screen. The scrub nurse is placed beside the surgeon and the anesthesiologist at the patient's left side.

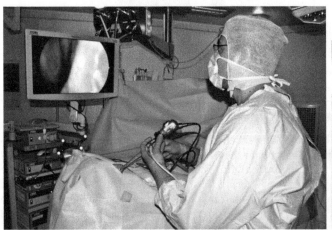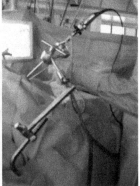

Fig. 9. Endoscope holding. Left: initial naso-sphenoidal step with a handed short endoscope. Right: Skull base opening and further steps with a rigid arm fixed to the operating table to hold the long endoscope. This allows a two hands working as with microscope. The tools are most of time introduced below the endoscope.

4.4 Surgical steps
4.4.1 Regular procedure for pituitary surgery

The choice of the side of the nasal fossa to be used is determined by the nasal anatomy (septal deviation, megaturbinate…), lateral extension (contralateral approach to a lateral extension) and size of the tumor (binostril approach for large tumors).

In most cases of pituitary adenomas, a unilateral approach is used except for large tumors. The entire endonasal procedure until the opening of the sellar floor is performed with a hand-held short 0° angle endoscope (4 mm, 18 cm, Karl Storz®, Tuttlingen, Germany). The superior and middle turbinates are identified and gently pushed laterally aside. It is very rare to have to remove the middle turbinate except in the case of hypertrophy as in some cases of acromegalic patient. The mucosa from the sphenoidal ostium to the choanae at the base of the vomer is coagulated and thereafter opened up pushing away the vomer until the contralateral ostium appears (figure 10). A large sphenoidotomy is performed by removing the posterior part of the vomer and the sella turcica aperture is done by performing a small bone flap from one cavernous sinus to the other, and from the tuberculum of the sella to the clivus with bone scissors (figure 11). This bone flap, kept in place at the bottom of the sphenoid sinus during the surgery, is used at the end of the surgical procedure to close the sella.

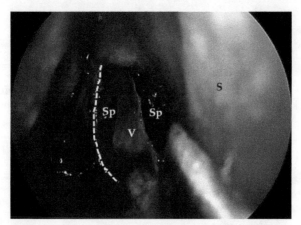

Fig. 10. Anterior sphenoidotomy via a right endonasal route. A 1 cm mucosa aperture (dotted white line) is done vertically after cauterization. After a sub-mucosa dissection pushing aside the bone septum (S), the vomer (V) appears and has to be removed to achieve the opening of the sphenoid sinus (Sp).

After opening of the dura mater, a long 0° endoscope (4 mm, 30 cm) fixed on a table-mounted endoscope holder is placed up into the nostril thus allowing the use of both hands for tumor dissection and removal (figure 9, right). The surgical tools are passed through the nose below the endoscope. Other teams work with four hands (neurosurgeon with ENT surgeon), an assistant playing the role of a smart holder. The latter can move freely to help more efficiently the operator without losing time but this needs 2 surgeons of the same level of experience, a condition not available in all institutions.

Adenomas are removed using a piecemeal technique similar to that used with microscopic surgery. In rare cases of firm adenomas, an en bloc removal with an extracapsular dissection may be used. At the end of the procedure, the sellar and suprasellar regions are explored using 0°, 30° and rarely 45° endoscopes pushed up within the sella turcica (figure 11).

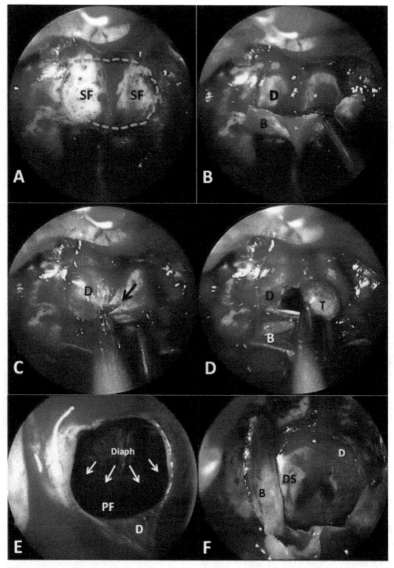

Fig. 11. Steps of the endoscopic endonasal approach to pituitary non-functioning adenoma.
A: Exposition of the sphenoid sinus and the sellar floor (SF)
B: Sellar floor craniotomy leaving a bone flap (B) and exposing pituitary dura (D)
C: Dural (D) opening with a blade knife
D: Piece-meal removal of the adenoma (T) with ring curettes
E: End of removal allowing a drop of the sellar diaphragm (Diaph) and verification of the vacuity of the pituitary fossa (PF)
F: End of the procedure after verification of the hemostasis, interposition of dural substitute (DS) before closure of the bony sellar floor (B)

A jugular compression is applied by the anesthesiologist at the patient's neck to detect a CSF leak before closure. Except in the case of a huge fistula, our preference is to avoid any plugging of the sella to facilitate the analysis of postoperative MRI. The closure technique did not differ from the one used during microscopic surgery with a combination of a dura mater substitute placed extradurally and covered by the bone flap embedded in fibrin glue. Should a peroperative CSF leak occurred, additional autologous material such as fat or fascia lata will be placed respectively into the sella and the sphenoid sinus with postoperative CSF lumbar drainage or puncture performed. The repositioning of the middle turbinate without any nasal packing ends the procedure.

4.4.2 Extended approaches

For anterior skull base tumors, a mucosa nasoseptal flap pediculated on the sphenopalatine artery or its posterior nasal branches is usually prepared and pushed down into the cavum during the surgery (Hadad et al., 2006). A Doppler probe can be used to find and keep intact the posterior nasal branches of the sphenopalatine artery which vascularize the mucosa flap. For suprasellar or retrochiasmatic tumors, an opening of the sella and the tuberculum of the sella is sufficient to expose the tumors as well as both the ICA and the optic tract. The surgeon may have to keep in mind that the wider the opening is, higher is the risk of postoperative CSF leak. We always try to perform a bone flap as we do for adenomas, to restore a rigid bone plane for the closure time. The dura mater is therefore incised on both parts of the anterior intercavernous sinus. The latter is coagulated, while small clips are placed on both extremities to prevent bleeding. The intradural time does not differ much from that of regular microsurgery.

Closure time is essential. A multilayer technique (refer to the closure paragraph), restoring all the anatomic planes, has to be done meticulously. Fibrin glue is injected onto the intradural space to seal the arachnoid. Others authors prefer to fill up the cavity with fat. Two layers of a bio-absorbable dura are thereafter placed extradurally and the bone flap flips back on the aperture sealed with fibrin glue. The mucosa flap is placed in such a manner to cover entirely the bone defect and glue is injected over to reinforce the watertight of the closure. A last layer with fat and/or fascia lata is finally used to fill up the sphenoid sinus. To prevent any layer migration during the first hours and days after surgery, an inflatable balloon can be placed inside the sphenoid sinus but only for patients who can be woken up rapidly to have their vision checked.

The same steps are respected for a transcribriform or transplanum surgery, the extension of the bone removal particularly the ethmoidectomy is dictated by the tumor extension and facilitated by the use of neuronavigation.

For parasellar approaches, after preparing the nasoseptal flap (if an intradural time or a CSF leak are expected), a lateral opening of the sphenoid sinus recess on the side of the lesion is done. The optic canal, the superior orbital fissure and orbital apex, the infratemporal fossa (behind, are Meckel's cave and the petrous apex) and medially, the cavernous sinus can be exposed, after opened up the bone, by drilling or with punches (Cebula et al., 2010). Working close to the cavernous sinus and to the Meckel's cave will require a proximal and distal control of the ICA from the C2 to the C5 segments. The C2 segment and the genu of the ICA at the foramen lacerum can be exposed following the vidian canal.

For transclival approaches, anatomical landmarks have been described previously. A midline access from the upper clivus to the superior part of C2 is possible and provides a useful corridor to the tumors located anteriorly to the brainstem.

4.5 Postoperative management

Extended approaches with grafts and/or recovering flaps are the only approaches requiring postoperative nasal packing. The latter may be uncomfortable and painful.

If a balloon is used at the end of the surgery to maintain the grafts, it will usually be remove after 3 to 5 days, depending on the degree of skull base bone removal.

Patients are asked to avoid nose blowing as well as any activities that may raise intracranial pressure for 2 or 3 weeks after surgery and not to wash their nostrils during the first week.

To avoid germ selection, we do not give any antibiotics postoperatively whatever the type of surgery (whether extended approach or not, with or without CSF leak).

After an extended approach with CSF cisterns' opening (or after a moderate to major CSF leak during adenoma surgery), a 3 to 5 days lumbar puncture or drainage is systematically done to prevent a permanent nasal CSF fistula. The first few days after the skull base reconstruction are critical but CSF leak can be observed as much as 8 to 10 days after surgery. In our own experience, there were very few problems thereafter. Thus, the patient is usually discharged on day 4 for pituitary surgery but not before day 8 for extended approaches.

For sellar or perisellar tumors surgery, blood and urinary parameters are closely monitored for 4 days following surgery to detect diabetes insipidus. Corticosteroids hormone substitution is kept until the results of the postoperative hormonal assessment.

It may be useful to control nasal healing under local anesthesia, washing and removing crusts for 2 or 3 weeks after surgery especially for extended approaches.

5. Classification of endoscopic endonasal approaches to skull base

Endoscopic endonasal skull base surgery (EESBS) was initially dedicated to treat anterior and middle skull base CSF leaks, mainly by ENT surgeons but also neurosurgeons. During the 1990's, EESBS indications extended to pituitary surgery and to anterior skull base tumors, parasellar tumors and clival lesions (figure 12), shifting to what is now called extended EESBS (Kassam et al., 2006, 2007a, 2007b, 2008; Schwartz et al., 2008). Even if it is very attractive because it is considered as less invasive and adds new routes for deeply located tumors, these techniques are limited by a long learning curve (Snyderman et al., 2007, 2008) and many closure challenges.

5.1 CSF leaks and skull base defects

Since the publication by Dandy in 1926, in which he reported the repair of a cranio-nasal fistula through a frontal craniotomy, few advances have been described in this field, until Malte Erik Wigand, a German ENT surgeon, opened the way to endoscopic endonasal skull base fistulas' management in the early 1980's (Hirsch, 1952). Nowadays, endoscopic endonasal approach is the gold standard in this field, regarding anterior, middle or posterior skull base defects (Castelnuovo et al., 2007, 2008; Martin & Loehrl, 2007; Nyquist et al., 2010). Closure techniques have recently benefited from biomaterial innovations (synthetic dura, fibrin glue) and pediculated flaps, and help to deal with closure issues in tumoral pathologies managed by EESBS.

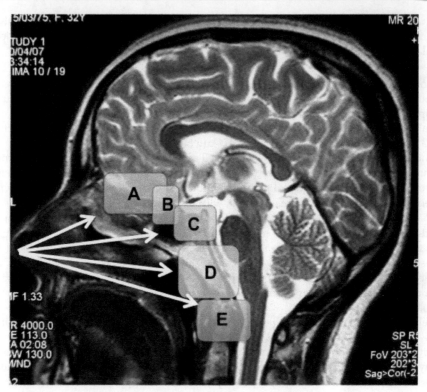

Fig. 12. Sagittal classification of endoscopic endonasal corridors.
A: Transcribriform transethmoidal
B: Transtubercular transplanum
C: Transsphenoidal sellar
D: Transclival
E: Transodontoid

5.2 Endoscopic endonasal pituitary surgery

The immediate position of the pituitary fossa posterior to the sphenoid sinus naturally led to the widespread use of the transsphenoidal route either by sublabial or by nasal corridors. One must keep in mind the pioneering influence of the Pittsburgh school (Jho and colleagues) and Neapolitan school (Paolo Cappabianca and colleagues) among others in the development of the endonasal endoscopic pituitary surgery during the last 2 decades (Cappabianca et al., 1998; Jankowski et al., 1992; Jho et al., 1996, 1997). Nowadays, this approach is becoming the first-line technique and most of pituitary surgeons are shifting to the endoscopic technique because of the excellent visualization of supra and para-sellar compartments it provides and a painless shorter postoperative course. Despite the absence of randomized studies proving definitely the superiority of endoscopic surgery upon microsurgery, the recent literature is accumulating evidence in favor of endoscopy especially for non-functioning pituitary adenomas (Dehdashti et al., 2008; Kassis et al. 2009 ; Frank et al., 2006, Higgins et al., 2008; Messerer et al., 2011; Schaberg et al., 2010). The rate of gross total removal is definitely higher in endoscopic series than in microscopic ones, for such adenomas. Data regarding functional adenomas are still debated and it seems that their results are at least comparable if not better with endoscopy (D'haens et al., 2009; Har-El, 2005).

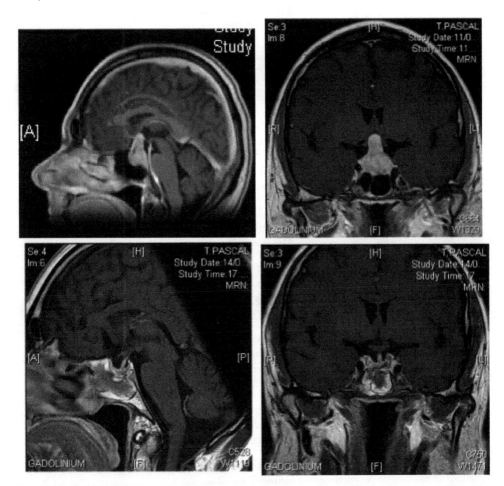

Fig. 13. Complete resection of non-functioning pituitary adenoma by endonasal endoscopic approach. Preoperative (up) and postoperative (down) MRI, T1 sequence with gadolinium.

It is important to consider that anatomic training in the lab followed by a regular practice of pituitary surgery is the first step towards endoscopic technique. The first level in the learning curve is obviously dealing with extradural cases, which have less closure and vascular issues. Surgeons will also have to learn to work with a 2D system and to watch a screen. After having gathered enough experience, (roughly more than 100 cases of endoscopic pituitary surgery according to almost all the renowned endoscopic experts), the training of the surgeon will enable him to perform further operations such as intradural works and extended approaches (Snyderman et al., 2007).

5.3 Extended endoscopic endonasal surgery

Anterior skull base	Olfactory groove meningioma Planum sphenoidale meningioma Tuberculum sellae meningioma Ethmoidal carcinoma Nasopharyngeal fibroma Esthesioneuroblastoma
Sellar and suprasellar regions	Diaphragm sellae meningioma Pituitary adenomas Craniopharyngiomas Rathke cleft cyst Inclusion tumors (epidermoids, dermoids, teratomas) Germinal tumors Suprasellar tumor, "(biopsy)"
Meckel's cave	Chondrosarcoma and Chondroma Trigeminal schwannoma Metastasis (biopsy in case of doubt)
Cavernous sinus	Extension of pituitary adenoma or of others soft tumors such as chondrosarcomas Meningioma or metastasis (biopsy in case of doubt)
Orbital apex and optic canal	Orbital tumor located medially to the optic nerve (biopsy or resection) Exophtalmos Canal optic decompression
Petrous apex and clivus	Chordoma Chondroma and chondrosarcoma Epidermoid cyst Meningiomas
Anterior craniocervical junction	Rheumatoid pannus Spondylodiscitis Malformative anomaly Bone tumors Chordoma

Table 1. Topographical classification of skull base lesions accessible to EESBS

5.3.1 Anterior skull base neoplasms

Meningiomas remain the more frequent neoplasms in this region, arising between the crista galli process and the tuberculum of the sella (Fernadez-Miranda et al., 2009). Herein, the true advantages of EESBS are to provide a direct devascularization of the tumor (cauterization of anterior and posterior ethmoidal arteries) and avoid any retraction of the frontal lobes. The limits are detailed further in the controversies' discussion and include a high risk of fistula, a higher risk of olfactory nerves injury and a lower control of the lateral margins of the tumor. For such a location, intracranial mini-invasive keyhole approaches represent serious alternatives.

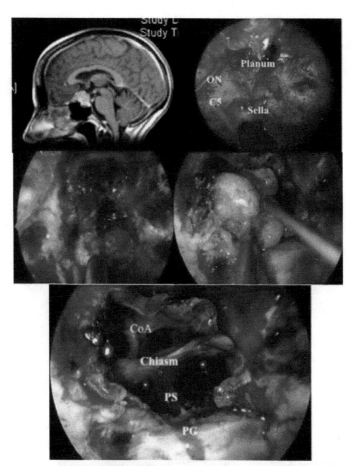

Fig. 14. Endonasal endoscopic resection of planum sphenoidale meningioma by a transtubercular approach. A one and half centimeter bone window is done with bone punch or by drilling to remove the roof of the sella, the tuberculum of the sella and the adjacent planum. After coagulation of the insertion basal dura, this latter is resected and the meningioma is progressively debulked and dissected from critical neurovascular structures (ON: optic nerve; Chiasm; CoA: anterior communicating artery; PS: pituitary stalk; PG: pituitary gland).

Many other neoplasms involving the anterior skull base have been approached through the endonasal route such as esthesioneuroblastomas (Suriano et al., 2007), nasopharyngeal fibromas and carcinomas (Batra et al., 2005).

5.3.2 Sellar and suprasellar non-adenomatous tumors

Endoscopic endonasal route has been naturally and progressively applied to the suprasellar lesions (craniopharyngiomas (Cavallo et al., 2009; Gardner et al., 2008a, 2008b), Rathke cleft cyst (Alfieri, 2002), epidermoid cysts, teratomas, etc,) with an obvious absence of frontal lobe retraction and a better corridor to the retro-chiasmatic region (de Divitiis et al, 2002). An approach from below provides a direct view of the tumor and its extension into the third ventricle (figures 15 & 16). Soft or non-adherent tumors can be more completely removed under direct visualization, what cannot be done through the intracranial route. However, identifying the tumor extension does not involve its systematic removal. Tumors adherent to the third ventricle like some craniopharyngiomas have to be kept in place considering the important risk of poor postoperative outcome.

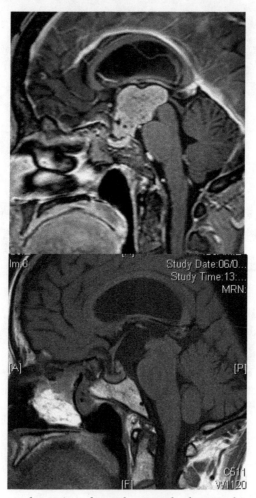

Fig. 15. Resection via an endoscopic endonasal approach of a retrochiasmatic and intraventricular suprasellar epidermoid cyst. Preoperative sagittal T1 gado MRI (left), postoperative control (right) with uneventful postoperative course.

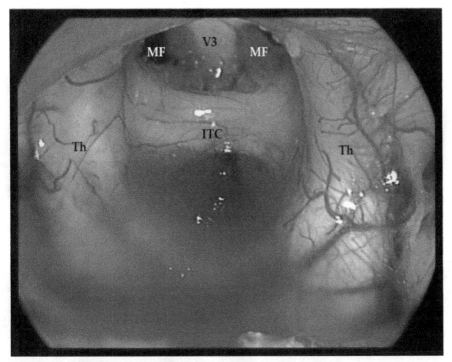

Fig. 16. Same patient as in figure 15. End of the resection showing the cavity of the 3rd ventricle, its roof (V3), both Monro foraminas (MF), and the 2 thalami bridged by the interthalamic commissure (ITC).

5.3.3 Meckel's cave tumors

Mainly represented by trigeminal shwannomas (figure 17), their approach requires classically an extensive orbitozygomatic frontopterional craniotomy. Meckel's cave can be approached by EESBS through its anterior aspect laterally to the para-clival portion of the internal carotid artery (Kassam et al., 2009). By this route, we can either remove the tumor or take a sample for a biopsy, the main advantage being not crossing cranial nerves, usually pushed laterally when the tumor grows.

5.3.4 Cavernous sinus lesions

There are very few indications of direct surgery for cavernous sinus tumors. Primarily represented by meningiomas, the current strategy is to treat them with radiotherapy or radiosurgery, when imaging is typical. However, when some soft tumors project into the cavernous sinus such as adenomas or chondrosarcomas, the panoramic view offered by the endoscopic endonasal route allows us to complete the removal safely. In our own experience (112 cases of pituitary adenomas extending into the cavernous sinus), the endoscope allowed us to cure more than one third of functioning or non-functioning adenomas without additional morbidity (figure 18). This route can also be used for biopsy when there is any doubt about the nature of a cavernous disease.

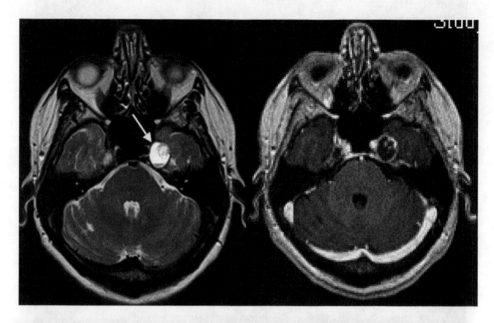

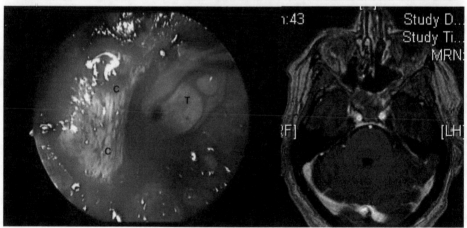

Fig. 17. Removal of a trigeminal schwannoma by an endoscopic endonasal approach. Top
pictures, axial T2 and gadolinium T1 MRI showing a partially cystic tumor. Anterior
approach of Meckel's cave with on the medial and the inferior side respectively the C3 and
C2 portion of the ICA (C) and a typical aspect of a schwannoma (T) (down left picture).
Down right: the postoperative MRI that shows a complete removal.

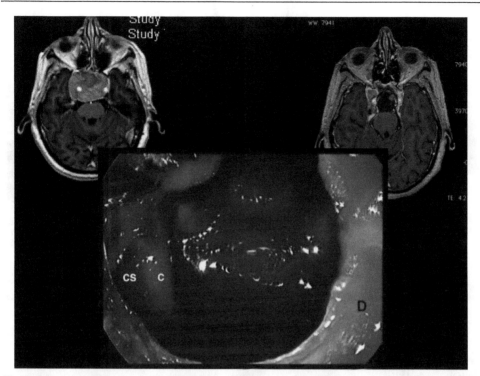

Fig. 18. Giant non-functioning adenoma invading the right cavernous sinus operated with a pure endoscopic endonasal approach (top left). During the surgery with a 30° angle endoscope pushed at the entry of the pituitary fossa (D), the cavernous portion of the carotid (C) was clearly seen with a perforation on the cavernous sinus wall (CS). Under visualization and with a two suction technique, a large part of the cavernous portion of the adenoma was removed without additional morbidity. The remnant tumor is therefore minimized and accessible to radiotherapy (top right).

5.3.5 Petrous apex and clival tumors
Petrous apexes as well as clival tumors are very challenging lesions because of their deepness and their neurovascular environment. EESBS provides a direct access to such tumors replacing progressively the traditional subtemporal, transpetrosal or retrosigmoid approaches (Griffith & Terrel, 1996; Kassam et al., 2005). Combination of both endonasal and intracranial procedures may be performed depending of the tumor conformation (figure 19).

5.3.6 Anterior craniocervical junction
Midline anterior lesions are good candidates for a direct approach by an endonasal endoscopic route, as standard far lateral approaches require crossing nerves and vessels before reaching the tumor. Rheumatoid pannus are fortunately rare with modern treatment but endoscopic endonasal resection has been described in the literature (Nayak et al., 2007). Skull base malformative anomalies and tumors can also be more easily approached through the endonasal route (Leng et al., 2009; Magrini et al., 2008).

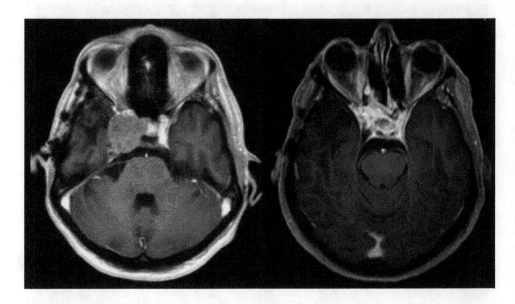

Fig. 19. Left: Petrocavernous chondrosarcoma operated on first via a subtemporal approach with a cavernous sinus tumor remnant. Right: A second step via a transsellar endonasal approach completed the removal without any postoperative cranial nerve or pituitary deficit.

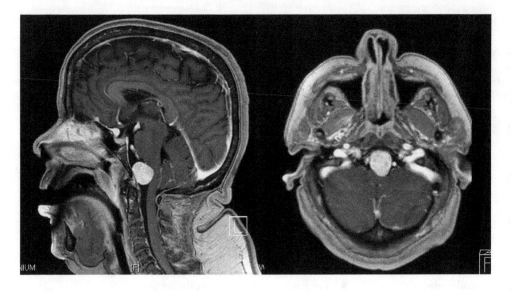

Fig. 20. Example of an anterior midline craniocervical meningioma that would be a good candidate for an endonasal endoscopic surgery because situated above the Kassam's line.

Drawing a line from the nasal bone to the palatine bone will help the surgeon to visualize the inferior limits of the surgical field (de Almeida et al., 2009). The endonasal route usually gives access to the odontoid and the upper third of C2 (figures 20 & 21). A lesion located inferiorly is an indication of a transoral surgery where the endoscope can also be useful as the surgical field is deep and narrow (Crockard, 1985).

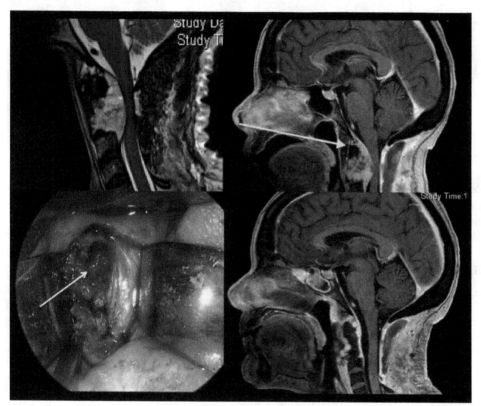

Fig. 21. Example of a C2 chordoma (top left). The tumor is located below Kassam's line indicating a transoral approach instead of the endonasal route (top right). The endoscope is a vast improvement on the microscope and provides a better visualization of this deep and narrow surgical field. Bottom left: an operative view with a typical aspect of chordoma, soft purplish tissue (white arrow). Bottom right, the postoperative MRI showing a macroscopic complete removal.

5.3.7 Infratemporal and pterygopalatine fossas

Herein, the endonasal approach competes with the usual transfacial approaches like Lefort I to remove tumors in this area (paragangliomas, shwannomas, meningiomas, juvenile nasopharyngeal angiofibromas) (figure 22). This region represents the lateral and inferior limits of endoscopic endonasal approaches with issues related to the multiples branches of the external carotid artery and the trigeminal nerve (Rivero-Serrano et al., 2010; Robinson et al., 2005).

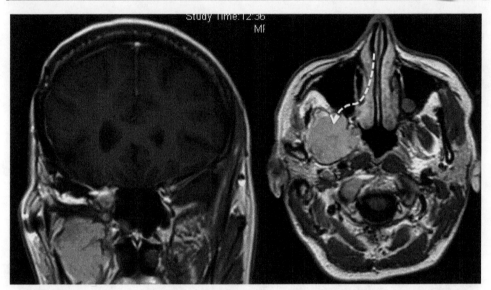

Fig. 22. Example of an extension of a sphenocavernous meningioma into the pterygopalatine fossa. Opening the maxillary sinus by an endonasal route will give a direct access to the lesion (white dotted arrow). It is a variant of the classic Lefort I approach.

6. Complications

6.1 Nasal morbidity

EESBS is constantly associated with postoperative nasal morbidity including mainly nasal crusting and blocked nose sensation lasting for the first few weeks. The intensity of these symptoms varies from one patient to another, and is usually moderate for pituitary surgery and perfectly managed by local treatments given to patients on discharge from hospital. Nasal consequences of extended approaches are far more complicated, with frequent chronic crusting rhinosinusitis. Indeed in such approaches, turbinectomies and wide sinus aperture impair the nasal airflow which leads to crusting and obstruction. With the spread of these kinds of approaches, many teams are studying the postoperative quality of life using questionnaires such as the SNOT-22 (Sino-Nasal Outcome Test-22) and the anterior skull base questionnaire. Nasal crusting remains the most frequent postoperative complaint while no risk factors have been identified (98 % of the patients had nasal crusting at one month in Almeida's series). According to Almeida *et al.*, the use of nasoseptal flap for skull base closure is not a significant risk factor of nasal morbidity (de Almeida et al., 2011).

Patients have to be informed preoperatively of this nasal morbidity and particularly the high rate of nasal crusting and possible loss of smell. They should also know that these morbidities are transitional in almost all cases and will improve within 3 to 6 months postoperatively. A postoperative nasal care including sinus humidification and saline irrigation is highly recommended.

Postoperative infectious sphenoid sinusitis may occur in about 2% of patients, while it can reach 9% in microsurgical series of pituitary adenomas. A large opening of the sphenoid sinus and a lesser use of artificial packing material within the sphenoid sinus may prevent these infections (Balaker et al., 2010).

6.2 CSF leak and meningitis

CSF leak is the most common complication during endoscopic endonasal approaches to the skull base, with initial high rates decreasing progressively with the learning curve and the closure methods with pediculated flaps. Higher experience in pituitary surgery means rarer CSF leaks, less than 5% (Messerer et al., 2011). Obviously, extensive approaches involving the anterior skull base are more likely to lead to per and postoperative CSF leaks. We also experienced more frequent CSF leaks for planum meningiomas than for other types of tumors. A postoperative leakage was observed in 15.9% of the 800 patients treated by Kassam *et al.*, but for anterior skull base meningiomas it can reach up to 50% of cases (Kassam et al., 2010). An accurate multilayer closure of the skull base is of a paramount importance to avoid postoperative CSF leaks, especially when a peroperative leak is observed. The use of pedicle flaps dramatically decreased the rate of these postoperative CSF leaks (Hadad et al., 2006; Kassam et al., 2005).

Postoperative infection risk is comparable to intracranial open skull base surgery with a rate reaching 1.8% of patients. Risk factors of meningitis are mainly peroperative CSF leaks and postoperative external ventricular or lumbar drains (Gondim et al., 2010, Kono et al., 2010).

6.3 Vascular complications

Early or delayed nasal hemorrhages may occur postoperatively in up to 7% of patients. These hemorrhages related to small mucosal arteries, are usually of small volume and respond easily to transitory nasal tamponade. An injury or insufficient coagulation of branches of the sphenopalatine artery in the sphenoethmoidal recess may rarely lead to important potentially life-threatening epistaxis, requiring reoperation and/or endovascular management (Gondim et al., 2010).

An internal carotid artery injury is a striking peroperative complication. This artery may be encased within an invasive skull base tumor as well as in redo surgeries, conditions in which neuronavigation and microdoppler probe are very useful tools. In such difficult cases of Meckel's cave or cavernous sinus surgery, a preoperative angiogram should be done and an extra-intracranial anastomosis discussed in the case of a non-functional Willis polygon.

One must be particularly aware of "kissing" carotid arteries sometimes observed in acromegalic patients.

Pseudoaneurysms and carotid-cavernous fistulas may result months or years after aggressive tumoral dissection and curettage within the cavernous sinuses (Cappabianca et al., 2001).

A careful analysis of preoperative MRI and eventually angiographic studies is mandatory to avoid such dramatic complications (Solares et al., 2010).

6.4 Endocrinological issues

Hydro-electrolytic balance monitoring is compulsory during the early postoperative course in order to detect diabetes insipidus, either transient (2–20% in pituitary adenomas) or permanent (1–5%), usually secondary to surgical manipulation or injury to posterior pituitary gland and/or pituitary stalk.

Postoperative anterior pituitary dysfunction may occur in 13% to one third of patients with pituitary adenomas managed endoscopically, depending of the preoperative condition (Messerer et al., 2011). Endocrine results are clearly poorer for craniopharyngiomas while unclear or sparse for the other sellar tumors.

6.5 Ocular complications

Orbital hemorrhages may be caused by an injury to the ethmoidal artery during an endoscopic endonasal approach, and subsequent retraction of this artery within the orbit may occur. In such a case, an emergency orbital decompression can be needed (Charalampaki et al., 2009). Elsewhere, a direct injury to the globe or to the medial rectus muscle or even to the nasolacrymal duct may occur, specially during the initial learning curve (May et al., 1994).

6.6 Pituitary apoplexy

Postoperative apoplexy usually occurs when an obvious suprasellar adenomatous remnant is left in place. The major risk of this complication is the acute compression of the visual apparatus, acute pituitary insufficiency and obstructive hydrocephalus. Emergent reoperation may be necessary, either by the same endonasal route or intra-cranial approach according to apoplexy configuration.

7. Closure techniques: The multilayer technique as key point

The CSF leak is the main issue of EESBS, thus making closure time as important as the tumor removal itself. Many studies have been pusblished on this topic, each progress leading to a decrease in the percentage of postoperative CSF leak. One must understand that each layer has to be rebuilt (figure 23).

The arachnoid plane can be reinforced with intradural injection of fibrin glue and/or using a soft inlay graft covering the dural aperture. Extraduraly, the removed dura mater has to be replaced by a substitute. We prefer a bio-absorbable one as we experienced 3 cases of sellar space-occupying infections following pituitary surgery, where the dural plane had been rebuilt with a non-resorbable dural substitute. The bone plane is recreated using synthetic material (titanium plate) or using autologous bone (ie what we called the bone flap previously). This latter has our preference, as the long term tolerance of synthetic material is not known. The turbinates can be also used specially in locations where a bone flap cannot be done (clivus for instance).

The bone flap has to be covered after its repositionning. Autologous but inert material such as fat graft and fascia lata alone are disapointing with 30 to 50% of postoperative CSF leaks (Kassam et al., 2008). Vascular pediculated flaps (figure 24) is the biggest advance in endoscopic surgery leading to a dramatic decrease in the rate of CSF leak from 30% to around 4% (Kassam et al., 2008). The most easy to prepare is the nasoseptal flap (Hadad et al., 2006) but many other flaps are possible: pericranial, buccinator and temporoparietal fascia flap (Caicedo-Granados et al., 2010 ; Patel et al., 2010 ; Rivera-Serrano et al., 2010). To reinforce the watertight of the reconstruction, a fibrin glue is applied all over the bone and mucosa. The sinus cavities are therefore filled up with fat embedded in glue.

When repairing the anterior skull base, the risk of graft migration is higher during the first few days. A balloon can be used in prevention, as a support kept in place for 3 or 5 days. This must not be used in patients where visual function cannot be monitored closely.

Finally, CSF drainage to decrease intracranial pressure is still being discussed. External drain should be avoided because of the risk of contamination but we perform 3 to 5 postoperative lumbar punctures for high-risk surgeries such as anterior skull base, meningiomas and intraventricular surgeries.

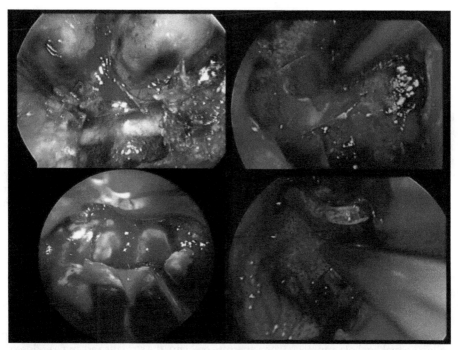

Fig. 23. Multilayered closure. Arachnoid with fibrin glue (top left), dura mater substitute (top right), bone flap positioning (bottom left) and mucosa flap(bottom right).

8. Controversies and limits: Extended endonasal approaches versus trans-eyebrow keyhole endoscopic approaches for anterior skull base tumors

If no one disputes the benefit of the endonasal endoscopic approach for retrochiasmatic parasellar or clival tumors, its use for anterior skull base tumors is still being discussed (i.e. from the cribriform plate to the tuberculum of the sella) (de Devitiis et al., 2008).

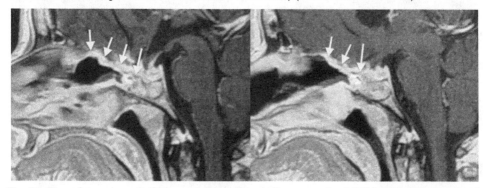

Fig. 24. Complete removal of planum meningioma. Postoperative MRI (sagittal T1 weighted sequence with gadolinium). The nasoseptal flap used to reconstruct the skull base is clearly visible enhanced after contrast injection (arrows).

Indeed, the endonasal route presents many advantages: no brain retraction, a useful suppression of the blood supplies of the tumour always interesting specially for meningiomas and a better control of the inferomedial part of the optic canal. Other arguments argue against the endonasal approach in case of anterior skull base tumors.

The first one is a risk of CSF fistula higher than in others locations as the dura mater and bone graft might migrate down more easily when repairing the anterior skull base compared to middle cranial base. As reported by others (de devitiis et al. 2008), in our own experience of extended approaches (more than 100 cases to date comprising all locations), around half of the procedures done for anterior skull base (20 cases) was complicated by postoperative CSF leaks. Even though, we obtain clearly better results when using the bone and nasal flaps, this point was the first to exhort us to find an alternative mini-invasive keyhole approach.

The second one was the absence of control of the tumor margins when tumors grow over the optic nerves and carotid arteries, a common feature of meningiomas that usually extend largely on the anterior skull base. This may lead to tumor remnant (figure 25). On that particular point, it will be interesting to consider the frequency of tumor recurrence in series of anterior skull base meningiomas operated from below with long-term follow up before giving a definitive conclusion.

Finally, anterior skull tumors without olfactory impairment are another reason to choose the intracranial instead of the endonasal route. There are, of course, better chances to preserve olfactory nerves by an intracranial route.

The supraorbital trans-eyebrow approach was initially introduced for vascular clipping or skull base tumors removal primarily with the use of microscope (Reisch et al., 2003).

Since 2010, we use this keyhole approach purely with the endoscope instead of microscope. This allows a real keyhole approach (bone aperture of 2 cm), the straight and angle endoscopes give a panoramic view of the entire anterior skull base but also of the opticocarotid recess and of the medial part of the optic canal (figure 26). With such a technique, we are able to remove meningiomas with as uneventful postoperative course as after endonasal endoscopic approaches (even with shorter hospital stay), without the risk of CSF fistula.

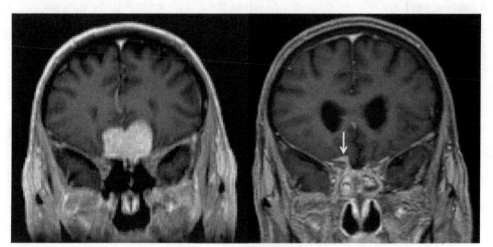

Fig. 25. Example of an anterior skull base meningioma removed from below. The postoperative MRI clearly indicated a tumor remnant on the top of the right clinoidal process (white arrow) that has not been seen during the endonasal route.

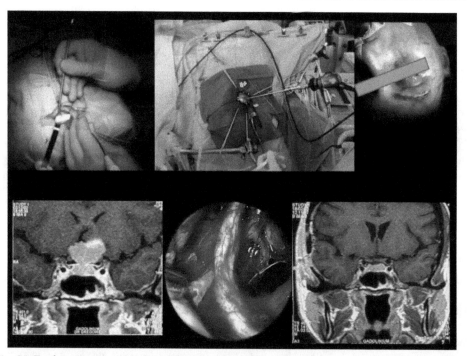

Fig. 26. Eyebrow supraorbital surgery for a suprasellar meningioma. This keyhole approach (frontal craniotomy of 2 cm, top left) can be done with the endoscope instead of the microscope (middle top). Angled endoscopes give the possibility of exploring all the corners of the surgical field like the medial opticocarotid recess (middle bottom) but also the entire anterior skull base, what cannot be done with the endonasal route.

For the authors, this mini invasive endoscopic eyebrow approach should be considered for large tumors grown beyond the suprasellar carotid arteries but also for small anteriorly based tumors, thus avoiding any CSF leak.

9. Conclusion

The part of the endoscopic endonasal approach is getting more and more important in skull base surgery since the beginning of the nineties. Under the impulsion of the Pittsburgh and Neapolitan neurosurgical teams, the last two decades saw an increasing number of publications on that topic either on anatomy or surgical techniques (more than 800 entries on Pubmed using 2 key words, "endoscopy" and "skull base"). Thus, new surgical corridors to approach especially midline skull base tumors have been described.

However, the exact role and indications of the endonasal endoscopic surgery are still being discussed in the absence of large or randomized series. Compared to intracranial microsurgical approaches, the endoscopic endonasal routes offer genuine benefits for pituitary surgery as well as for retrochiasmatic or midline clival tumors. For parasellar lesions, the endonasal endoscopic technique is also interesting to remove or to biopsy Meckel's cave lesions or tumors extending into the cavernous sinus. This will not change much the current management of cavernous sinus lesions where most of the time radiotherapy is the treatment of choice and for which no biopsy is required when imaging is typical.

Its use for anterior skull base tumors is more controversial. Indeed, the high percentage of CSF leaks, specially for meningiomas, and the absence of control of the lateral tumour margins raise interrogation about the real benefit of this endonasal approach. In their experience, the authors think that other mini-invasive approaches such as the supraorbital eyebrow one are likely to be more seductive.

To date, the endonasal endoscopic surgery provides interesting and complementary routes for skull base tumors but will not replace the standard intracranial approaches. Large multicentric studies with long-term follow up are being done to define precisely the real indications and benefits of such endonasal surgery. Technical refinements are also expected in a close future using 3D endoscope and robotics (Hanna et al., 2007; Levy et al., 2006; O'Malley & Weinstein, 2007).

10. References

Alfieri A, Jho HD. (2001). Endoscopic endonasal cavernous sinus surgery: an anatomic study. *Neurosurgery* 48: 827-836; discussion 836-837.

Alfieri A, Jho HD. (2001). Endoscopic endonasal approaches to the cavernous sinus: surgical approaches. *Neurosurgery* 49: 354-360; discussion 360-362.

Alfieri A, Jho H, Tschabitscher M. (2002). Endoscopic endonasal approach to the ventral cranio-cervical junction: anatomical study. *Acta Neurochir (Wien)* 144: 219-225; discussion 225.

Alfieri A, Schettino R, Tarfani A, Bonzi O, Rossi GA, Monolo L. (2002). Endoscopic endonasal removal of an intra-suprasellar Rathke's cleft cyst: case report and surgical considerations. *Minim Invasive Neurosurg* 45: 47-51.

de Almeida JR, Zanation AM, Snyderman CH, Carrau RL, Prevedello DM, Gardner PA, et al. (2009). Defining the nasopalatine line: the limit for endonasal surgery of the spine. *Laryngoscope* 119: 239-244.

de Almeida JR, Snyderman CH, Gardner PA, Carrau RL, Vescan AD. (2011). Nasal morbidity following endoscopic skull base surgery: A prospective cohort study. *Head Neck* 33(4):547-51.

Balaker AE, Bergsneider M, Martin NA, Wang MB. (2010). Evolution of sinonasal symptoms following endoscopic anterior skull base surgery. *Skull Base* 20(4):245-51.

Batra PS, Citardi MJ, Worley S, Lee J, Lanza DC. (2005). Resection of anterior skull base tumors: comparison of combined traditional and endoscopic techniques. *Am J Rhinol* 19: 521-528.

Caicedo-Granados E, Carrau R, Snyderman CH, Prevedello D, Fernandez-Miranda J, Gardner P, et al. (2010). Reverse rotation flap for reconstruction of donor site after vascular pedicled nasoseptal flap in skull base surgery. *Laryngoscope* 120: 1550-1552.

Cappabianca P, Alfieri A, de Divitiis E. (1998). Endoscopic endonasal transsphenoidal approach to the sella: towards functional endoscopic pituitary surgery (FEPS). *Minim Invasive Neurosurg* 41: 66-73.

Cappabianca P, Briganti F, Cavallo LM, de Divitiis E. (2001). Pseudoaneurysm of the intracavernous carotid artery following endoscopic endonasal transsphenoidal surgery, treated by endovascular approach. *Acta Neurochir (Wien)* 143: 95-96.

Carrau RL, Kassam AB, Snyderman CH. (2001). Pituitary surgery. *Otolaryngol. Clin. North Am* 34: 1143-1155, ix.

Castelnuovo P, Dallan I, Pistochini A, Battaglia P, Locatelli D, Bignami M. (2007). Endonasal endoscopic repair of Sternberg's canal cerebrospinal fluid leaks. *Laryngoscope* 117: 345-349.

Castelnuovo P, Dallan I, Bignami M, Pistochini A, Battaglia P, Tschabitscher M. (2008). Endonasal endoscopic management of petroclival cerebrospinal fluid leaks: anatomical study and preliminary clinical experience. *Minim Invasive Neurosurg* 51: 336-339.

Castelnuovo P, Dallan I, Battaglia P, Bignami M. (2010). Endoscopic endonasal skull base surgery: past, present and future. *Eur Arch Otorhinolaryngol* 267: 649-663.

Caton R. (1893). Notes of a case of acromegaly treated by operation. *Br Med J* 2: 1421-1423.

Cavallo LM, Cappabianca P, Messina A, Esposito F, Stella L, de Divitiis E, et al. (2007). The extended endoscopic endonasal approach to the clivus and cranio-vertebral junction: anatomical study. *Childs Nerv Syst* 23: 665-671.

Cavallo LM, Prevedello DM, Solari D, Gardner PA, Esposito F, Snyderman CH, et al. (2009). Extended endoscopic endonasal transsphenoidal approach for residual or recurrent craniopharyngiomas. *J Neurosurg* 111: 578-589.

Charalampaki P, Ayyad A, Kockro RA, Perneczky A. (2009). Surgical complications after endoscopic transsphenoidal pituitary surgery. *J Clin Neurosci.* 16(6):786-9.

Cebula H, Lahlou A, De Battista JC, Debry C, Froelich S. (2010). [Endoscopic approaches to the orbit]. *Neurochirurgie* 56: 230-235.

Crockard HA. (1985). The transoral approach to the base of the brain and upper cervical cord. *Ann R Coll Surg Engl* 67: 321-325.

Cushing H.(1909). III. Partial Hypophysectomy for Acromegaly: With Remarks on the Function of the Hypophysis. *Ann. Surg* 50: 1002-1017.

Dandy W. (1926). Pneumocephalus (intracranial pneumatocoele or aerocoele). *Arch Surg* 12: 949-982.

Dandy W. (1932). Practice of surgery. Dans: The brain. Hagerstown; p. 247-252.

de Divitiis E, Cappabianca P, Cavallo LM. (2002). Endoscopic transsphenoidal approach: adaptability of the procedure to different sellar lesions. *Neurosurgery* 51: 699-705; discussion 705-707.

de Divitiis E, Esposito F, Cappabianca P, Cavallo LM, de Divitiis O, Esposito I. (2008). Endoscopic transnasal resection of anterior cranial fossa meningiomas. *Neurosurg Focus* 25(6):E8.

Dehdashti AR, Ganna A, Karabatsou K, Gentili F. (2008). Pure endoscopic endonasal approach for pituitary adenomas: early surgical results in 200 patients and comparison with previous microsurgical series. *Neurosurgery.* 62(5):1006-15; discussion 1015-7.

D'Haens J, Van Rompaey K, Stadnik T, Haentjens P, Poppe K, Velkeniers B. (2009). Fully endoscopic transsphenoidal surgery for functioning pituitary adenomas: a retrospective comparison with traditional transsphenoidal microsurgery in the same institution. *Surg Neurol.* 72(4):336-40. Epub 2009 Jul 14.

Draf W. (1973). [Clinical value of sinus endoscopy (author's transl)]. *Z Laryngol Rhinol Otol* 52: 890-896.

Fernandez-Miranda JC, Gardner PA, Prevedello DM, Kassam AB. (2009). Expanded endonasal approach for olfactory groove meningioma. *Acta Neurochir (Wien)* 151: 287-288; author reply 289-290.

Frank G, Pasquini E. (2003). Approach to the cavernous sinus. Dans: *Endoscopic endonasal transsphenoidal surgery.* Vienna: de Devitiis E, Cappabianca P; p. 159-175.

Frank G, Pasquini E, Farneti G, Mazzatenta D, Sciarretta V, Grasso V, et al. (2006). The endoscopic versus the traditional approach in pituitary surgery. *Neuroendocrinology* 83: 240-248.

Gardner PA, Kassam AB, Rothfus WE, Snyderman CH, Carrau RL. (2008). Preoperative and intraoperative imaging for endoscopic endonasal approaches to the skull base. *Otolaryngol. Clin. North Am* 41: 215-230, vii.

Gardner PA, Kassam AB, Snyderman CH, Carrau RL, Mintz AH, Grahovac S, Stefko S. (2008). Outcomes following endoscopic, expanded endonasal resection of suprasellar craniopharyngiomas: a case series. *J. Neurosurg* 109: 6-16.

Gardner PA, Prevedello DM, Kassam AB, Snyderman CH, Carrau RL, Mintz AH. (2008). The evolution of the endonasal approach for craniopharyngiomas. *J. Neurosurg* 108: 1043-1047.

Gondim JA, Almeida JP, Albuquerque LA, Schops M, Gomes E, Ferraz T, Sobreira W, Kretzmann MT. (2010). Endoscopic endonasal approach for pituitary adenoma: surgical complications in 301 patients. *Pituitary.* 2010 Dec 23. [Epub ahead of print]

Grant JA. (1996). Victor Darwin Lespinasse: a biographical sketch. *Neurosurgery* 39: 1232-1233.

Griffith AJ, Terrell JE. (1996). Transsphenoid endoscopic management of petrous apex cholesterol granuloma. *Otolaryngol Head Neck Surg* 114: 91-94.

Guiot G, Bouche J, Hertzog E, Vourc'h G, Hardy J. (1963). [Hypophysectomy by trans-sphenoidal route.]. *Ann Radiol (Paris)* 6: 187-192.

Guiot J, Rougerie J, Fourestier M, Fournier A, Comoy C, Vulmiere J, et al. (1963). [Intracranial endoscopic explorations.]. *Presse Med* 71: 1225-1228.

Hadad G, Bassagasteguy L, Carrau RL, Mataza JC, Kassam A, Snyderman CH, et al. (2006). A novel reconstructive technique after endoscopic expanded endonasal approaches: vascular pedicle nasoseptal flap. *Laryngoscope* 116: 1882-1886.

Hanna EY, Holsinger C, DeMonte F, Kupferman M. (2007). Robotic endoscopic surgery of the skull base: a novel surgical approach. *Arch. Otolaryngol. Head Neck Surg* 133: 1209-1214.

Har-El G. (2005). Endoscopic transnasal transsphenoidal pituitary surgery--comparison with the traditional sublabial transseptal approach. *Otolaryngol. Clin. North Am* 38: 723-735.

Hardy J. (2010). [History of pituitary surgery]. *Neurochirurgie* 56: 358-362.

Herr HW. (2006). Max Nitze, the cystoscope and urology. *J. Urol* 176: 1313-1316.

Higgins TS, Courtemanche C, Karakla D, Strasnick B, Singh RV, Koen JL, et al. (2008). Analysis of transnasal endoscopic versus transseptal microscopic approach for excision of pituitary tumors. *Am J Rhinol* 22: 649-652.

Hirsch O. (1952). Successful closure of cerebrospinal fluid rhinorrhea by endonasal surgery. *AMA Arch Otolaryngol* 56: 1-12.

Jankowski R, Auque J, Simon C, Marchal JC, Hepner H, Wayoff M. (1992). Endoscopic pituitary tumor surgery. *Laryngoscope* 102: 198-202.

Jho HD, Carrau RL, McLaughlin ML, Somaza SC. (1996). Endoscopic transsphenoidal resection of a large chordoma in the posterior fossa. Case report. *Neurosurg Focus* 1: e3; discussion 1p following e3.

Jho HD, Carrau RL. (1997). Endoscopic endonasal transsphenoidal surgery: experience with 50 patients. *J. Neurosurg* 87: 44-51.

Kassam A, Carrau RL, Snyderman CH, Gardner P, Mintz A. (2005). Evolution of reconstructive techniques following endoscopic expanded endonasal approaches. *Neurosurg Focus* 19: E8.

Kassam AB, Gardner P, Snyderman C, Mintz A, Carrau R. (2005). Expanded endonasal approach: fully endoscopic, completely transnasal approach to the middle third of the clivus, petrous bone, middle cranial fossa, and infratemporal fossa. *Neurosurg Focus* 19: E6.

Kassam AB, Mintz AH, Gardner PA, Horowitz MB, Carrau RL, Snyderman CH. (2006). The expanded endonasal approach for an endoscopic transnasal clipping and aneurysmorrhaphy of a large vertebral artery aneurysm: technical case report. *Neurosurgery* 59: ONSE162-165; discussion ONSE162-165.

Kassam AB, Thomas AJ, Zimmer LA, Snyderman CH, Carrau RL, Mintz A, et al. (2007). Expanded endonasal approach: a fully endoscopic completely transnasal resection of a skull base arteriovenous malformation. *Childs Nerv Syst* 23: 491-498.

Kassam AB, Gardner PA, Mintz A, Snyderman CH, Carrau RL, Horowitz M. (2007). Endoscopic endonasal clipping of an unsecured superior hypophyseal artery aneurysm. Technical note. *J. Neurosurg* 107: 1047-1052.

Kassam AB, Gardner PA, Snyderman CH, Carrau RL, Mintz AH, Prevedello DM. (2008). Expanded endonasal approach, a fully endoscopic transnasal approach for the resection of midline suprasellar craniopharyngiomas: a new classification based on the infundibulum. *J. Neurosurg* 108: 715-728.

Kassam AB, Prevedello DM, Carrau RL, Snyderman CH, Gardner P, Osawa S, et al. (2009). The front door to meckel's cave: an anteromedial corridor via expanded endoscopic endonasal approach- technical considerations and clinical series. *Neurosurgery* 64: 71-82; discussion 82-83.

Kassam AB, Prevedello DM, Carrau RL, Snyderman CH, Thomas A, Gardner P, Zanation A, Duz B, Stefko ST, Byers K, Horowitz MB. (2010). Endoscopic endonasal skull base surgery: analysis of complications in the authors' initial 800 patients. *J Neurosurg*. 2010 Dec 17. [Epub ahead of print]

Kassis S, De Battista JC, Raverot G, Jacob M, Simon E, Rabilloud M, Froehlich P, Trouillas J, Borson-Chazot F, Perrin G, Jouanneau E. (2009). [Endoscopy versus microsurgery:

results in a consecutive series of nonfunctioning pituitary adenomas]. *Neurochirurgie* 55: 607-615.

Kono Y, Prevedello DM, Snyderman CH, Gardner PA, Kassam AB, Carrau RL, Byers KE. (2011). One thousand endoscopic skull base surgical procedures demystifying the infection potential: incidence and description of postoperative meningitis and brain abscesses. *Infect Control Hosp Epidemiol.* 32(1):77-83. Epub 2010 Dec 1.

Landolt AM. (2001). History of pituitary surgery from the technical aspect. *Neurosurg. Clin. N. Am* 12: 37-44, vii-viii.

Leng LZ, Anand VK, Hartl R, Schwartz TH. (2009). Endonasal endoscopic resection of an os odontoideum to decompress the cervicomedullary junction: a minimal access surgical technique. *Spine* 34: E139-143.

Levy ML, Nguyen A, Aryan H, Jandial R, Meltzer HS, Apuzzo MLJ. (2006). Robotic virtual endoscopy: development of a multidirectional rigid endoscope. *Neurosurgery* 59: ONS134-141; discussion ONS134-141.

Léger P. (2004). [Antonin Jean Desormeaux]. *Prog. Urol* 14: 1231-1238.

Lindholm J. (2007). A century of pituitary surgery: Schloffer's legacy. *Neurosurgery* 61: 865-867; discussion 867-868.

Litynski GS. (1999). Endoscopic surgery: the history, the pioneers. *World J Surg* 23: 745-753.

Liu JK, Das K, Weiss MH, Laws ER, Couldwell WT. (2001). The history and evolution of transsphenoidal surgery. *J. Neurosurg* 95: 1083-1096.

Magrini S, Pasquini E, Mazzatenta D, Mascari C, Galassi E, Frank G. (2008). Endoscopic endonasal odontoidectomy in a patient affected by Down syndrome: technical case report. *Neurosurgery* 63: E373-374; discussion E374.

Martin TJ, Loehrl TA. (2007). Endoscopic CSF leak repair. *Curr Opin Otolaryngol Head Neck Surg* 15: 35-39.

May M, Levine HL, Mester SJ, Schaitkin B. (1994). Complications of endoscopic sinus surgery: analysis of 2108 patients--incidence and prevention. *Laryngoscope* 104: 1080-1083.

Messerer M, De Battista JC, Raverot G, Kassis S, Dubourg J, Lapras V, Trouillas J, Perrin G, Jouanneau E. (2011). Evidence of improved surgical outcome following endoscopy for nonfunctioning pituitary adenoma removal. *Neurosurg Focus.* 30(4):E11.

Nayak JV, Gardner PA, Vescan AD, Carrau RL, Kassam AB, Snyderman CH. (2007). Experience with the expanded endonasal approach for resection of the odontoid process in rheumatoid disease. *Am J Rhinol* 21: 601-606.

Nyquist GG, Anand VK, Mehra S, Kacker A, Schwartz TH. (2010). Endoscopic endonasal repair of anterior skull base non-traumatic cerebrospinal fluid leaks, meningoceles, and encephaloceles. *J. Neurosurg* 113: 961-966.

O'Malley BW, Weinstein GS. (2007). Robotic skull base surgery: preclinical investigations to human clinical application. *Arch. Otolaryngol. Head Neck Surg* 133: 1215-1219.

Patel MR, Shah RN, Snyderman CH, Carrau RL, Germanwala AV, Kassam AB, et al. (2010). Pericranial flap for endoscopic anterior skull-base reconstruction: clinical outcomes and radioanatomic analysis of preoperative planning. *Neurosurgery* 66: 506-512; discussion 512.

Pollock JR, Akinwunmi J, Scaravilli F, Powell MP. (2003). Transcranial surgery for pituitary tumors performed by Sir Victor Horsley. *Neurosurgery* 52: 914-925; discussion 925-926.

Prevedello DM, Pinheiro-Neto CD, Fernandez-Miranda JC, Carrau RL, Snyderman CH, Gardner PA, Kassam AB. (2010). Vidian nerve transposition for endoscopic endonasal middle fossa approaches. *Neurosurgery.* 67(2 Suppl Operative):478-84.

Ramachandran R, Singh PM, Batra M, Pahwa D. (2011). Anaesthesia for endoscopic endonasal surgery. *Trends in Anaesthesia and Critical Care* 1 : 79-83

Rathert P. (1967). Max Nitze (1848-1906). *Invest Urol* 5: 327-330.

Reisch R, Perneczky A, Filippi R. (2003). Surgical technique of the supraorbital key-hole craniotomy. *Surg Neurol* 59: 223-227.

Reuter M. (2000). The historical development of endophotography. *World J Urol* 18: 299-302.

Rivera-Serrano CM, Oliver CL, Sok J, Prevedello DM, Gardner P, Snyderman CH, et al. (2010). Pedicled facial buccinator (FAB) flap: a new flap for reconstruction of skull base defects. *Laryngoscope* 120: 1922-1930.

Rivera-Serrano CM, Terre-Falcon R, Fernandez-Miranda J, Prevedello D, Snyderman CH, Gardner P, Kassam A, Carrau RL. (2010). Endoscopic endonasal dissection of the pterygopalatine fossa, infratemporal fossa, and post-styloid compartment. Anatomical relationships and importance of eustachian tube in the endoscopic skull base surgery. *Laryngoscope.* 120 Suppl 4:S244.

Robinson S, Patel N, Wormald PJ. (2005). Endoscopic management of benign tumors extending into the infratemporal fossa: a two-surgeon transnasal approach. *Laryngoscope* 115: 1818-1822.

Schaberg MR, Anand VK, Schwartz TH, Cobb W. (2010). Microscopic versus endoscopic transnasal pituitary surgery. *Curr Opin Otolaryngol Head Neck Surg* 18: 8-14.

Schwartz TH, Fraser JF, Brown S, Tabaee A, Kacker A, Anand VK. (2008). Endoscopic cranial base surgery: classification of operative approaches. *Neurosurgery* 62: 991-1002; discussion 1002-1005.

Snyderman C, Kassam A, Carrau R, Mintz A, Gardner P, Prevedello DM. (2007). Acquisition of surgical skills for endonasal skull base surgery: a training program. *Laryngoscope* 117: 699-705.

Snyderman CH, Carrau RL, Kassam AB, Zanation A, Prevedello D, Gardner P, et al. (2008). Endoscopic skull base surgery: principles of endonasal oncological surgery. *J Surg Oncol* 97: 658-664.

Solares CA, Ong YK, Carrau RL, Fernandez-Miranda J, Prevedello DM, Snyderman CH, et al. (2010). Prevention and management of vascular injuries in endoscopic surgery of the sinonasal tract and skull base. *Otolaryngol. Clin. North Am* 43: 817-825.

Suriano M, De Vincentiis M, Colli A, Benfari G, Mascelli A, Gallo A. (2007). Endoscopic treatment of esthesioneuroblastoma: a minimally invasive approach combined with radiation therapy. *Otolaryngol Head Neck Surg* 136: 104-107.

Wigand ME. (1981). Transnasal ethmoidectomy under endoscopical control. *Rhinology* 19: 7-15.

2

Objective Outcomes in Endoscopic Sinus Surgery

David W.J. Côté and Erin D. Wright
University of Alberta
Canada

1. Introduction

Use of endoscopes in the sinonasal cavity dates as far back as the turn of the 20th century with Hirschmann and Reichert performing the first sino-endoscopies and sinus surgeries, respectively. Widespread use was limited until H.H. Hopkins helped address illumination difficulties with the rod optic system in the 1960s and Walter Messerklinger began systematic use of the endoscope to evaluate the lateral nasal wall and mucociliary clearance in the late 1970s (Lee & Kennedy 2006). With the advent of modern endoscopic sinus surgery instruments and techniques in the 1980s, the endoscope has radically altered the surgical approach and management of inflammatory and neoplastic sinonasal disease rendering many of the open approaches nearly obsolete.

Successful outcomes in endoscopic sinus surgery have often been largely based on subjective qualifiers by the patient. Significant improvements in patient perceived nasal congestion, obstruction, facial pressure, rhinorrhea, headache, postnasal drainage have been the impetus for the widespread growth of functional endoscopic sinus surgery, while modest improvements in olfaction, taste, allergic symptoms and tooth pain have also been reported. (Lee & Kennedy 2006). Some objective measures of outcomes previously proposed include acoustic rhinometry, mucociliary measures using saccharine transit times and ciliary beat clearance, and olfactory thresholds using butanol testing and the UPSIT-University of Pennsylvania Smell Identification Test (Min et al 1995; Lund & Scadding 1994). Radiologic evidence of polyp disease on CT scanning has also been studied with validated scoring systems, but with poor correlation with clinical symptoms and as such a poor indicator of outcomes (Newman et al 1994; Friedman 1990; Giklich 1994; Jorgensen 1991; Browne et al 2006; Newton & Ah-See 2008). Increasingly, the rhinologic community looks to standardized objective endoscopic measures in scientific communications to evaluate success in managing sinonasal disease. These various grading schemes have been targeted at eliciting objective reproducible measures of: (1) polyp grade, (2) sinus cavity status, and (3) surgical field visibility. We present the first complete review of all objective published endoscopic scoring schemes for sinonasal disease.

2. Objective endoscopic measures of polyp disease

2.1 Objective endoscopic measures of polyp disease

Objective, standardized endoscoping scoring systems to communicate disease burden of nasal polyposis dates back at least to the late 1980s with staging systems being proposed by various international clinical groups over the years (Table 1).

YEAR	AUTHOR(S)	COUNTRY	SCALE	TYPE
1990	Levine	United States of America	6 point	Polyp staging
1992	Kennedy	United States of America	5 point	Sinus cavity staging
1992	Gaskins	United States of America	5 point	Sinus cavity staging
1993	Johansen et al.	Denmark	5 point inflammation	Sinus cavity staging
			5 point previous surgery	
			5 point infection	
			4 point polyp staging	
1993	Lund & Mackay	United Kingdom	3 point including polyp, discharge, edema, scars, crusting	Sinus cavity staging
1993	May & Levine	United States of America	5 point	Polyp staging
1995	Lildholdt et al.	Sweden	4 point	Polyp staging
1995	Lund & Kennedy	United Kingdom, United States of America	3 point polyp edema discharge, scarring crusting	Sinus cavity staging
1996	Mackay & Nacleiro	United Kingdom	4 point	Polyp staging
2000	Johansson et al.	Sweden	0-100 VAS	Polyp staging
2000	Rasp	Germany	4 point	Polyp staging
2003	Passali et al	Italy	4 point	Polyp staging
2006	Meltzer et al	United States of America	5 point	Polyp staging
2007	Wright & Agrawal	Canada	20 point	Sinus cavity staging
2009	de Sousa et al	Brazil	4 point horizontal	Polyp staging
			5 point vertical	
			5 point AP	

Table 1. Staging Systems for Endoscopic Polyp Disease and Sinonasal Cavaties.

Howard Levine from Cleveland presented his 6 point staging system at the *VIIth International Symposium on Infection and Allergy of the Nose* in Baltimore, 1989 (Table 2). This system was employed to evaluate outcome in a series of 250 patients undergoing endoscopic sinus surgery and followed long term up to 42 months post-operatively to advocate for the utility of nasal endoscopy to diagnose and monitor sinonasal disease (Levine, 1990).

0	no polyps
1	polyps totally confined to the middle meatus
2	anterior to the turbinate, extending inferiorly to the inferior turbinate but not covering it
3	medial and posterior to the middle turbinate in addition to being anterior to it
4	extending to the floor of the nose, but with parts of the turbinates visible
5	filling the nasal cavity with no portion of the turbinate visible
Adapted from Levine HL. Functional endoscopic sinus surgery: evaluation, surgery, and follow-up of 250 patients. *Laryngoscope* 1990; 100:79-84.	

Table 2. Endoscopic grading of polyp systems proposed by Levine, 1990

In 1993, a group from Aarhus, Denmark, under Lars Johansen proposed a 4-point staging system they employed in their study to evaluate the efficacy of intranasal budesonide in treating small and medium sized nasal polyps (See table 3) (Johansen et al, 1993). Simpler than the system proposed by Levine in 1989, the Johansen system outlined parameters to divide eosinophilic sinonasal polyp disease between mild, moderate and severe.

0	*no polyps*
1	*mild polyposis-* small polyps not reaching the upper edge of the inferior turbinate, causing only slight obstruction
2	*moderate polyposis-* medium-sized polyps reaching between the upper and the lower edge of the inferior turbinate and causing troublesome obstruction
3	*severe polyposis-* large polyps reaching below the lower edge of the inferior turbinate and causing total or almost total obstruction
*total score = sum of scores for each nasal cavity	
Adapted from Johansen VL, Illum P, Kristensen S, Winther L, Petersen S, Synnerstad B. The effect of Budesonide (Rhinocort®) in the treatment of small and medium sized nadal polyps. *Clin Otolaryngol* 1993; 18: 524-7.	

Table 3. Endoscopic grading of polyp systems proposed by Johansen et al, 1993.

That same year, Howard Levine along with Mark May published staging systems aimed at facilitating quantifying objectively outcomes in sinus surgery (May et al, 1993). Among the various staging systems proposed including staging of the endoscopic sinus surgical intervention, anatomical abnormalities on CT scans, patient subjective measures, etc., a five point scheme was proposed (table 4).

Also in 1993, an overall staging system for sinonasal disease was published by Lund and Mackay from University College of London. In addition to scoring systems for the nasal cavity and of the radiographic appearance on sinus CT, a simple 3 point staging system for endoscopic appearance of nasal polyps was proposed with 0 correlating to no polyps, 1 for polyps confined to the middle meatus and 2 for polyps beyond the middle meatus (Lund & Mackay, 1993). Moreover, the *Danish/Swedish Study Group* carried out a double-blind placebo-controlled study of topical budesonide for nasal polyps and presented a 4 point scoring scheme (table 5) which expanded on the simple classification presented by Lund and Mackay (Lildholdt et al, 1995).

1+	anterior attachment of middle turbinate visible
2+	anterior attachment of middle turbinate obscured
3+	nasal cavity filled to vestibule
4+	nasal cavity filled to nares
5+	nasal cavity filed to lip
Adapted from May M, Levine HL, Schaitkin B, Mester SJ. Results of surgery. In: Levine H, May M, editors. Endoscopic sinus surgery. New York: Thieme Medical Publishers, Inc., 1993:176-92.	

Table 4. Endoscopic grading of polyp systems proposed by May and Levine, 1993

0	no polyposis
1	*mild polyposis* - (small polyps not reaching the upper edge of the inferior turbinate)
2	*moderate polyposis* - (medium sized polyps reaching between the upper and lower edge of the inferior turbinate)
3	*severe polyposis* - (large polyps reaching below the lower edge of the inferior turbinate)
Adapted from Lildholdt T, Rundkrantz H, Lindqvist N. Efficacy of topical corticosteroid powder for nasal polyps: a double-blind, placebo-controlled study of budesonide. *Clin Otolaryngol* 1995; 20(1): 26-30.	

Table 5. Endoscopic grading of polyp systems proposed by Lildholdt et al., 1995

In March 1996, an international workshop on nasal polyposis in Davos, Switzerland, *the International Conference on Sinus Disease,* proposed a polyp staging scheme somewhat adapted from the polyp staging system based on Lund and MacKay (Lund & MacKay 1993; Lund & Kennedy 1995). This staging system, sometimes referred to as Mackay & Nacleiro, includes an endoscopic polyp grading system with grading from 0 to 3 depending upon the polyp burden (table 6) where a score of 0 indicates to visible polyp disease on endoscopy, 1 polyps confined to the middle meatus, 2 polyps not completely obstructing the nasal cavity and 3 polyps completely obstructing the nasal cavity (Malm, 1997). This system has since been employed several times in the rhinology literature as a validated scale for outcomes measures (Andrews et al, 2005; Browne et al, 2006). Multicentre validation of this system demonstrated a strong correlation between its scores and symptom reduction using the 22-question Sinonasal Outcome Test-SNOT 22, as well as a correlation with complication rates and revision rates (Hopkins et al, 2007).

Johansson et al from the Central Hospital in Skövde, Sweden conducted an evaluation of 5 various endoscopic measures of polyp burden and proposed their own Visual Analog Scale from 0-100 where 0 refers to a total absence of polyps and 100 a nasal cavity completely filled with polyps. They conducted a study to evaluate the reproducibility of this system along with evauation of the Lildholdt scoring system and the Lund-Mackay scoring systems as well as lateral imaging (where polyps are expressed on a schematic picture of the lateral nasal wall and expressed as a percentage of total area) and their 0-100 visual analog scale for nasal patency. They found that their visual analog scale, along with the Lund-Mackay, and nasal patency score yielded poor inter-rater reproducibility; rather, the Lildholdt score and

0	absence of polyps
1	polyps that do not prolapse beyond the middle turbinate and may require an endoscope for visualization
2	polyps that are extended below the middle turbinate and are visible with a nasal speculum
3	polyps are massive and occlude the entire nasal cavity
Adapted from Malm L. Assessment and staging of nasal polyposis. *Acta Otolaryngol (Stockh)* 1997; 117:465-467.	

Table 6. Endoscopic grading of polyp systems proposed by Mackay & Nacleiro, 1996

lateral imaging were found to be superior for reliability and reproducibility (Johansson et al, 2000). After finding poor inter-rater agreement using the Lund-Mackay polyp scoring but a high correlation using lateral imaging and the four step scoring system proposed by Lildholdt et al, that same group then conducted a study in 2002 to identify the sensitivity of grading systems for detect early changes in polyp disease with topical budesonide treatments in a prospective, randomized placebo controlled trial. Lateral imaging showed statistically significant changes in polyp size was detectable after 14 days of topical corticosteroid use and found to be more sensitive than the Lildholdt staging (Johansson et al, 2002).

Rasp et al from the Ludwig-Maximilians-Universität in Munich proposed a four grade polyp score to include early polypoid changes and was again validated and employed to evaluate effect of topical and systemic steroid therapy (see table 7) (Rasp et al, 2000, Kramer&Rasp, 1999).

I	polyposal swelling of the mucosa of the middle meatus
II	nasal polyps within the middle or lower meatus
III	polyps extending over the middle turbinate
IV	nasal polyposis with protrusion into the anterior nose
Adapted from Kramer MF, Rasp G. Nasal polyposis: eosinophils and interleukin-5. *Allergy* 1999; 54:669-680.	

Table 7. Endoscopic grading of polyp systems proposed by Rasp 1999.

Passali et al from the University of Siena conducted a prospective randomized controlled study of 170 patients evaluating the efficacy of intranasal furosemide compared to intranasal mometasone for chronic sinusitis with polyposis. They evaluated subjective patient outcomes and for quantifying objective outcomes proposed a four point staging system very much like the Mackay – Nacleiro system, but taking into account endoscopic appearance as well as nasal volumes on acoustic rhinomanomatry (Table 8) (Passali et al 2003).

The multinational *Rhinosinusitis Initiative* with representation from national societies of the USA, Belgium, Netherlands, United Kingdom and Japan, in 2006 developed guidelines for facilitating clinical trials for rhinosinusitis. Among the recommendations put forth by the guidelines was a 5-point polyp grading (table 9) scheme which the group advocated to be used in all subsequent rhinologic literature (Meltzer et al, 2006).

0	no polyps seen
1	polyps confined to the middle meatus with AR values in normal range
2	polyps prolapsing beyond the middle turbinate, with less than 10% reduction in volume by AR
3	subobstructive forms requiring another operation (>50% reduction of nasal volumes)
Adapted from Passali D, Bernstein JM, Passali FM, Damiani V, Passali GC, Bellusi L. Treatment of recurrent chronic hyperplastic sinusitis with nasal polyposis. *Arch Otol Head Neck* 2003; 129: 656-659.	

Table 8. Grading of polyp system proposed by Passali et al, 2003.

0	no visible polyps seen
1	small amount of polypoid disease confined within the middle meatus
2	multiple polyps occupying the middle meatus
3	polyps extending beyond the middle meatus, within the sphenoethmoid recess but not totally obstructing, or both
4	polyps completely obstructing the nasal cavity
Adapted from Meltzer et al. Rhinosinusitis: developing guidance for clinical trials. *J All Clin Immun* 2006; 118(suppl): 17-61.	

Table 9. Grading of polyps system proposed by Meltzer et al, 2006.

A group from Brazil proposed a novel endoscopic staging system using three-dimensional nasal polyp assessment and nasal endoscopy with polyp scales in vertical, horizontal and antero-posterior planes (see Table 10) but in the end was found to show less inter-rater agreement than the polyp systems of Johanssen et al and the Lund-Mackay polyp scores (de Sousa et al, 2009).

Overall, a common theme seems to emerge amongst all polyp scores regarding the degree polyp disease obstructs the middle meatus and the overall nasal cavity. Agreeing upon a single polyp system that is reliable, reproducible with high intra and inter-rater reliability and touches on clinically important factors pertaining to extent of polyp disease continues to challenge the rhinologic community.

Horizontal Plane (H)	
H0	no polyps
H1	polyps restricted to the middle meatus
H2	polyps expand beyond the middle meatus
HT	polyps expand beyond the middle meatus and touch the septum
Vertical Place (V)	
V0	no polyps
V1	polyps in the middle meatus only
VI	polyps extending inferiorly to the middle meatus, going beyond the upper border of the inferior turbinate
VS	polyps extending superiorly to the middle meatus, between the septum and the middle turbinate
VT	polyps occupying the entire vertical aspect of the nasal cavity
Antero-posterior plane (P)	
P0	no polyps
P1	polyps in the middle meatus only
PA	polyps extending anteriorly to the middle meatus, reaching the head of the inferior turbinate
PP	polyps extending posterior to the middle meatus, reaching the tail of the inferior and middle turbinate
PT	polyps occupying the entire antero-posterior aspect of the nasal cavity
Adapted from de Sousa, MCA, Becker HMG, Becker CG, de Castro MM, de Sousa NJA, dos Santos Guimaraes RE. Reproducibility of the three-dimensional endoscopic staging system for nasal polyposis. Braz J Otorhinolaryngol 2009;75(6):814-20.	

Table 10. Grading of polyps system proposed by de Sousa et al, 2009.

2.2 Objective endoscopic measures of the sinonasal cavity

Scoring systems for endoscopic findings in the sinonasal cavity beyond simple polyp grading schemes have been used increasingly in the literature to objectively measure outcomes in interventions involving sinonasal disease (Cote & Wright, 2010). As early as the late 1980's, efforts to classify severity of sinus pathology based on endoscopic findings was attempted. A rudimentary staging system was proposed by Jacobs et al relying on CT and endoscopic findings to classify severity of chronic sinusitis (Jacobs et al, 1990). At the first *International Symposium: Contemporary Sinus Surgery* in Pittsburgh, 1990, Ralph Gaskins of Atlanta, GA, presented a staging system for chronic sinusitis that incorporated endoscopic, radiologic findings, and patient immunologic factors, polyp severity, prior surgeries, and infection history into a complex staging system (table 11) to facilitate prediction of surgical response and guide selection of surgical procedure. Gaskins et al recommended Messerklinger technique functional endoscopic middle meatal surgery for stages 1 and early stage 2, with a Wigand total sphenoethmoidectomy for late stage 2 and stage 3 disease and external techniques for stage 4 disease (Gaskins, 1990).

Stage	
0	No surgical sinus disease
I	Score: <1.3
Site	Inflammation limited to the ostiomeatal area
Surgery	No prior sinus/nasal surgery except septoplasty and/or inferior metal antrostomies
Polyps	No polyps or localized to <10% of the sinus space
Infection	Well-controlled infection with no active mucopurulen drainage
Immune status	No underlying immunologic disease except well-controlled allergy
II	Score: 1.3-2.3
Site	Inflammation confined to the maxillary/ethmoid/ostiomeatal areas
Surgery	Prior Caldwell-Luc or polypectomy
Polyps	Polyp disease, with involvement of 10%-50% of the nasal/sinus cavities
Infection	Persistent, localized infection with some active purulent drainage
Immune status	Low-grade immune disorder or fair allergy control
III	Score: >2.3
Site	Pansinus involvement, unilateral or bilateral; isolated sphenoid disease
Surgery	Prior anterior ethmoidectomy/middle turbinate surgery
Polyps	Nasal/sinus polyposis filling more than 50% of the nasal and sinus cavities
Infection	Poorly controlled multisinus infection with active mucopurulent drainage; active fungal disease
Immune status	Poorly controlled allergic rhinitis or significant immune disorder; history of long term steroid treatment
IV	Any score: 4
Site	Sinus disease with extranasal/sinus extension; orbital or intracranial; frontal disease above the nasofrontal duct
Surgery	Prior complete ethmoidectomy or sphenoidectomy
Polyps	Inverting papilloma or other potentially malignant nasal/sinus neoplasm
Infection	Osteomyelitis or infection eroding into the orbit or cranium; mucormycosis
Immune status	Endstage immunologic disease/profoundly immunocompromised patient.
Adapted from Gaskins RE. A surgical staging system for chronic sinusitis. Am J Rhinol 1992; 6:5-12.	

Table 11. Stages of Surgical Sinus Disease by Gaskins, 1990

The University of Pennsylvania's David Kennedy, in his 1992 thesis to the American Laryngological, Rhinological and Otological Society, attempted to classify extent of sinonasal inflammatory disease into 8 groups based on disease found at time of endoscopic surgery (see Table 12). In his study, he reviewed over 240 data fields for each of the 120 patient subjects to establish correlation with outcomes. Extent of preoperative disease and

1	Unilateral or bilateral anatomic abnormality
2	Unilateral ethmoid disease
3	Unilateral ethmoid diseas and involvement of 1 dependent sinus
4	Bilateral ethmoid disease
5	Unilateral ethmoid disease and involvement of 2 or 3 dependent sinuses
6	Bilateral ethmoid disease and involvement of 1 dependent sinus
7	Bilateral ethmoid disease and involvement of 2 or more dependent sinuses
8	Diffuse sinonasal polyposis
Adapted from Kennedy DW. Prognostic factors, outcomes and staging in ethmoid sinus surgery. *Laryngoscope* 1992;102(Suppl 57):1-18.	

Table 12. Classification of the extent of disease by Kennedy, 1992.

surgical outcomes was found to be strongly correlated and as such, a staging system for chronic sinusitis was presented to help facilitate prognosis and comparison in inflammatory sinus disease (Table 13).

I	Anatomic abnormailities
	All unilateral sinus disease
	Bilateral disease limited to ethmoid sinuses
II	Bilateral ethmoid disease with involvement of one dependent sinus
III	Bilateral ethmoid disease with involvement of two or more dependent sinuses on each side
IV	Diffuse sinonasal polyposis
Adapted from Kennedy DW. Prognostic factors, outcomes and staging in ethmoid sinus surgery. *Laryngoscope* 1992;102(Suppl 57):1-18.	

Table 13. Chronic sinusitus staging system proposed by Kennedy, 1992.

Other endoscopic fields including mucosal hypertrophy, inflammation, discharge, crusting adhesions and polyp recurrence were examined but not incorporated into the staging scheme (Kennedy, 1992). Valerie Lund and Ian Mackay of University College London, in 1993, proposed a preoperative and postoperative inventory of the endoscopic appearance of the nasal cavities with a score of 0-2 for polyps (0: none; 1: confined to middle meatus; 2: polyps beyond the middle meatus), as well as 0-2 for discharge (0: none; 1: clear and thin; 2: thick and purulent) as well as observations for edema, scarring and crusting (Lund-Mackay, 1993). In 1995, the *Staging and Therapy Group*, headed by Valerie Lund and David Kennedy, proposed an endoscopic staging system for non-neoplastic sinonasal to evaluate therapeutic outcomes that was complex enough to incorporate the most important measures of the sinonasal cavity but simple enough to facilitate regular clinical use. Characteristics are assessed endoscopically of each sinonasal cavity to provide a score – polyp disease, mucosal edema/crusting/scarring and nasal secretion each receiving a score from 0 to 2 (Table 14)(Lund & Kennedy, 1997).

This scoring system has since been the instrument of choice to endoscopically evaluate outcomes of interventions in non-neoplastic sinonasal disease prospectively over time in research and clinical practice.

Polyp	0=absence of polyp, 1=polyps in middle meatus only, 2=beyond middle meatus
Edema	0=absent, 1=mild, 2=severe
Discharge	0=no discharge, 1=clear, thin discharge, 2=thick, purulent discharge
Scarring	0=absent, 1=mild, 2=severe
Crusting	0=absent, 1=mild, 2=severe
Adapted from Lund VJ, Kennedy DW. Quantification for staging sinusitis. In: Kennedy DW, editor. International Conference on Sinus Disease: Terminology, Staging, Therapy. Ann Otol Rhinol Laryngol 1995; 104(Suppl 167):17-21.	

Table 14. Sinus endoscopy scoring system proposed by Lund and Kennedy, 1995.

A newer sinonasal scoring system, the Perioperative Sinus Endoscopy (POSE) scoring system was employed by Wright & Agrawal to evaluate the outcomes in a randomized trial of perioperative systemic steroids on surgical patients with chronic rhinosinusits with polyposis (Wright & Agrawal, 2007). POSE scoring was introduced to enhance face validity and responsiveness to change by providing richer measures of the inflammation in the ethmoid cavity, scarring and obstruction in outflow, as well as evaluation of secondary sinuses and included instructions for baseline assessments (table 15).

Middle Turbinate		Right	Left
Normal	0		
Synechia/Lateralized	1-2		
Middle Meatus/MMA		Right	Left
Healthy	0		
Narrowing/Closure	1-2		
Maxillary Sinus Contents	1-2		
Ethmoid Cavity		Right	Left
Healthy	0		
Crusting	1-2		
Mucosal Edema	1-2		
Polypoid Change	1-2		
Polyposis	1-2		
Secretions	1-2		
Total (16)			
Secondary Sinuses			
Frontal Recess/Sinus	0-2		
Sphenoid Sinus	0-2		
Overall Total	16 18F 18S 20		
18F = middle meatal antrostomy + ethmoidectomy + frontal sinusotomy; 18S = middle meatal antrostomy + ethmoidectomy + sphenoidotomy 20 = middle meatal antrostomy + ethmoidectomy + sphenoidotomy + frontal sinusotomy			
Adapted from Wright ED, Agrawal S. Impact of perioperative systemic steroids on surgical outcomes in patients with chronic rhinosinusitis with polyposis: evaluation with the novel perioperative sinus endoscopy (POSE) scoring system. *Laryngoscope* 2007; 117(suppl):1-28.			

Table 15. Peri-Operative Sinus Endoscopy (Pose) Score by Wright and Agrawal, 2007.

In that study, both the Lund – Kennedy Endoscopic score and POSE score were shown to be sensitive to changes over time but the POSE seemed to be more sensitive to subtle changes over time (fig 1) and correlated better with symptom scores. (Wright & Agrawal, 2007). We found employing both measures simultaneously has merit in exploiting the established reliability of the Lund-Kennedy score while benefiting from the added information gleaned from the POSE score (Cote & Wright, 2010). With further use and validation of the POSE score, it may perhaps become the staging system of choice to prospectively stage sinonasal cavities over time.

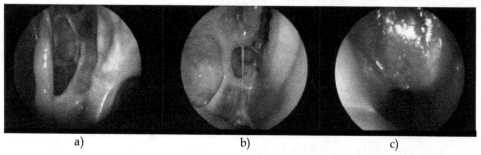

a)   b)   c)

Fig. 1. Three cavites: a) Left cavity, POSE = 0 (normal middle turbinate, healthy middle meatal antrostomy, healthy ethmoid cavity); b) Right cavity, POSE = 3 (2 points for edema, 1 point for mild secretions); c) Right cavity, POSE = 10 (2 points for closure of middle meatus 2 for edema, 2 for polypoid changes, 2 for polyposis,2 for secretions)

2.3 Objective endoscopic measures of surgical field visibility

With novel technologies and procedures being developed with the aim of facilitating visibility during endoscopic surgery, objective measures to evaluate such techniques are being proposed. The first proposed endoscopic surgical field grading scale (table 16) was published by Boerzaart et al in 1995 to objectively evaluate controlled hypotension with sodium nitroprusside in esmolol to facilitate sinus surgery and found that controlled esmolol-induce hypotension yielded superior surgical conditions.

0	No bleeding.
1	Slight bleeding - no suctioning of blood required.
2	Slight bleeding- occasional suctioning required. Surgical field not threatened.
3	Slight bleeding- frequent suctioning required. Bleeding threatens surgical field a few seconds after suction is removed.
4	Moderate bleeding- frequent suctioning required. Bleeding threatens surgical field directly after suction is removed.
5	Severe bleeding- constant suctioning required. Bleeding appears faster than can be removed by suction. Surgical field severely threatened and surgery not possible.
Adapted from Boerzaart AP, van der Merwe J. Comparison of sodium nitroprusside- and esmolol-induced controlled hypotension for functional endoscopic sinus surgery. Can J Anaesth 1995;42:373-376.	

Table 16. Assessment of intra-operative surgical field by Boezaart et al, 1995

This six point scale was aimed at quantifying the amount of bleeding in the surgical field that hindered progression of the surgical intervention – 0 no bleeding, 1 slight bleeding no suctioning, 2 slight bleeding occasional suctioning, 3 slight bleeding frequent suctioning, 4 moderate bleeding frequent suctioning with bleeding threatening the surgical field, 5 severe bleeding constant suctioning (Boezaart 1995).

An eleven point grading scale was then proposed by PJ Wormald's group from Adelaide which sought to address some of the limitations with the Boezaart scale with grades 1-6 varying by number of points of ooze and 7-10 by severity of hemorrhage .

0	No bleeding.
1	1-2 points of ooze
2	3-4 points of ooze
3	5-6 points of ooze
4	7-8 points of ooze
5	9-10 points of ooze (sphenoid fills in 60 seconds)
6	>10 points of ooze, obscuring surface (sphenoid fills in 50 seconds)
7	Mild bleeding/oozing from entire surgical surface with slow accumulation of blood in the post nasal space (sphenoid fills by 40 seconds)
8	Moderate bleeding from entire surgical surface with moderate accumulation of blood in the post nasal space (sphenoid fills by 30 seconds)
9	Moderately severe bleeding with rapid accumulation of blood in the post nasal space (sphenoid fills by 20 seconds)
10	Severe bleeding with nasal cavity filling rapidly (sphenoid fills in <10 seconds)
Adapted from Athanasiadis T, Beule A, Embate J, Steinmeier E, Field J, Wormald PJ. Standardized video-endoscopy and surgical field grading scale for endoscopic sinus surgery: a multi-centre study. *Laryngoscope* 2008; 118:314-319.	

Table 17. Intra-operative surgical field grading by Wormald, 2008

By employing a standardized video-endoscopy technique both the Boerzaart and Wormald scores were found to have improved intra and inter-rater reliability; the Wormald scale, however, was found to be more sensitive to bleeding changes in endoscopic sinus surgery and demonstrated slightly better inter-rater reliability (Athanasiadis 2008). Further application and evaluation of these two systems must be undertaken before the rhinologic community decides a gold standard and establishes their strengths and limitations.

3. Conclusion

With increased refinement of endoscopic interventions for sino-nasal disease, there is simultaneous refinement in objective measures to audit the outcomes of these interventions. While each grading system has inherent limitations, they represent efforts to create a means to objectively communicate a richness in observations and outcomes that is both reliable and reproducible by practitioners treating sinonasal disease. In addition, many centres around the world are using these objective measures to monitor inflammatory sinus disease that, based simply on subjective measures, would be occult. This provides the opportunity to intervene with topical or less invasive therapies at a point where the disease may be more easily managed.

4. References

Andrews AE, Bryson JM, Rowe-Jones JM. Site of origin of nasal polyps: Relevance toPathogenesis and management. *Rhinology* 2005; 43(3) 180-184.

Athanasiadis T, Beule A, Embate J, Steinmeier E, Field J, Wormald PJ. Standardized video-endoscopy and surgical field grading scale for endoscopic sinus surgery: a multi-centre study. *Laryngoscope* 2008; 118:314-319.

Boerzaart AP, van der Merwe J. Comparison of sodium nitroprusside- and esmolol-induced controlled hypotension for functional endoscopic sinus surgery. *Can J Anaesth* 1995;42:373-376.

Browne JP, Hopkins C, Slack R et al. Health related quality of life after polypectomy with and without additional surgery. *Laryngoscope* 2006; 116:297-302.

Cote DWJ, Wright ED. Triamcinolone-impregnated nasal dressing following endoscopic sinus surgery: a randomized, double-blind, placebo-controlled study. *Laryngoscope* 2010; 120:1269-1273. de Sousa, MCA, Becker HMG, Becker CG, de Castro MM, de Sousa NJA, dos Santos

Guimaraes RE. Reproducibility of the three-dimensional endoscopic staging system for nasal polyposis. *Braz J Otorhinolaryngol* 2009;75(6):814-20.

Friedman WH, Katsantonis GP, Sivore M, Kay S. Computed tomography staging of the paranasal sinuses in chronic hyperplastic rhinosinusitis. *Laryngoscope* 1990; 100:1161-1665.

Gaskins RE. A surgical staging system for chronic sinusitis. *Am J Rhinol* 1992; 6:5-12.

Giklich RE, Metson R. A comparision of sinus computed tomography (CT) staging systems for outcomes research. *Am J Rhinol* 1994; 8:291-7.

Hopkins C, Browne JP, Slack R, Lund V, Brown P. The Lund-Mackay staging system for chronic rhinosinusitis: How is it used and what does it predict? *Otolaryngol Head Neck Surg* 2007; 137(4):555-61.

Jacobs JB, Gittelman P, Holliday R. Endoscopic sinus surgery for ostiomeatal disease. *Am J Rhinol* 1990; 4:41-43.

Johansen VL, Illum P, Kristensen S, Winther L, Petersen S, Synnerstad B. The effect of Budesonide (Rhinocort®) in the treatment of small and medium sized nasal polyps. *Clin Otolaryngol* 1993; 18: 524-7.

Johansson L, Akerlund A, Holmberg K, MelenI, Stierna P, Bende M. Evaluation of methods for endoscopic staging of nasal polyposis. *Acta Otolaryngol* 2000; 120(1):72-6.

Johansson L, Holmberg K, Melen I, Stierna P, Bende M. Sensitivity of a new grading system for studying nasal polyps with the potential to detect early changes in polyp size after treatment with a topical corticosteroid (budesonide). *Acta Otolaryngol* 2002; 122:49-53.

Jorgensen RA. Endoscopic and computed tomographic findings in ostiomeatal sinus disease. *Arch Otolaryng Head Neck Surg* 1991; 117: 279-287.

Kennedy DW. Prognostic factors, outcomes and staging in ethmoid sinus surgery. *Laryngoscope* 1992;102(Suppl 57):1-18.

Kramer MF, Rasp G. Nasal polyposis: eosinophils and interleukin-5. *Allergy* 1999; 54:669-680.

Lee JT, Kennedy DW. Endoscopic sinus surgery. In: Bailey B, Johnson J, Newlands SD, editors. *Head & Neck Surgery – Otolaryngology, 4th Edition*. Lippincott Williams & Wilkins, 2006: 459-475.

Levine HL. Functional endoscopic sinus surgery: evaluation, surgery, and follow-up of 250 patients. *Laryngoscope* 1990; 100:79-84.

Lildholdt T, Rundkrantz H, Lindqvist N. Efficacy of topical corticosteroid powder for nasal polyps: a double-blind, placebo-controlled study of budesonide. *Clin Otolaryngol* 1995; 20(1): 26-30.

Lund V, Mackay IS. Staging in chronic rhinosinusitis. *Rhinology* 1993; 31: 183-4.

Lund VJ, Scadding GK. Objective assessment of endoscopic sinus surgery in themanagement of chronic rhinosinusitis: an update. *J Laryngol Otol* 1994; 108(9): 749-53.

Lund VJ, Kennedy DW. Quantification for staging sinusitis. In: Kennedy DW, editor. International Conference on Sinus Disease: Terminology, Staging, Therapy. *Ann Otol Rhinol Laryngol* 1995; 104(Suppl 167):17-21.

Lund VJ, Kennedy DW. Staging for rhinosinustis. *Otolaryngol Head Neck Surg* 1997; 117:S35-S40.

Malm L. Assessment and staging of nasal polyposis. *Acta Otolaryngol (Stockh)* 1997; 117:465-467.

May M, Levine HL, Schaitkin B, Mester SJ. Results of surgery. In: Levine H, May M, editors. *Endoscopic sinus surgery.* New York: Thieme Medical Publishers, Inc., 1993:176-92.

Meltzer EO, Hamilos DL, Hadley JA, Lanza DC, Marple BF, Nicklas RA, Adinoff AD,Bachert C, Borish L, Chinchilli VM, Danzig MR, Ferguson BJ, Fokkens WJ, Jenkins SG, Lund VJ, Mafee MF, Nacleiro RM, Pawankar R, Ponikau JU, Schubert MS, Slavin RG, Stewart MG, Togias A, Wald ER, Winther B. Rhinosinusitis: developing guidance for clinical trials. *J All Clin Immun* 2006; 118(suppl): 17-61.

Min Y, Yun Y, Song B et al. Recovery of nasal physiology after functional endoscopic sinus surgery: olfaction and mucociliary transport. *Otorhinolaryngology* 1995; 57:264-268.

Newton JR, Ah-See KW. A review of nasal polyposis. *Therapeutics and Clinical Management*2008; 4(2): 507-512.

Newman LJ Platts-Mills TAE, Phillips CD, Hazen KC, Gross CW. Chronic sinusitis: relationship of computed tomographic findings to allergy, asthma, and eosinophilia. *JAMA* 1994;271(5): 363-367.

Passali D, Bernstein JM, Passali FM, Damiani V, Passali GC, Bellusi L. Treatment of recurrent chronic hyperplastic sinusitis with nasal polyposis. *Arch Otol Head Neck* 2003; 129: 656-659.

Rasp. [A new system for he classification of ethmoid polyposis. Effect of combined local and systemic steroid theray]. *Laryngorhinootologie.* 2000; 79(5):266-72.

Wright ED, Agrawal S. Impact of perioperative systemic steroids on surgical outcomes in patients with chronic rhinosinusitis with polyposis: evaluation with the novel perioperative sinus endoscopy (POSE) scoring system. *Laryngoscope* 2007; 117(suppl):1-28.

3

Endoscopy in Nasopharyngeal Adenoid Surgery

W. F. Ezzat
ORL- Head and Neck Surgery,
Consultant Pediatric Otolaryngologist,
Ain-Shams University, Cairo
Egypt

1. Introduction

Adenoid diseases include acute adenoiditis, recurrent acute adenoiditis, chronic adenoiditis, and obstructive adenoid hyperplasia. The latter, that constitutes a triad of symptoms including chronic nasal obstruction (with snoring and obligate oral breathing), nasal discharge, and nasal intonation of voice, is the most common cause necessitating surgical intervention. Differentiating adenoid infection from that of the sinuses may be challenging due to similarity of signs and symptoms, and the high incidence of coexistence of both diseases adds to the dilemma, as one may even lead to the other. An additional factor that has been recently recognized is the effect of extraesophageal reflux disease and its role in inducing both adenoid and sinus infection, when this is identified and treated, and treatment fails, surgery should intervene, usually adenoidectomy, putting in mind that the associated sinus affection may take a few weeks to months to clear out.

The diagnosis of adenoid hyperplasia and hypertrophy needing surgery is best achieved by both history and physical examination, the aforementioned triad of symptoms is quite non-specific, as it may be present in other conditions, as allergic rhinitis, non allergic rhinitis, sinusitis, and reflux esophagitis. The physical examination should guide to the possible disease, and indicate if further investigations are needed. The classic "adenoid facies" appearance, luckily enough, is rarely seen now, as both the parents and physicians diagnose and treat such conditions early enough to avoid such drastic affection of prolonged nasal obstruction. One of the important investigations that are frequently needed is a sleep study, and a variety of tests are used according to need and facilities, starting from simple overnight oximetry, to a full sleep laboratory test, but these are used only in cases where more severe conditions are suspected, such as in cases of resistant nocturnal enuresis without definite history or physical findings of obstructive condition. When the condition is also not clear cut, a CT scan of the nasopharynx and sinuses may be done. It is the authors personal experience that for symptoms of nasal obstruction to occur in the very young child (below one year of age), to be attributed to simple adenoid hypertrophy, and to be severe enough to need surgery, a lateral radiograph of the nasopharynx would not suffice, but a CT scan should be done to exclude other more serious conditions that can cause nasal obstruction, as –and not restricted to- meningeocles, encephaloceles, dermoid cysts, and unilateral cases of choanal atresia. These conditions may present by mild nasal obstruction since birth but become aggravated during the next few months of life.

Till relatively recent, the well decided upon treatment to adenoid hypertrophy was surgical removal, but the understanding of the role of environmental inflammation from allergies and reflux, understanding the role of chronic infection, alterations in the relationship with commensal microorganisms, and the appearance of alternative therapeutic modalities has led us to revisit this concept. Alternatives to surgical interference in mild to moderate cases of adenoid hypertrophy implies judicious use of antibiotics and other possible contributing factors as allergy or reflux. The antibiotics used usually involve those acting on beta lactamase producing organisms, aiming to regain normal nasopharyngeal flora, and this was found very useful in some studies, especially when there is associated otitis media with effusion (Bernstein et al., 2002), of course this should not give the impression that adenoidectomy should be postponed as much as possible, but a judicious assessment should be done, to avoid the known "adenoid facies" of chronic nasal obstruction, which –as aforementioned- luckily enough is rarely encountered nowadays.

Adenoidectomy may be the most widely performed otolaryngologic procedure done worldwide, whether alone or in combination with other procedures, with rates reaching 65 per 10,000 children in England, and 50 per 10,000 children in the United States (Van Den Akker et al., 2004). Although it might seem as a very simple procedure, it is not without complications. Changes in technique have progressed over the years parallel to the advances in instrumentation and technology used in surgery.

Still, the classic technique of adenoidectomy is widely performed and adopted by many, if not most, otolaryngologic surgeons all over the world, regardless the economic status. This classic technique of adenoidectomy implies blind curettage of the adenoid tissue, which may or may not be followed by digital –still blind- palpation of the nasopharynx by the surgeon, to assure removal. A survey was performed among otolaryngologic surgeons in the United Kingdom, and showed –despite all the facilities and the total coverage of health services by insurance- that still approximately 80% of the surgeons performed this blind adenoidectomy, and approximately 70% performed digital palpation of the nasopharynx at the end of the procedure, even though about 40% of them recognize a possible need for revision surgery (Dhanasekar et al., 2010). Even mirror examination during or after the curettage procedure is not agreed upon nor done universally.

The most common complication of adenoidectomy is recurrence. The recurrence rates of adenoid regrowth needing revision surgery are so diverse and un-agreed upon, Tolczynski (1955) published a paper in 1955 reviewing earlier studies which showed recordings or recurrence ranging from as low as 4-8% as reported by Lundgren, to 23.7-50% according to Hill's investigation, and may even reach above 70% according to Crowe!!!

Residual adenoid tissue is now becoming to be recognized as a cause of persistence of symptoms, or early recurrence of symptoms with regrowth of adenoid tissue. Several studies have shown significant remaining adenoid tissue after the classic "blind" adenoid curettage technique, and Ark (2010) reported that only about 20% of patients had complete removal of their adenoid tissue when only digital palpation was done without any type of visualization. A study conducted by Saxby and Chappel (2009), where they performed nasopharyngoscopic examination postoperatively, showed that 68% of cases had some residual adenoid tissue evident of which 24% had significant obstruction (grade 2 or 3), Bross-Soriano D et al. (2004) even stated that less than 30% of adenoidectomies are complete in absence of use of endoscopy!

The place of residual adenoid tissue with conventional curettage is also controversial, and Regmi et al (2011) reported that when curettage was used alone, it failed to completely remove adenoid tissue from the superiomedial choanae and anterior vault in all cases; incomplete removal was also seen in other parts of the choanae in 67.2% of patients, the Eustachian tube opening in 63 %, the nasopharyngeal roof in 61.78% and the fossa of Rosenmuller in 61%. Ezzat (2010) reported that even with the aid of a mirror, 14.5% of patients had residual adenoid tissue, 35% of which had remnants at the vault of the nasopharynx, 47% at the lateral walls of the nasopharynx (peritubal), and 18% at the posterior choana.

Although the rates of residual adenoid tissue, even in modern literature when postoperative assessment is done, is relatively significant, the number or incidence of patients actually needing revision surgery is not as high as would be expected, thus other factors must be present that would favor or induce further regrowth of the residual adenoid tissue, but to date these factors are still to be determined, although theories as reflux or infection by Helicobacter pylori have been proposed by some as Bulut et al., (2006).

Although the history of endoscopy goes back to the early nineteenth century when it was introduced by Bozzini, it was not practically used for nasal and nasopharyngeal assessment until the early nineteen seventies, and the earliest published papers in this field addressed the use of endoscopy in merely assessing the size of the adenoid tissue as a survey (Weymuller E, 1974), later on with advancement of scopes and refinement of technique the uses were widened.

Adenoidectomy is not only indicated in cases of enlarged and obstructing adenoid tissue, other indications may be any type of chronic otitis media, resistant to treatment, whether secretory otitis media, or chronic suppurative otitis media, where any adenoid tissue should be removed, and especially from the area of the opening of the nasopharynx. Also in cases of sinusitis, especially in children, whether recurrent or chronic, adenoid enlargement must be suspected. Other conditions where adenoid tissue is suspected and should be excluded or removed even if not extensively enlarged are cases of obstructive sleep apnoea, or nocturnal enuresis.

Evaluation of the adenoid status includes symptoms, signs and some investigations (outlined in table 1), in order to differentiate adenoid hyperplasia from other causes presenting with similar symptoms such as rhinitis, sinusitis, deviated septum, reflux disease, or even lymphoproliferative disorders.

The general indications for adenoidectomy are usually classified into obstructive, infective, and neoplastic, the various indications are enumerated in table 2.

Preoperative preparation of a candidate for adenoidectomy does not differ than any other type of surgery, the general status of the patient should be assessed for any contraindications of surgery, but otherwise, especially in children, a blood picture and the bleeding profile usually suffices, although it is still a controversial matter (Hartnick and Ruben, 2000; Wei et al., 2000)

Since most patients are children, an addition to the preoperative assessment is to check the status of teeth, as the mouth gag may dislodge loose teeth, and risk of aspiration may occur. Also checking for overt or submucous cleft palate should be done preoperatively, even by simple palpation, to avoid the risk of developing velopharyngeal insufficiency if a complete adenoidectomy is done in presence of such condition.

Cause	Symptoms	Signs	Investigations
Obstruction	-Obligate oral breather -Sleep disordered breathing -Change in tone of voice	-Hyponasality -Adenoid facies	-Endoscopy of the nose and nasopharynx -X-ray lateral view skull -Polysomnography
Infection	-Nasal and postnasal discharge -Halitosis -Recurrent cough (increase at night) -Possible recurrent vomiting and gastric upset	-Nasal and postnasal discharge, clear or colored -Possible cobblestone appearance of posterior pharyngeal wall	-CT scan, nasopharynx and sinuses -24-h pH probe acid monitoring

Table 1. Evaluation of adenoid status

A factor that seems overt but sometimes missed by junior staff is putting in mind the status of the atlantoaxial joint and the cervical spine, which can be affected by the hyper extension done during exposure, and the author has personally seen two cases with postoperative acute disc prolapse of the cervical spine in adults undergoing adenoidectomy. In young patients this is quite rare except in cases with congenital laxity of the ligaments, which is usually overt and diagnosed previously, or in cases of Down's syndrome.

Depending on the type of adenoidectomy to be performed, one or more techniques can be used for tissue removal:

- Primary adenoidectomy can be performed using a curette, suction coagulator, or a microdebrider. The suction coagulator is ideal for small adenoids, although it can be used routinely regardless of adenoid size.
- Secondary (revision) adenoidectomy can also be performed using curette, suction coagulator, or microdebrider; however, greater precision is achieved by the latter two methods. The suction coagulator generally results in the least bleeding.
- Partial superior adenoidectomy is performed in children at risk for Velo-Pharyngeal-Insufficiency. The suction coagulator and microdebrider are best suited for this procedure (Kakani et al., 2000).

- OBSTRUCTIVE
  - o Chronic nasal obstruction attributed to adenoid tissue hyperplasia, proven by endoscopy, X –ray, or CT scan
  - o Obligate nasal breathing attributed to adenoid tissue hyperplasia, proven by endoscopy, X –ray, or CT scan.
  - o Sleep disordered breathing attributed to adenoid tissue hyperplasia
    - ▪ Obstructive sleep apnoea/hypopnoea syndrome
    - ▪ Obstructive hypoventilation syndrome
    - ▪ Upper airway resistance syndrome
  - o Speech abnormalities (closed nasality) attributed to adenoid tissue hypertrophy.
  - o Dental and orofacial abnormalities attributed to chronic nasal obstruction
  - o Failure to thrive attributed to chronic nasal obstruction
  - o Cor-pulmonale attributed to chronic nasal obstruction
  - o Lymphoproliferative disorders

- INFECTIVE
  - o Repeated, or chronic adenoiditis
  - o Recurrent otitis media
  - o Chronic otitis media with effusion, non responsive to medical treatment
  - o Chronic suppurative otitis media
  - o Chronic sinusitis

- NEOPLASTIC
  - o Documented or suspected tumor, benign or malignant

Table 2. Indications for adenoidectomy

2. Endoscopy in nasopharyngeal adenoid surgery

Indications, uses and benefits of endoscopic use in nasopharyngeal adenoid surgery have varied over the years, but still to date, it has not become routine in this type of surgery, in spite of all the evidence and published studies that show the benefit of such use!!!

The uses of uses of endoscopy in nasopharyngeal adenoid surgery imply use in diagnosis, during surgery, and in follow up.

The types of rigid endoscopes used in adenoid surgery are illustrated in figure 1, and an example of the photo documentation systems that is optional but very beneficial is illustrated in figure 2.

2.1 Use of endoscopy in diagnosis of nasopharyngeal adenoid size

Although the most important factor in diagnosing adenoid size is the symptomatology the patient presents with, which is mainly nasal obstruction, mouth breathing, and/or snoring, other tools have been used to verify or exclude adenoid as the cause of nasal obstruction, the most commonly used is the X-ray of a lateral view of the skull, but this is not flawless. X-rays have over and under estimated sizes of adenoid tissue in many instances. Another issue is that adenoid tissue may be present in areas causing obstruction and not that well apparent in the X-ray, especially in recurrent or persistent cases after adenoidectomy, such as choanal adenoids. Therefore, a more realistic and accurate estimate is to perform an office endoscopy by a rigid sinoscope or flexible nasopharyngoscope, this is quite simple and applicable in adults, adolescents and cooperative older children, which are rarely the case where adenoid hypertrophy is a major problem. In younger children, which compromise most cases, to perform such office type endoscopy is quite difficult and challenging, but it can be used using short acting sedatives such as chloral hydrate which has been used safely in children and infants since 1869 (Buck, 1992), the recommended dose of chloral hydrate is 50 to 75 mg/kg given orally or rectally. In other studies, higher single doses of up to 100 mg/kg have been used with increased success in children and infants over 1 month of age (Steinberg, 1993). It is the author's belief that such endoscopy is much more beneficial in assessing the whole upper airway for proper planning of the treatment modality, whether surgical, medical or both.

Endoscopy is also valuable in case symptoms are present other than obstruction, such as loss of appetite, slower development than peers, and decreased hearing which is related to Eustachian Tube dysfunction, in absence of apparent X-ray enlargement of the adenoid tissue, in such cases surgery may be indicated to remove tubal adenoid tissue even in absence of X-ray evidence of enlargement or significant nasal obstruction. Another important issue to be addressed is that there may be an element of septal deviation that is causing the obstruction, which was be missed by anterior rhinoscopy and X-ray, although this is quite rare below the age of 5 (Reitzen et al. 2011).

2.2 Use of endoscopy in nasopharyngeal adenoid surgery

Although many studies have reached a prevailed conclusion that endoscopic aided adenoidectomy has benefits covering any added cost or time, in terms of better exposure or complete removal, still regrettably it is not the standard teaching in many parts of the world, not only in developing countries, which might have some concern for cost, but also in developed countries. The application of endoscopy in adenoidectomy has several techniques, from full endoscopic power aided adenoidectomy to adenoidectomy by conventional curettage but with endoscopic visualization, to simple endoscopic examination at the end of conventional adenoidectomy to assess complete excision.

2.2.1 Simple endoscopic examination after conventional adenoidectomy

One of the simplest ways of using an endoscope for assurance of complete surgery and total removal of adenoid tissue is the mere transnasal endoscopic examination of the posterior choanal and the nasopharynx after conventional curettage adenoidectomy, with or without mirror assistance, and to proceed with completion adenoidectomy –if needed- under endoscopic guidance. In such case, after the surgeon has removed the main bulk of the adenoid tissue and established hemostasis, the endoscope -size of which is determined by age of patient- is introduced through BOTH SIDES of the nasal fossae to visualize the posterior choana and the nasopharynx (Ezzat 2010) (figure 3), and if any adenoid tissue is found it is removed either with a smaller adenoid curette, with a Blakesly-Wigand Nasal Forceps ® (figure 4), or a Blakesly Rhinoforce ® Ethmoid forceps (figure 5), straight or with upward curve. Further hemostasis should be accomplished if needed. An important sign of complete adenoid removal, without injury of the underlying pharyngeal bed, at least to the author's experience, is the lack of need for packing the nasopharyngeal bed after surgery, although there has been no published literature highlighting this fact

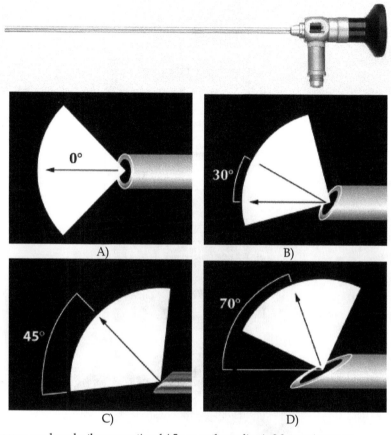

The endoscope used can be the conventional 4.5mm or the pediatric 2.3 mm sinoscope.

The angulations of the endoscope used is determined by the approach it is used in, when the endoscope is introduced and used through the nasal fossa, a $0°$, or $30°$ endoscope can be used, as they give a more direct view of the nasopharynx (A, and B), but when the endoscope is used transorally, a $45°$ or $70°$ endoscope is needed to obtain a better view by angulating the view (C, and D)

Fig. 1. Endoscopes used in adenoid surgery

2.2.2 Endoscopic visualization with routine curettage adenoidectomy

To start the surgery of adenoidectomy under direct endoscopic visualization has been described by many (Wan et al, 2005, Songu et al, 2010), this technique implies the introduction of the endoscope endonasally at the beginning of surgery, attachment to a monitor, then using the regular mouth gag and conventional curette in excision of the adenoid tissue.

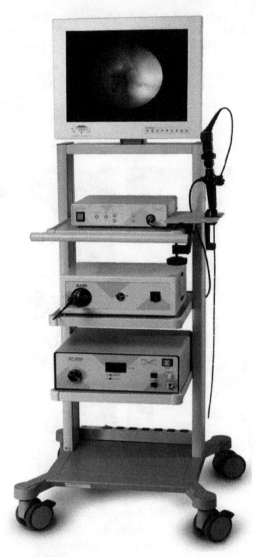

The system is optional, but helps in documentation, illustration to the patient and for teaching purposes.

Fig. 2. The photo documentation system of use with endoscopes.

According to the size of the adenoid tissue as assessed endoscopically, a curette is chosen and should fit snugly over the adenoid and is inserted up to the septal vomer , the curette is swept inferiorly with a side-to-side rocking motion to completely remove all adenoid tissue. Care is taken to avoid deep muscular or vertebral injury, injury to the torus region, and injury to the choana. Again, if endoscopy reveals any residual tissue, a smaller curette or a St Clair adenoid forceps or a Blakesly-Wigand Nasal Forceps ® (figure 4), or a Blakesly

Rhinoforce ® Ethmoid forceps (figure 5), straight or with upward curve is used to remove any retained tissue noted.

Although this technique might seem appealing, in practice it is quite cumbersome, too many instruments and connections, and lack of direct eye-to-hand sense is difficult for beginners, although it is very useful in teaching and monitoring trainees. The cost of such a setting might also be a burden in less funded establishments, and no additional benefit over the routine adenoidectomy followed by mere examination by the endoscope at the end of surgery has been documented in any study published over the past years.

Some have described using the a 45° or 70° endoscope through the oral cavity to guide the excision of adenoid tissue all through the surgical procedure (Jong & Gendeh, 2008), this might seems more appealing, especially in younger children, as their nasal cavities are smaller, but even with the transoral approach to insert the endoscope, the field may be somewhat narrow.

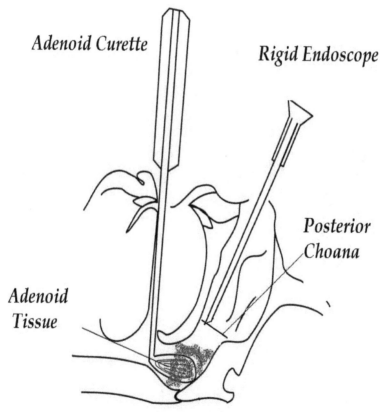

Fig. 3. Simultaneous use of the endoscope and adenoid curette

2.2.3 Fully endoscopic diathermy aided ablation adenoidectomy

The use of diathermy in adenoidectomy has been used since the nineteen sixties (Remington-Hobbs C, 1968), but with the regular monopolar blade, and was not widely used, as issues of pharyngeal stenosis and post operative pain were addressed, and many used such a technique for control of bleeding in cases where simple packing was not enough. The suction diathermy was introduced in the late nineteen nineties and gained popularity rapidly due to several reasons, the procedure is simple, with minimal blood loss, not associated way any risk of pharyngeal stenosis (Walker P., 2001) or recurrence, although it is repeatedly reported to have longer working time than conventional curettage adenoidectomy (Jonas NE., 2007). The price is not an issue, as the disposable hand piece is relatively cheap, and is even cheaper than other disposable more sophisticated instruments used (Walker P., 2001). (figure 6)

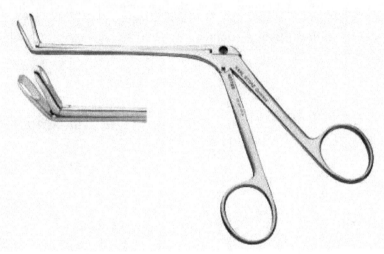

Fig. 4. Blakesly- Wigand Nasal Forceps

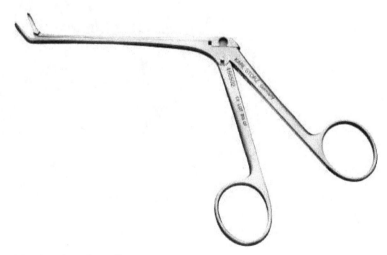

Fig. 5. Blakesly- Rhinoforce Forceps

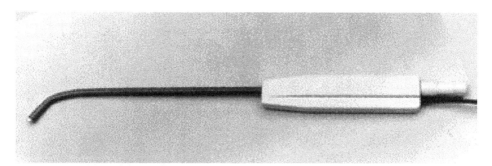

The tip of the handpiece is flexible and can be manipulated according to need

Fig. 6. The suction diathermy handpiece

The original description of such use dictated that the nasopharynx is exposed by means of two catheters introduced through the nose, and brought out of the mouth, retracting the soft palate. Often, a mirror was used to guide the suction diathermy to visualize the adenoid tissue, but the use of endoscopes with this suction diathermy technique is very beneficial. Endoscopes have been used by two approaches, the first of which a 45° endoscope is introduced ORALLY for visualization, and then with the other hand the suction is introduced and surgery completed (Lo and Rowe-Jones, 2006), the second of which a fully transnasal endoscopic ablation adenoidectomy is done (Shin and Hartnick, 2003). Although this second type has the benefit of not needing hyperextension of the neck, it is not suitable for all age groups as it requires a certain wideness of the nasal fossa, but it is optimal in certain situations –if applicable- such as lack of neck stability as in children with Down's syndrome.

2.2.4 Endoscopic coblation (hydrodebrider) adenoidectomy
Coblation adenoidectomy (figure 7) is a relatively recent introduction in the field of otolaryngologic surgery. Coblation, that uses lower temperatures than electrocautery to remove tissue and achieve hemostasis, has been shown to reduce pain and decrease postoperative narcotic use, leading to shorter recovery times and a quicker return to normal in children (Benninger M and Walner D, 2007). The use of coblation can be used by guidance of mirror viewing, but of course endoscopic guidance gives much more accurate view, whether used transnasally to transorally, and does not add any cumbersome to the surgical field, as the hand that uses the mirror uses the endoscope. As with most guided techniques, this approach dictates the partial exposure of the surgical field by using 2 catheters introduced transnasal and delivered orally, to retract the soft palate.

2.2.5 Endoscopic micro-debrider-aided adenoidectomy
Microdebrider (power) aided adenoidectomy was introduced and started to be common in the early 21st century, the use of the microdebrider (figure 8) has been used for adenoidectomy in several modes and approaches, the more common approach and practical one is introduction of the endoscope through the nasal fossa and the hand piece of the microdebrider through the mouth, and under endoscopic vision, shaving the adenoid tissue piece by piece. Both the hand piece and the endoscope can be introduced through the oral cavity if the nasal fossa is too narrow, in younger children.

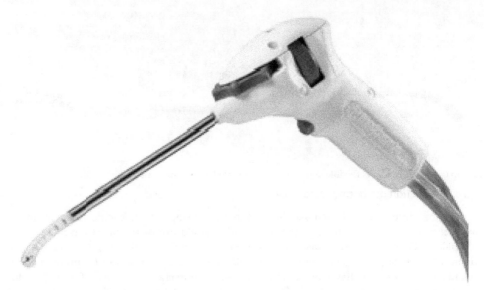

Fig. 7. Hydrodebrider Hand piece

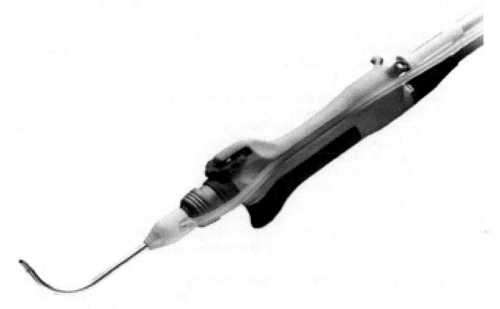

Fig. 8. Microdebrider hand piece

One of the major advantages of using the microdebrider is having the option to remove adenoid tissue only partially (Rodriguez et al., 2002; Koltai et al., 2002), as in cases of insufficient velopharyngeal valve, in cases of repaired cleft palate, and those with submucous cleft palate.

Blood loss is comparable to other methods used, and although the time used may be more than with conventional curette adenoidectomy, the clearer filed and more complete surgery seems to justify the extra time, to save time, some have used such powered instrumentation after removal of the main bulk of the adenoid tissue by conventional curettage (Pagella F et al., 2009). The main limitation is the price of the disposable hand piece that exceeds by far all other modes of adenoidectomy. Figure 9 shows the typical setting for use of combined endoscopic and powered instrumentation adenoidectomy.

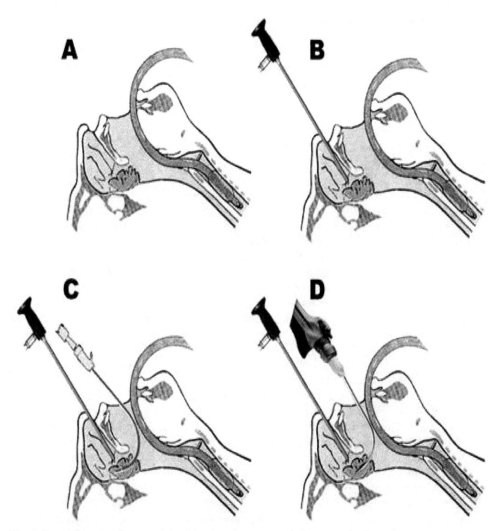

Fig. 9. Typical setting for use of combined endocopic guided powered adenoidectomy a; positioning of the patient with endotracheal tube inserted orally, b; introduction of the endoscope trans-nasally, c; introduction of the microdebrider hand piece, d; attachment of the hand piece to the micromotor and commencing surgery *(Courtsy of Prof Dr MZ Helal with permission)*

2.3 Follow up after adenoidectomy

Postoperative follow up after adenoidectomy does not entail any special proceedings; the child is usually discharge from the hospital on the same day of surgery. The usual regime is to advice soft diet for 24 hours, and then regular diet allowed after that, usually no antibiotics are used. A mild analgesic may be prescribed. Nasal decongestant drops may be used with caution for 2-3 days, as the child is more liable to toxicity from the raw surface of the adenoid bed. The child is usually scheduled for a post operative visit after 3-4 days to assure that everything is going in order. Some have advised postoperative endoscopy to assess any residual adenoid tissue, but this is of no value except if the patient develops symptoms of regrowth of the adenoid.

2.4 Limitations of use of endoscopy in adenoid surgery

In younger children with small nasal fossae, the introduction of the endoscope nasally can by quite difficult, if not impossible, but this can be overcomed if the endoscope is used trans-oral, otherwise there are no limitations. Excessive bleeding in the operative field may limit the view, but this should not be an indication to abort the surgery except in very rare cases, and if such case occurs it can be managed by regular packing for a few minutes, and then continuing surgery.

2.5 Complications of endoscopy use in adenoid surgery

No additional complications during adenoid surgery have been recorded with the additional use of endoscopy to guide the surgical procedure. Complications –if occur- would be those of the technique, and not from use of endoscopy. Complications related to surgery are outlined in table 3, with their presentation and possible management lines.

Noniatrogenic complications after adenoidectomy include (Randall and Hoffer, 1998)

- Regrowth of adenoid tissue, particularly in very young children, which may require revision (secondary) adenoidectomy.
- Hypernasality, because of temporary pain splinting. Persistent hypernasality is rare and probably caused by unrecognized pre-existing velopharyngeal weakness. Management includes speech therapy or a sphincter pharyngoplasty, if refractory.
- Atlantoaxial subluxation (Grisel's syndrome), which presents with persistent torticollis 1-2 weeks after surgery. Neurological or orthopedic consultation may be required.

Iatrogenic complications after adenoidectomy include

- Dental injury, from intubation or the mouth gag. Dentition should be checked prior to inserting and removing the mouth gag. Urgent laryngoscopy and bronchoscopy must be performed for any newly discovered missing teeth.
- Nasopharyngeal stenosis, caused by excessive tissue removal. Repair is difficult and may include dilation, steroid injection, or a tissue flap (rotational, advancement, or free flap) (Giannoni et al., 1998).
- Eustachian tube injury, if the torus tubarius is cauterized or denuded
- Meningitis, after injecting lidocaine and epinephrine into the posterior nasopharynx prior to adenoidectomy. Injections are unnecessary and should be avoided.
- Lingual nerve palsy, caused by pressure from the tongue blade of the mouth gag.
- Cautery burns, caused by operator error or equipment malfunction. (Zinder and Parker, 1996).

Complication	Presentation	Management
Hemorrhage	Bleeding from mouth or nose	Local control (vasoconstricting agents, cautery)
Airway obstruction	Stridor/stertor, palatal swelling	Nasopharyngeal airway +/- steroids
Dehydration	Dry mucous membrane	Hydration
Persistent velopharygneal valve insufficiency	Hypernasal speech (>2 months postoperative)	Speech therapy/ palatal surgery
Pulmonary edema	Difficult oxygenation and pink secretions from endotracheal tube	Posetive end expiratory ventilaton
Nasopharyngeal stenosis	Progressive nasal difficult breathing and closed nasality	Palatal surgery
Torticollis	Neck pain and deviation to one side	Physiotherapy/ surgery
Cervical spine sublaxation	Neck pain +/- neurologic deficit	Neurological/ orthopedic consultation
Dental injury	Defective teeth	?? reinmplantation
Eustachian Tube injury	Hearing loss and otitis media	?? Ventilation tube
Lingual nerve palsy	Poor tongue movement	Conservative
Cautery burns	Burning sensation and ulcers	Surface anesthetics
Nasal adhesions	Nasal bleeding and obstruction later on	?? Lysis
Recurrence	Progressive nasal obstruction	Revision surgery

Table 3. Complications related to adenoidectomy

Complications related to use of endoscope
- Nasal mucosal injury, with subsequent scarring and adhesions, this is very rare, and occurs only after rough manipulation.

3. Conclusion

Adenoidectomy is a very widely and commonly performed surgery, although the standards for surgery have changed due to the better understanding of the etiopathology. There is no worldwide agreement on the "typical technique" for adenoidectomy, thus various procedures and aids for such surgery have been used, all aiming at better removal and reducing recurrence rates. The use of endoscopy to guide adenoidectomy aids in achieving better results –in terms of complete surgery- with all techniques of adenoidectomy, whether conventional curettage, or with more recent methods, and whether for obstructive or non obstructive causes, and whether for complete or partial adenoidectomies. It is simple to use, does not add to time or expenses of surgery.

4. Acknowledgment

- The companies of Storz, and Medtronic for supplying their catalogues for use of pictures.
- Professor MZ Helal for supplying the diagram for use of combined endocopic guided powered adenoidectomy.

5. References

Ark N., Kurtaran H., Ugur K.S., Yilmaz T., Ozboduroglu A.A., & Mutlu C. (2010). Comparison of adenoidectomy methods: examining with digital palpation vs. visualizing the placement of the curette. *International Journal of Pediatric Otorhinolaryngology*. Jun;74(6):649-51.

Benninger M. & Walner D. (2007). Coblation improving outcomes for children following adenotonsillectomy. *Clinical Cornerstone*. ;9 Suppl 1:S13-23.

Bernstein JM, Faden HS, Scannapieco E, et al (2002). Interference of non-typeable Haemophilus Influenzae and MOraxella Catarrhalis by Streptococcus oralis in adenoid organ culture; possible strategy for the treatment of otitis prone child. *Annals of Otorhinolaryngology*; 111:696-700.

Bozzini. In, Nezhat's *History of Endoscopy*, Available from, http://laparoscopy.blogs.com/endoscopyhistory/chapter_06/

Bross-Soriano D., Schimelmitz-Idi J., & Arrieta-Gómez J.R. (2004). Endoscopic adenoidectomy; use or abuse of the technology. *Cirugia Y Ciruganos*. Jan-Feb;72(1):15-9; discussion 21-2.

Buck M.L. (1992). Chloral hydrate use during infancy. *Neonatal Pharmacology Quarterly*, 1:31-7

Bulut Y., Agacayak A., Karlidag T., Toraman Z.A., & Yilmaz M. (2006). Association of cagA+ Helicobacter pylori with Adenotonsillar Hypertrophy, *Tohoku Journal of Experimental Medicine*. 209;229–233.

Carr MM, Poje CP, Ehrig D, Brodsky LS. (2001). Incidence of reflux in young children undergoing adenoidectomy. *Laryngoscope*. Dec;111(12):2170-2.

Dhanasekar G., Liapi A., & Turner N.(2010). Adenoidectomy techniques: UK survey. *Journal of Laryngology and Otology*. Feb;124(2):199-203.

Ezzat W.F., (2010) Role of endoscopic nasal examination in reduction of nasopharyngeal adenoid recurrence rates. *International Journal of Pediatric Otorhinolaryngology*, 74; 404–406

Giannoni C, Sulek M, Friedman EM, Duncan NO.(1998) Acquired nasopharyngeal stenosis. *Archives of Otolaryngology Head & Neck Surgery*;124:163–7.

Hartnick CJ, Ruben RJ. (2000) Preoperative coagulation studies prior to tonsillectomy. *Archives of Otolaryngology Head & Neck Surgery*, 126:684–6.

Jonas N.E., Sayed R., & Prescott C.A. (2007). Prospective, randomized, single-blind, controlled study to compare two methods of performing adenoidectomy. *International Journal of Pediatric Otorhinolaryngology*. Oct;71(10):1555-62.

Jong YH, Gendeh BS. (2008) Transoral endoscopic adenoidectomy: initial experience. *Medical Journal of Malaysia* 63:81.

Kakani RS, Callan ND, April MM. (2000) Superior adenoidectomy in children with palatal abnormalities. *Ear Nose & Throat Journal*; 79:300–5.

Koltai P.J., Chan J., & Younes A. (2002). Power-assisted adenoidectomy: total and partial resection. *Laryngoscope*. Aug;112(8 Pt 2 Suppl 100):29-31.

Lo S., & Rowe-Jones J. (2006). How we do it: Transoral suction diathermy adenoid ablation under direct vision using a 45 degree endoscope. *Clinical Otolaryngology*. Oct;31(5):440-2.

Pagella F., Matti E., Colombo A., Giourgos G., & Mira E. (2009). How we do it: a combined method of traditional curette and power-assisted endoscopic adenoidectomy. *Acta Otolaryngolgica*. May;129(5):556-9.

Randall DA, Hoffer ME. (1998) Complications of tonsillectomy and adenoidectomy. *Otolaryngology Head & Neck Surgery*;118:61–8.

Regmi D., Mathur N.N., & Bhattarai M. (2011). Rigid endoscopic evaluation of conventional curettage adenoidectomy. *Journal of Laryngology and Otology*. Jan;125(1):53-8.

Reitzen S.D., Chung W., & Shah A.R. (2011). Nasal septal deviation in the pediatric and adult populations. *Ear Nose and Throat Journal*. Mar;90(3):112-5.

Remington-Hobbs C. (1968) Diathermy in dissection tonsillectomy and retrograde dissection adenoidectomy. *Journal of Laryngology and Otology*. Nov;82(11):953-62.

Rodriguez K., Murray N., & Guarisco J.L. (2002). Power-assisted partial adenoidectomy. *Laryngoscope*. Aug;112(8 Pt 2 Suppl 100):26-8.

Saxby A.J., & Chappel C.A. (2009). Residual adenoid tissue post-curettage: role of nasopharyngoscopy in adenoidectomy ANZ J Surg. Nov;79(11):809-11.

Shin J.J., & Hartnick C.J. (2003). Pediatric endoscopic transnasal adenoid ablation. *Annals of Otology Rhinology and Laryngology*. Jun;112(6):511-4.

Songu M., Altay C., Adibelli Z.H., & Adibelli H. (2010). Endoscopic-assisted versus curettage adenoidectomy: a prospective, randomized, double-blind study with objective outcome measures. *Laryngoscope*. Sep;120(9):1895-9.

Steinberg A.D. (1993). Should chloral hydrate be banned? Pediatrics;92:442-6.

Tolczynski B., The recurrence of adenoids, *Canadian Medical Association Journal*. 72 (December) (1955) 672–673, Quoted from.

Van Den Akker E.H., Hoes A.W., Burton M.J., & Schilder A.G. (2004). Large international differences in adenotonsillectomy rates, *Clinical Otolaryngology and Allied Sciences*. 29 (2) 161–164.

Walker P. (2001). Pediatric adenoidectomy under vision using suction-diathermy ablation. *Laryngoscope*. Dec;111(12):2173-7.

Wan YM, Wong KC, Ma KH, (2005) Endoscopic guided adenoidectomy using a classic adenoid curette: a simple way to improve adenoidectomy Hong Kong Med J;11:42-4

Wei JL, Beatty CW, Gustafson RO. (2000). Evaluation of post tonsillectomy hemorrhage and risk factors. *Otolaryngology Head & Neck Surgery*, 2000;123:229–35.

Weymuller E. (1974) Nasopharyngoscopic observations in the Alaskan native. *Laryngoscope* May;84(5):864-8.

Zinder DJ, Parker GS. (1996), Electrocautery burns and operator ignorance. *Otolaryngology Head & Neck Surgery*;115:145–9.

4

Endoscopic Surgery of Maxillary Sinuses in Oral Surgery and Implantology

Miroslav Andrić
University of Belgrade, Faculty of Dentistry
Serbia

1. Introduction

Due to the close anatomical relationship of the maxillary sinuses to the dentoalveolar complex, surgical procedures involving these anatomical structures represent a part of a everyday practice in oral surgery and implantology. Those interventions are directed mainly towards the treatment of odontogenic infections of the sinuses as well as surgical treatment of oroantral fistulae and odontogenic cysts and tumors of the upper jaw invading the antrum. Traditional approach under such circumstances is a Caldwell-Luc type of surgery, comprising osteotomy of the anterior sinus wall and creation of artificial opening of the sinus into the inferior nasal meatus. Although high success rates are reported, this kind of surgery may result in significant long-term complications, such as sclerosis of the antral walls, collapse of the sinus and creation of the postoperative cysts of maxilla (Nemec at al., 2009).

Also, widespread use of dental implants resulted in development of numerous techniques of alveolar bone augmentation in order to provide adequate amount of bone for implant placement. Many of those techniques involve the maxillary sinuses. However, complications of dental implant placement and augmentation procedures may include injuries to the maxillary sinuses, infections of the sinuses and displacement of augmentation material or implants themselves into the sinus. Again, the primary treatment of those complications includes surgery of the sinus, most commonly a Caldwell-Luc procedure.

Recent technological advances in field of endoscopy resulted in substantial improvement in techniques of endoscope–controlled surgery of nose and paranasal sinuses. Those techniques proved to be very useful in this area of complex anatomy and limited access to the surgical field. In particular, endoscopic surgery of the maxillary sinuses is widespread and has a long track of good results in ENT surgery. This is especially true for functional endoscopic sinus surgery (FESS). This technique, proved to be safe and effective for treatment of both chronic rhino-sinusitis and nasal polyposis (Chiu & Kennedy, 2004), nowadays is widely accepted as a standard of care for patients who require surgical treatment of chronic rhino-sinusitis.

In contrast to this, surgical treatment of odontogenic diseases of the maxillary sinus still predominantly comprises traditional surgical techniques. Recently, several studies reported results of FESS for treatment of odontogenic sinusitis. Also, new techniques of endoscope-assisted surgery of odontogenic cysts and tumors were described. Finally, endoscope-controlled sinus augmentation and endoscopic treatment of implant–related complications involving the maxillary sinuses were reported in the literature.

Therefore, the aim of this article was to describe clinical problems encountered in this field, to briefly discuss indications for the surgery and to analyze available treatment options and criteria for selection of optimal treatment modality. Also, a literature review will present available data on endoscopic surgery for treatment of odontogenic diseases of the maxillary sinuses, as well as for sinus augmentation procedures and treatment of implant–related complications affecting the maxillary sinuses. Finally, the level of current scientific evidence on these issues will be evaluated.

2. Odontogenic maxillary sinusitis

Apart from more common rhinogenic sinusitis, some cases of maxillary sinus infections are related to odontogenic sources. This entity, designated as odontogenic maxillary sinusitis (OMS) accounts for approximately 10-12% of all cases of maxillary sinusitis (Mehra & Murad, 2004).

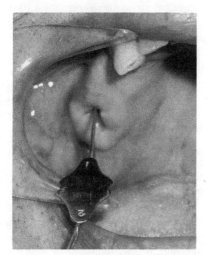 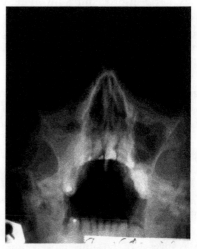

Fig. 1. a. Clinical photograph of a right oroantral fistula. A probe is inserted through the fistula into the sinus. b. Waters' view of the same patient indicating acute maxillary sinusitis.

The most common cause of OMS are oroantral fistulae (OAF) (Figures 1a and 1b) which are defined as pathological communications between the oral cavity and the maxillary sinus (Brook, 2006). Usually, they result from unsuccessful healing of Schneidarian membrane perforations that occur during tooth extractions and other surgical procedures involving alveolar processes of the upper jaw. In contrast to oroantral communications, which occasionally may heal spontaneously, most cases of OAF and subsequent maxillary sinusitis will require some kind of surgical treatment. This treatment varies from simple fistula closure by local flap to endoscopically assisted surgery of the maxillary sinus.

Besides oroantral fistulae, other common causes of OMS are chronic periapical or periodontal odontogenic infections, odontogenic cysts of the maxilla and iatrogenic factors, including placement of dental implants, sinus augmentations and intra-antral foreign bodies

(Brook, 2006; Zimbler et al., 1998) (Figure 2). What is common for all these conditions is that disruption of the sinus membrane results in creation of a pathway through which oral microorganisms invade the antrum, resulting in sinus inflammation.

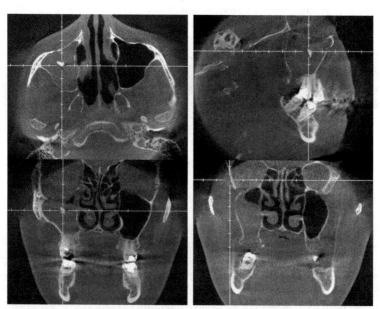

Fig. 2. Cone-beam CT of a patient with OAF and a root tip pushed into the sinus. Such situation is usually followed by pronounced inflammatory reaction.

Traditionally, OMS is treated by a Caldwell-Luc type of surgery (Guven, 1998) or by conservative procedures, including antibiotics and sinus irrigation, followed by surgical treatment of odontogenic source of infection (Dolanmaz et al., 2004). Caldwell-Luc operation is criticized as aggressive surgery with relatively high incidence of complications (De Freiatas & Lucente, 1988; Ikeda et al., 1996). Most important of all, efficacy of inferior meatal antrostomy, typically performed in this kind of surgery, is doubtful, as the mucociliary clearance remains directed toward the natural sinus ostium in the middle meatus (Kennedy & Shaalan, 1989). Car & Juretić (1998) and Al-Belasy (2004), showed that inferior meatal antrostomy might be avoided, at least in some patients. Nevertheless, opening of the sinus on its anterior wall has to be performed, which results in permanent defect of anterior maxilla, sclerosis of the antral walls and collapse of the sinus cavity (Nemec at al., 2009). This kind of defect could complicate future prosthetic rehabilitation of these patients, regarding possible use of dental implants.

3. Functional endoscopic sinus surgery for treatment of odontogenic sinusitis

Principles of functional endoscopic sinus surgery (FESS) are based on actual understanding of sinus physiology, particularly regarding mucociliary clearance of the sinus. If effective drainage of the maxillary sinus is to be established, the optimal location to do so is at the level of the natural sinus ostium, in the middle nasal meatus. Therefore, FESS is directed towards establishment and preservation of osteomeatal complex patency. It aims to restore sinus ventilation and reestablish mucociliary clearance, which in turn results in resolution of sinus disease and maintenance of healthy sinus mucosa (Stammberger, 1986; Kennedy, 1985). It was demonstrated that such therapeutical approach is a viable option for treatment of both maxillary sinusitis and other inflammatory conditions affecting this anatomical structure (Busaba & Kieff, 2002). In contrast to rhino-sinusitis, most cases of OMS are still treated by a Caldwell-Luc type of surgery. However, several studies were published, reporting results of FESS for treatment of chronic odontogenic sinusitis (Lopatin et al., 2002; Costa et al., 2007; Andric et al., 2010; Albu & Baciut, 2010; Hajiioannou et al., 2010), which will be discussed in details later in this chapter.

3.1 Surgical technique

Endoscopic surgery of the maxillary sinuses is most commonly based on usage of rigid endoscopes, usually of 4.0 mm diameter. These endoscopes, providing different angles of vision, from 0 to 120 degrees, allow for good visualization of all parts of the osteomeatal complex, sinus ostium and sinus itself. Also, a set of specially designed surgical instruments includes different biting and grasping forceps, cutting knives and microdebriders.

This kind of surgery is usually done with patient under the general anesthesia. If possible, carefully controlled hypotension is useful to minimize bleeding during the procedure (Eberhart et al., 2007) since it was shown that pronounced intraoperative bleeding correlates with higher failure rates in endoscopic sinus surgery (Albu & Baciut, 2010). Also, infiltration of surgical field with local anesthetic solution containing epinephrine is very helpful for this purpose.

Procedures starts with careful medial dislocation of the middle turbinate which allows good visualization of the middle nasal meatus, uncinate process and ethmoidal bulla. Uncinate process is cut by a sickle-knife in a direction parallel to its upper edge and removed by grasping forceps (Figures 3a, 3b and 3c).

After that, natural sinus ostium is identified and subsequently enlarged in a postero-inferior direction. Ostium is enlarged to the size that should allow access to the sinus with appropriate instruments and also effective drainage of the sinus after the surgery (Figure 4). At this point care must be taken, as extremely anterior enlargement of the ostium might result in an injury to the nasolacrimal duct. Through this enlarged ostium it is possible to inspect entire maxillary sinus, particularly when angled-view endoscopes are used (Figure 5). Also, using long curved antrum forceps and suction tips, most of intra-antral pathology and foreign bodies can be removed by this approach too.

What is specific for odontogenic sinusitis is that most of mucosal inflammation, as well as majority of foreign bodies of dental origin, are located in the alveolar recess of the sinus. Depending on local anatomy and position of sinus ostium, access to this part of the sinus might be difficult, even when large middle meatal antrostomy is performed. Still, in cases with OAF it is possible to reach alveolar recess through the fistula itself. Beside this, additional small puncture of the sinus in canine fossa, with an endoscope introduced through it, can provide better visualization of this part of the sinus. However, in most of the cases, angled view endoscopes will ensure good visual control in the entire sinus, even through middle meatal antrostomy.

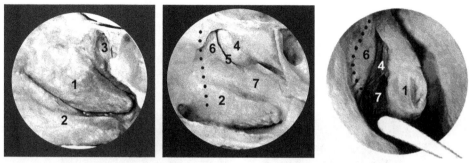

Fig. 3. Schematic presentation of the right lateral nasal wall. a. Middle turbinate (1), inferior turbinate (2) and spheno-ethmoidal recess (3) are seen. b. Upon removal of the middle turbinate, middle nasal meatus (7) is visible. Semilunar hiatus (5) is bounded by ethmoidal bulla (4) and uncinate process (6). Aperture of the maxillary sinus can not be seen, as it is located behind these structures. Dotted line illustrates path of the nasolacrimal duct. c. The same anatomic structures as seen through a 0° endoscope. Middle turbinate (1) is dislocated medially by a Freer elevator. Dotted line represents line of resection of the uncinate process (6). Previously published in ref: Andric et al, 2010.

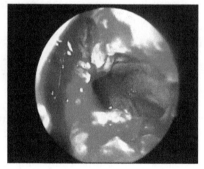

Fig. 4. A view of the enlarged natural ostium of the left maxillary sinus (0° endoscope). Previously published in ref: Andric et al, 2010.

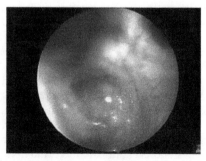

Fig. 5. A view of the alveolar recess of the maxillary sinus through the enlarged ostium (70° endoscope). Previously published in ref: Andric et al, 2010.

The most important advantage of FESS, compared to other treatment options for odontogenic sinusitis, is a possibility to surgically treat inflammation of other paranasal sinuses as well, in particular that of anterior ethmoidal cells. Residual inflammation in this area is one of common causes of failure in treatment of odontogenic sinusitis. Therefore, if necessary, removal of ethmoidal bulla and opening of the anterior ethmoidal cells may be performed too (Figures 6a and 6b).

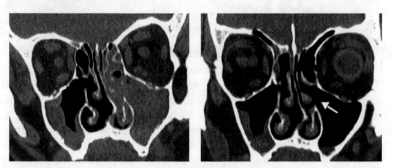

Fig. 6. a. Coronal CT scan of odontogenic sinusitis demonstrating pronounced inflammation of left maxillary sinus and anterior ethmodial cells. b. Six months postoperatively reduction in extent of sinus inflammation, as well as resection of the uncinate process (arrow) are clearly visible. Previously published in ref: Andric et al, 2010.

Finally, successful treatment of odontogenic sinusitis is based on efficient elimination of odontogenic source of infection. Therefore, closure of oroantral fistula (if present) and extraction of causative teeth should be performed in the same surgical act.

3.2 Literature data
Recently, several authors reported results of FESS for treatment of chronic odontogenic sinusitis (Lopatin et al., 2002; Costa et al., 2007; Andric et al., 2010; Albu & Baciut, 2010; Hajiioannou et al., 2010). Although there were some technical differences, all studies have reported essentially the same surgical procedure, comprising middle meatal antrostomy, access to the maxillary sinus through enlarged natural sinus ostium and endonasal approach for removal of intra-antral foreign bodies, such are root tips and dental implants. The most important results of these studies are summarized in table 1.

Lopatin (Lopatin et al., 2002) was the first who reported 70 cases of odontogenic sinusitis treated by endoscopic sinus surgery. Apart from 39 cases with OAF, he presented 10 cases with odontogenic cysts and 6 with fungal balls in the sinuses. Also, he presented 21 cases with foreign bodies inside the sinus. Surgical technique included usage of microdebrider, resection of the uncinate process and removal of ethmoidal bulla. Removal of foreign bodies was accomplished by curved suction tip through enlarged sinus ostium. Authors commented on difficulty in reaching alveolar recess of the sinus through middle meatal antrostomy. In initial cases they used additional puncture in canine fossa, and later on, access to alveolar recess was established through OAF itself. Out of 70 cases, after the follow-up period of up to three years, there were 4 failures. In 3 patients recurrence of OAF was noticed and in one patient stenosis of antrostomy resulted in recurrent sinusitis. Besides facial edema and nasal discharge, which were described as less pronounced compared to Caldwell-Luc procedure, no other complications were reported.

	Total cases (n)	Cases with OAF (n)	OAF reccurence n (%)	Revision surgery n (%)	Follow up period	Overall sucess rate n/all cases (%)
Lopatin et al., 2002	**70**	39	3 (8%)	3 (4%)	1 – 3 yr	**66 / 70 (95%)**
Costa et al., 2007	**17**	5	No	No	6 mo – 2 yr	**17 / 17 (100%)**
Andric et al., 2010	**14**	14	No	No	6 mo – 2 yr	**14 / 14 (100%)**
Albu & Baicut, 2010	**104**	30	4 (13%)	9 (9%)	Min. 6 mo	**95 / 104 (91%)**
Hajiioannou et al., 2010	**4**	4	No	No	6 mo – 3 yr	**4 / 4 (100%)**

Table 1. Results of clinical studies on FESS for treatment of odontogenic sinusitis. Mo – months, Yr – years. Previously published in ref: Andric, 2010.

Costa (Costa et al., 2007) presented 17 cases of OMS, including 5 OAF, 7 cases with odontogenic cysts, 2 cases of sinusitis related to placement of dental implants and 3 patients with root-canal sealing materials pushed into the sinus. Again, microdebrider was used and access to alveolar recess was obtained through OAF. In cases with odontogenic cysts, a bone window in the anterior sinus wall was created for removal of the cyst, while middle meatal antrostomy was performed to enhance resolution of corresponding sinus inflammation. After a 2-years follow up period, good long - term results (defined as absence of sinusitis symptoms and healing of OAF) were obtained in all cases. In one case nasal synechiae were observed postoperatively, which was corrected under the local anesthesia.

Another retrospective study (Andric et al., 2010) reported results of FESS in 14 patients with OAF and corresponding OMS. Similarly to previous studies, middle meatal antrostomy was performed by resection of the uncinate process, and most of instrumentation inside the sinus was accomplished through the enlarged sinus ostium, including removal of intra-antral foreign bodies. Closure of OAF was achieved by Rehrmann's buccal advancement flap or buccal fat pad. During the follow up period of up to two years, clinical examination and control CT scans showed good results in all cases. No significant complications were reported.

The only prospective study on this issue included 104 patients with OMS and 307 with rhinogenic sinusitis (Albu & Baciut, 2010). It is of interest that no statistically significant differences in failure rates was noted comparing these two groups of patients (7% in odontogenic *vs.* 9% in rhinogenic group). Still, somewhat higher failures rates (13%) were noticed in cases with OAF. Surgical technique was similar to other studies, including puncture of the sinus in the canine fossa for better visualization of the alveolar recess. Again, there were not significant intraoperative and postoperative complications.

Finally, in a case series from Hajiioannou, four cases of odontogenic sinusitis with OAF were successfully treated by endoscopic sinus surgery and fistula closure by synthetic surgical glue and buccal advancement flap (Hajiioannou et al., 2010). Also, retrospective analysis of 27 cases of odontogenic sinusitis revealed that most common causes of this condition were complications of dental implants placement and tooth extraction. Treatment included transnasal endoscopic sinus surgery in 19 (70.4%) patients, Caldwell-Luc operation in two (7.4%) patients and only antibiotics in 4 (14.8%) cases. During the follow-up period of two to six months, no recurrences were recorded (Lee, KC. & Lee, SJ., 2010).

In summary, all these studies reported essentially the same surgical procedure, applying principles of FESS for treatment of rhinogenic sinusitis in patients with OMS. In all cases middle meatal antrostomy was performed which presents substantial difference to Caldwell-Luc procedure. It is interesting that most of the surgeons, at least in some cases, used additional puncture of the sinus in canine fossa, creating better access to the alveolar recess of the sinus. This is very specific for treatment of odontogenic sinusitis in which most of the intra-antral pathology is located in the lower third of the sinus. Still, it was also demonstrated that access to this part of the maxillary sinus can be achieved through oroantral fistula, if present.

It is important that practically no significant intraoperative or postoperative complications occurred in any case. Although endoscopic sinus surgery might result in broad range of major and minor complications (McMains, 2008), rare occurrence of complications in the treatment of odontogenic maxillary sinusitis might be related to the relatively limited extent of endo-nasal surgery, compared to the treatment of rhinosinusitis and nasal polyps.

Although all studies presented very good short to mid-term results (follow up period lasted up to three years), there is a lack of objective measures of improvement in patients condition after the surgery. All studies reported lack of symptoms and subjective patients' perception of improvement as outcome measures. In one study (Andric et al., 2010) control CT scans were performed, but without attempt to use some scoring system of CT findings in sinusitis. The only result which can be objectively validated is recurrence rate of OAF. It ranged from 0 to 13% which is similar or somewhat higher comparing to Caldwell-Luc procedure (Guven, 1998; Yilmaz et al., 2003). Still, it has to be addressed that closure of OAF is a delicate procedure, requiring vast experience specific to this kind of surgery. Although it is a common procedure for oral and maxillofacial surgeons, some of otorhinolaryngologists rarely perform this intervention. In fact, in a study with highest recurrence rate reported (Albu & Baciut, 2010), authors were able to demonstrate "learning curve" since three recurrences occurred in the first 15 cases and only one in remaining patients.

Finally, it can be concluded that use of FESS for treatment of OMS is clinically well documented procedure with good results and low incidence of complications. Still, from the scientific point of view, the main shortcoming of all these studies is that results of FESS are not compared with results of some traditional treatment options for odontogenic sinusitis, such is Caldwell-Luc procedure. Therefore, prospective and randomized studies are needed to establish efficacy of this kind of treatment, as well to provide criteria for individual selection of most suitable treatment of odontogenic sinusitis.

4. Endoscopic surgery for treatment of odontogenic cysts and tumors

The most common odontogenic cysts and tumors involving the upper jaw include periapical and dentigerous cysts, keratocystic odontogenic tumors (previously known as odontogenic keratocysts) and ameloblastomas. Their expansive growth within the upper jaw might result in destruction of the bony walls of the sinus and subsequent sinus infection (Figure 7).

Clinical course of these lesions tends to be relatively asymptomatic and it is not uncommon that symptoms of maxillary sinusitis are among the first signs indicating the presence of an odontogenic cyst or tumor.

Selection of the most appropriate surgical treatment is based on hystological type of the lesion, but also having in mind its size and relationship to the neighboring anatomical structures, including maxillary sinuses. Inflammatory periapical and residual cysts, as well as dentigerous cysts are effectively treated by simple enucleation and extraction or endodontic treatment of the causative tooth. On the other hand, keratocystic odontogenic tumors (KCOT) and ameloblastomas require more aggressive type of surgery due to infiltrative growth and high recurrence rates. Still, while most of ameloblastomas of the upper jaw are treated by partial maxillectomy, surgical options for KCOT include decompression followed by complete enucleation, enucleation in combination with Carnoy solution or cryosurgery and, finally, resection of the involved jaw (Ghali & Connor, 2003).

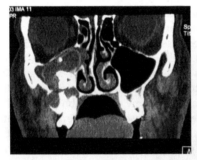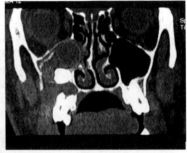

Fig. 7. Coronal CT scan of keratocystic odontogenic tumor of the right maxilla invading the maxillary sinus and resulting in secondary inflammation of antral mucosa.

In cases of odontogenic cysts or tumors occupying the sinus, common surgical approach includes removal of the lesion by a Caldwell-Luc type of surgery. Still, while such procedure results in permanent defect of anterior maxilla, visualization of the postero-inferior part of the upper jaw (which is a common site of occurrence of odontogenic lesions) might be difficult even when large antrostomy in the canine fossa is performed. Endoscope-assisted surgery for those lesions has a potential to provide better overview of the surgical field and still to allow less aggressive surgical approach.

Few articles were published describing techniques of endoscope-assisted removal of odontogenic cysts from the maxillary sinus. Cedin (Cedin et al., 2005) presented 4 cases of periapical cysts with oroantral fistulae, occupying alveolar recess of the sinus. Surgical technique comprised combined approach through canine fossa and inferior meatal antrostomy, cystectomy under the endoscopic control and closure of oroantral fistula by local flaps. Successful closure of OAF was obtained in all cases and there were no recurrences during the 2-years follow- up period.

In a case-series including 10 periapical and 3 dentigerous cysts (Seno et al., 2009), after partial resection of anterior portion of the inferior turbinate, inferior meatal antrostomy was performed to gain access to the alveolar recess and to allow removal of the cyst. Interestingly, although authors stated that in five cases of periapical cysts only partial resection of the cystic wall was performed, in a follow–up period ranging from 11 to 72 months no recurrences were noted. Also, several case reports were published, describing similar surgical techniques (Micozkadioglu & Erkan, 2007; Lamb et al., 2009; Di Pasquale & Shermetaro, 2006; Hasbini et al., 2001; Christmas et al., 2008).

It is interesting that in this studies access to the sinus was obtained through inferior nasal meatus, which reflects difficulties in reaching inferior portion of the maxillary sinus through middle meatal antrostomy. Such difficulties are best described in an article from Lamb and coworkers (Lamb et al., 2009), who reported that attempt to remove odontogenic cyst and the tooth from the sinus through middle meatal antrostomy was unsuccessful, so conversion to Caldwell-Luc approach had to be performed. On the other hand, several authors reported successful removal of dentigerous cysts through middle meatal antrostomy (Di Pasquale & Shermetaro, 2006; Hasbini et al., 2001; Christmas et al., 2008). As an alternative technique, Costa (Costa et al., 2007) used intraoral approach for removal of the cyst and middle meatal antrostomy was performed to treat corresponding sinusitis.

At this point, it seems reasonable to use inferior meatal antrostomy for removal of cysts from the sinus, if patency of natural sinus ostium is preserved. If not, widening of the natural sinus ostium, according to FESS principles, should enhance resolution of sinus inflammation. However, there is some concern that simultaneous persistence of more than one opening of the sinus might actually decrease its drainage, due to "circular flow" phenomenon (Coleman & Duncavage, 1996). Still, in a prospective study including 72 patients with severe maxillary sinusitis (as determined by Lund–Mackay CT score), combined inferior and middle meatal antrostomy shown superior results in reduction of sinus inflammation, compared to middle meatal antrostomy alone (Albu et al., 2011).

Regarding odontogenic tumors, several cases of endoscopic surgery for treatment of ameloblastomas of the upper jaw were reported (London & Schlosser, 2002; Bray et al., 2007; Leong et al., 2010). Although in most of them entire tumor was removed by an endoscopic approach, a technique of combined maxillectomy and endoscopic ethmoidectomy was described, too (Bray et al., 2007).

Also, few cases of fibro–osseous lesions involving ethmoidal region were presented (Akao et al 2003, Cansiz et al 2004, Lopatin and Kapitanov 2005). In all of them transnasal endoscopic approach was used with variable success, since in one case only reduction of tumor was achieved which required additional surgery for complete removal of the lesion (Akao et al, 2003).

At this point it has to be noted that follow up periods for cases of odontogenic tumors were variable in these reports, which rises the question of possible recurrences. While an average time for diagnosis of ameloblastoma recurrence is approximately 5 years, late recurrences are well documented in the literature (Carlson & Marx, 2006). Therefore, long term follow-up, as well as prospective studies comparing endoscopic and traditional surgical techniques for removal of odontogenic tumors are needed.

5. Endoscopic sinus surgery and dental implant treatment

An increasing number of dental implants is placed in posterior parts of the upper jaw. Although advances in surgical techniques and implant design resulted in high success rates, complications are still encountered, many of them involving maxillary sinuses. Such complications include creation of oroantral fistulae, sinus infections and displacement of implants or grafting material into the sinus. Also, in unfavorable anatomical situations, sinus augmentation procedures are needed prior or simultaneously to implant placement.

Recently, endoscopic techniques were described, both for treatment of sinus related complications of dental implants and for sinus augmentation.

5.1 Endoscopic surgery for treatment of implant-related complications

Occasionally, displacement of implants into the sinus may occur, either during implant insertion or during functional loading period. Although some of cases may remain asymptomatic, such situation usually results in inflammation of the corresponding sinus, obviously requiring some kind of treatment. Even in asymptomatic cases, removal of displaced implant should not be postponed, since it may result in migration of implant into distant spaces, such are nasal cavity (Kitamura, 2007), sphenoid sinus (Felisati et al., 2007), orbit (Griffa et al., 2010) or even anterior cranial fossa (Cascone et al., 2010).

Once the diagnosis has been made, surgical procedure for implant removal may include opening of the anterior sinus wall *via* Caldwell-Luc approach, or endoscopic sinus surgery. In available literature, two endoscopic techniques for removal of implants were described, creating access to the sinus through canine fossa or through middle meatal antrostomy.

Nakamura (Nakamura et al., 2004) reported endoscopic removal of displaced implant through a 10 x 10 mm window in the anterior sinus wall, using urological retrieval basket. Similar technique was described by Varol and colleagues in a series of 3 cases, except that curved hemostat was used for implant removal (Varol et al., 2006). Also, it was shown that endoscopic removal of implant from the sinus can be successfully combined with simultaneous sinus lift procedure (Ucer, 2009), facilitating future placement of a new implant. What is common for all these reports is that essentially conventional approach through canine fossa was used, but due to the use of endoscopes much smaller opening of the sinus wall had to be performed, compared to traditional Caldwell-Luc procedure.

Another possibility is to remove the implant by transnasal approach, usually through middle meatal antrostomy (Ramotar et al., 2010; Lubbe 2008). Such approach is particularly indicated if concomitant sinusitis is present, since it provides both an opportunity to remove displaced implant and to improve ventilation and drainage of affected sinus (Kim et al., 2007). Still, actual position of an implant has to be determined when decision regarding access through canine fossa or middle meatal antrostomy is to be made. In a case report from El Charkawi et al. (2005), it was shown that when an implant was in a more anterior and medial position in the maxillary sinus, transnasal access was unsuccessful so a Caldwell-Luc approach had to be used. Besides this, a clinician should have in mind that position of an implant within the sinus might change in a short period of time, so once appropriate radiographs are taken, surgery should not be delayed.

In a retrospective multi-center report of 27 patients with implants displaced into the sinus, Chiapasco proposed a treatment protocol based on presence of sinusitis and oroantral communication (OAC). In 17 patients who didn't have signs of sinusitis and in whom patency of the sinus ostium was preserved, intraoral approach through canine fossa was used for retrieval of implant and closure of OAC. In 6 patients who presented with maxillary sinusitis and obstruction of the sinus ostium, but without OAC, treatment consisted of partial uncinectomy, middle meatal antrostomy and removal of implant through enlarged ostium. Finally in 4 cases with sinusitis, ostium obstruction and oroantral communication, operative procedure comprised combined FESS and intraoral approach for closure of OAC by buccal advancement flap (Chiapasco et al., 2009).

It seems that in cases of sinus related complications in implantology, several factors have to be considered before the decision regarding the most suitable treatment option can be made. Chronic sinusitis with obstruction of the sinus ostium probably should be treated by FESS, and middle meatal antrostomy can be used for removal of foreign bodies, including implants and grafting material, as well. In situations with no or minimal signs of sinusitis and with preserved patency of the ostium, access via canine fossa is simple and effective for retrieval of displaced implants. When such an intervention is performed under the endoscopic control, it is possible to create significantly smaller bony window in the sinus wall, which should provide uneventful healing of the defect, without long-term effect on the corresponding sinus health. Finally, in a study from Aimeti and colleagues, it was shown that inferior meatal antrostomy and insertion of nasosinus tube might be useful in treatment of sinus lift complications (Aimeti et al, 2001).

5.2 Endoscopic surgery for sinus augmentation procedures

Reduction in hight of residual alveolar ridge of posterior maxilla might be the result of either increased pneumatization of the upper jaw or pronounced resorption of alveolar process following tooth extraction. Whatever is the reason, such situation must be resolved before placement of implants is considered. Regarding this, several sinus augmentation techniques are used, comprising crestal or lateral approach to the sinus. Although these techniques are well established, use of endoscopes has a potential to further improve results of this procedures.

A prospective study on osteotome sinus floor elevation under the endoscopic control was published in 2002 (Nkenke at al., 2002). In 14 patients a total of 22 implants were placed and the endoscopes with view angles of 70, 90 and 120 degrees were inserted through the canine fossa. After sinus floor elevation with appropriate osteotomes, β-tricalcium phosphate or autogenous bone from the retromolar region were used for sinus augmentation. At a second stage surgery, 6 months after the implant placement, follow–up sinusoscopy was performed. Out of 22 implant sites, perforation on sinus membrane was noted in one case, which was immediately repaired by periosteal patch. In all patients postoperative course was uneventful, without signs of sinusitis. However, at a second stage surgery mobility of 2 implants was noted (in a same patient who had sinus perforation) and implants were removed, while control sinusoscopy revealed migration of grafting material into the sinus. Also, in one patient polyposis of antral mucosa was noted in control endoscopy, but the implants were stable and the patient was free of symptoms, so no further treatment was performed. Authors commented on complexity of procedure and extended length of surgery (average time of surgery was 67 minutes), so they concluded that such approach is more of scientific than clinical interest.

Berengo and colleagues reported results of endoscopic controlled osteotome sinus floor elevation in 8 patients in whom 16 Osseotite implants were placed (Berengo et al., 2004). Endoscopes were introduced through a 4 mm diameter opening in the canine fossa and BioOss® particles were used for sinus augmentation. Lacerations of sinus membrane with minimal displacement of grafting material were noted in 2 cases. Authors commented on pattern of sinus membrane distension and concluded that it is possible that mucosal lacerations are more likely to occur when detachment of sinus membrane is confined to the small area around the implant site in contrast to situations when mucosa is elevated on the broader base. It is important that after a 14 months follow–up period all implants were considered to be successful, including two cases in whom membrane lacerations had occurred. Also, no signs of sinusitis were noted in these cases.

Apart from endoscope–controlled osteotome sinus lift procedure, a technique of minimally invasive lateral–window sinus augmentation was described by Engelke and colleagues (Engelke & Deckwer, 1997; Engelke et al., 2003). Basically, surgical technique comprised only a small 5 mm–diameter osteotomy at the lateral sinus wall, through which elevation of sinus membrane and placement of augmentation material was performed under the control of a 2,7 mm–diameter endoscope. A total of 118 sinus augmentations were performed in 83 patients and 211 implants were placed, most of them simultaneously with augmentation procedure. Perforation of sinus membrane was noted in 28 cases, which were repaired immediately using polyglactine mesh except of 1 case with large perforation, who required second surgical intervention. Postoperatively, one case of wound dehiscence was noted, resulting in creation of oroantral fistula and concomitant sinusitis. Out of 211 implants, 11 implants were lost, most of them before the prosthetic loading (Engelke et al., 2003). Same author (Engelke & Capobianco, 2005) described technique of flapless sinus augmentation and simultaneous implant placement using three-dimensional surgical template. Twenty one implants were placed in six patients using this approach. One case of sinus perforation was noted and out of 21 implants one failure occurred during the healing period.

Based on pertinent literature, it seems that endoscope–controlled sinus augmentation yields similarly good results compared to conventional approach. However, need for expensive equipment and prolonged time of surgery are the factors that have to be considered when discussing this issue. Also, regarding minimally invasive lateral window augmentation, prospective study comparing this technique to the traditional surgical procedure will be necessary before its clinical use can be recommended.

6. Conclusion

Functional endoscopic sinus surgery for treatment of odontogenic sinusitis seems as a safe and predictable treatment option. Although scientific evidence is low (since there are not any studies comparing FESS to other treatment possibilities), this is a clinically well documented procedure with low incidence of complications. Also, it has to be noted that criteria for selection of optimal treatment modality for specific clinical situations are not established. Regarding this, FESS might be particularly indicated in cases of odontogenic sinusitis with severe ethmoidal inflammation and/or obstruction of sinus ostium. On the other hand, if patency of osteomeatal complex is preserved, which is not a rarity with odontogenic sinusitis, it is questionable if middle meatal antrostomy is of any benefit for the patient. Still, available scientific data are not sufficient to answer these questions.

In contrast to odontogenic sinusitis, endoscopic surgery for odontogenic cysts and tumors is documented only in limited case series reports, so at this moment it is difficult to discuss possible advantages and shortcomings of such procedures. However, it is clear that endoscope–assisted removal of these lesions should provide better visualization of the surgical field which is very important for prevention of recurrences. Until more scientific data are available, traditional treatment options with endoscopic control of poorly visualized regions (such is postero–inferior part of the sinus) can be recommended.

Also, regarding treatment of implant–related complications involving the maxillary sinus, endoscopic surgery has a potential to provide effective treatment of those cases, similarly to treatment of odontogenic sinusitis of non–implant etiology. On the other hand, endoscopic sinus augmentation needs scientific evidence of superiority to conventional techniques before it can be introduced into clinical practice.

7. Acknowledgment

This work was supported by grant no. 175021 from The Ministry of science of Republic of Serbia.

8. References

Aimetti, M., Romagnoli, R., Ricci, G. & Massei, G. (2001). Maxillary sinus elevation: the effect of macrolacerations and microlacerations of the sinus membrane as determined by endoscopy. *The International journal of periodontics & restorative dentistry*, Vol.21, No.6, (December 2001), pp. 581-589, ISSN 0198-7569

Akao, I., Ohashi, T., Imokawa, H., Otsuka, T., Taguchi, Y. & Takagi, M. (2003). Cementifying fibroma in the ethmoidal sinus extending to the anterior cranial base in an 11-year-old girl: a case report. *Auris Nasus Larynx*, Vol.30, Suppl.1, (15 February 2003), pp. 123-126, ISSN 0385-8146

Al-Belasy, FA. (2004). Inferior meatal antrostomy: is it necessary after radical sinus surgery through the Caldwell-Luc approach? *Journal of oral and maxillofacial surgery : official journal of the American Association of Oral and Maxillofacial Surgeons* Vol.62, No.5, (May 2004), pp. 559-562, ISSN 0278-2391

Albu, S. & Baciut, M. (2010). Failures in endoscopic surgery of the maxillary sinus. *Otolaryngology--head and neck surgery: official journal of American Academy of Otolaryngology-Head and Neck Surgery*, Vol.142, No.2, (February 2010), pp. 196-201, ISSN 0194-5998

Albu, S., Gocea, A. & Necula, S. (2011). Simultaneous inferior and middle meatus antrostomies in the treatment of the severely diseased maxillary sinus. *American journal of rhinology & allergy*. Vol.25, No.2, (March/April 2011), pp. e80-e85(6), ISSN 1945-8924

Andric, M. (2010). Endoscopic surgery of the maxillary sinuses in oral and maxillofacial surgery practice: a literature review. *Hellenic Archives of Oral & Maxillofacial Surgery*, Vol.2, No.2, (August 2010), pp. 57-68, ISSN 1108-829 X

Andric, M., Saranovic, V., Drazic, R., Brkovic, B. & Todorovic L. (2010). Functional endoscopic sinus surgery as an adjunctive treatment for closure of oroantral fistulae: a retrospective analysis. *Oral surgery, oral medicine, oral pathology, oral radiology, and endodontics*, Vol.109, No.4, (April 2010), pp. 510-516. ISSN 1079-2104

Berengo, M., Sivolella, S., Majzoub, Z. & Cordioli, G. (2004). Endoscopic evaluation of the bone-added osteotome sinus floor elevation procedure. *International journal of oral and maxillofacial surgery*, Vol.33, No.2, (March 2004), pp. 189-194, ISSN 0901-5027

Bray, D., Michael, A., Falconer, DT & Kaddour, HS. (2007). Ameloblastoma: a rare nasal polyp. *The Journal of laryngology and otology*, Vol.121, No.1, (January 2007), pp. 72-75, ISSN 0022-2151

Brook I. (2006). Sinusitis of odontogenic origin. *Otolaryngology--head and neck surgery: official journal of American Academy of Otolaryngology-Head and Neck Surgery*, Vol.135, No.3, (September 2006), pp. 349-355, ISSN 0194-5998

Busaba, NY. & Kieff, D. (2002). Endoscopic sinus surgery for inflammatory maxillary sinus disease. *Laryngoscope*, Vol.112, No.8, (August 2002), pp. 1378-1383. ISSN 0023-852X

Cansiz, H., Tuskan, K., Karaman, E. & DervisoÄŸlu, S. (2004). Endoscope assisted removal of cementoossifying fibroma in the paranasal sinuses in a five-year-old girl. *International journal of pediatric otorhinolaryngology*, Vol.68, No.4, (April 2004), pp. 489-493, ISSN 0165-5876

Car, M. & Juretić, M. (1998) Treatment of oroantral communications after tooth extraction. Is drainage into the nose necessary or not? *Acta oto-laryngologica*, Vol.118, No.6, (November 1998), pp. 844-846. ISSN 0001-6489

Carlson, ER. & Marx, RE. (2006). The ameloblastoma: primary, curative surgical management. *Journal of oral and maxillofacial surgery: official journal of the American Association of Oral and Maxillofacial Surgeons*, Vol.64, No.3, (March 2006), pp. 484-494, ISSN 0278-2391

Cascone P., Ungari, C., Filiaci, F., Gabriele, G. & Ramieri, V. (2010). A dental implant in the anterior cranial fossae. *International journal of oral and maxillofacial surgery*, Vol.39, No.1, (January 2010), pp. 92-93, ISSN 0901-5027

Chiapasco, M., Felisati, G., Maccari, A., Borloni, R., Gatti, F. & Di Leo, F. (2009). The management of complications following displacement of oral implants in the paranasal sinuses: a multicenter clinical report and proposed treatment protocols. *International journal of oral and maxillofacial surgery*, Vol.38, No.12, (December 2009), pp. 1273-1278, ISSN 0901-5027

Chiu, AG. & Kennedy, DW. (2004) Surgical management of chronic rhinosinusitis and nasal polyposis: a review of the evidence. *Current allergy and asthma reports*, Vol.4, No.6, (November 2004), pp. 486-489, ISSN 1529-7322

Christmas DA, Mirante JP, Yanagisawa E. (2008). Endoscopic view of a maxillary dentigerous cyst. *Ear, nose, & throat journal*, Vol.87, No.6, (June 2008), pp. 316, ISSN 0145-5613

Coleman, JR Jr. & Duncavage, JA. (1996). Extended middle meatal antrostomy: the treatment of circular flow. *Laryngoscope*, 1996; Vol.106, No.10, (October 1996), pp. 1214-1217, ISSN 0023-852X

Costa, F., Emanuelli, E., Robiony, M., Zerman, N., Polini, F. & Politi, M. (2007). Endoscopic surgical treatment of chronic maxillary sinusitis of dental origin. *Journal of oral and maxillofacial surgery: official journal of the American Association of Oral and Maxillofacial Surgeons*, Vol.65, No.2, (February 2007), pp. 223-228. ISSN 0278-2391

DeFreitas, J. & Lucente, FE. (1988). The Caldwell-Luc procedure: institutional review of 670 cases: 1975-1985. *Laryngoscope*, Vol.98, No.12, (December 1988), pp. 1297-1300, ISSN 0023-852X

Di Pasquale, P. & Shermetaro, C. (2006). Endoscopic removal of a dentigerous cyst producing unilateral maxillary sinus opacification on computed tomography. *Ear, nose, & throat journal*, Vol.85, No.11, (November 2006), pp. 747-748, ISSN 0145-5613

Dolanmaz, D., Tuz, H., Bayraktar, S., Metin, M., Erdem, E. & Baykul, T. (2004). Use of pedicled buccal fat pad in the closure of oroantral communication: analysis of 75 cases. *Quintessence international*, Vol. 35, No.3, (March 2004), pp. 241-246, ISSN 0033-6572

Eberhart, LH., Kussin, A., Arndt, C., Lange, H., Folz, BJ., Werner, JA., Wulf H. & Kill, C. (2007). Effect of a balanced anaesthetic technique using desflurane and remifentanil on surgical conditions during microscopic and endoscopic sinus surgery. *Rhinology*, Vol.45, No.1, (March 2007), pp. 72-78, ISSN 0300-0729

El Charkawi, HG., El Askary, AS & Ragab, A (2005). Endoscopic removal of an implant from the maxillary sinus: a case report. *Implant dentistry*, Vol.14, No.1, (March 2005), pp. 30–35, ISSN 1056-6163

Engelke, W. & Capobianco, M. (2005). Flapless sinus floor augmentation using endoscopy combined with CT scan-designed surgical templates: method and report of 6 consecutive cases. *The International journal of oral & maxillofacial implants*, Vol.20, No.6, (November – December 2005), pp. 891-897, ISSN 0882-2786

Engelke, W. & Deckwer, I. (1997). Endoscopically controlled sinus floor augmentation. A preliminary report. *Clinical oral implants research*, Vol.8, No.6, (December 1997), pp. 527-531, ISSN 0905-7161

Engelke, W., Schwarzwäller, W., Behnsen, A. & Jacobs, HG. (2003). Subantroscopic laterobasal sinus floor augmentation (SALSA): an up-to-5-year clinical study. *The International journal of oral & maxillofacial implants*, Vol.18, No.1, (January – February 2003), pp. 135-143, ISSN 0882-2786

Felisati, G., Lozza, P., Chiapasco, M. & Borloni, R. (2007). Endoscopic removal of an unusual foreign body in the sphenoid sinus: an oral implant. *Clinical oral implants research*, 2007; Vol.18, No.6, (December 2007), pp. 776-780, ISSN 0905-7161

Ghali, GE. & Connor, MS. (2003). Surgical management of the odontogenic keratocyst. *Oral and maxillofacial surgery clinics of North America*, Vol.15, No.3, (August 2003), pp. 383-392. ISSN 1042-3699

Griffa A., Viterbo, S. & Boffano, P. (2010). Endoscopic-assisted removal of an intraorbital dislocated dental implant. *Clinical oral implants research*, Vol.21, No.7, (July 2010), pp. 778–780, ISSN 0905-7161

Güven O. (1998). A clinical study on oroantral fistulae. *Journal of cranio-maxillofacial surgery*, Vol.26, No.4, (August 1998), pp. 267-271, ISSN 1010-5182

Hajiioannou, J., Koudounarakis, E., Alexopoulos, K., Kotsani, A. & Kyrmizakis, DE. (2010). Maxillary sinusitis of dental origin due to oroantral fistula, treated by endoscopic sinus surgery and primary fistula closure. *The Journal of laryngology and otology*, Vol.124, No.9, (September 2010), pp. 986-989, ISSN 0022-2151

Hasbini, AS., Hadi, U. & Ghafari, J. (2001). Endoscopic removal of an ectopic third molar obstructing the osteomeatal complex. *Ear, nose, & throat journal*, Vol.80, No.9, (September 2001), pp. 667-670. ISSN 0145-5613

Ikeda, K., Hirano, K., Oshima, T., Shimomura, A., Suzuki, H., Sunose, H., Kondo, Y. & Takasaka, T. (1996). Comparison of complications between endoscopic sinus surgery and Caldwell-Luc operation. *The Tohoku journal of experimental medicine*, Vol.180, No.1, (September 1996), pp. 27-31, ISSN 0040-8727

Kennedy, DW. & Shaalan, H. (1989). Reevaluation of maxillary sinus surgery: experimental study in rabbits. *The Annals of otology, rhinology, and laryngology*, Vol.98, No.11, (November 1989), pp. 901-906, ISSN 0003-489

Kennedy, DW. (1985). Functional endoscopic sinus surgery: technique. *Archives of otolaryngology*, Vol.111, No.10, (October 1985), pp. 643–649. ISSN 0003-9977

Kim, JW., Lee, CH., Kwon, TK. & Kim, DK. (2007). Endoscopic removal of a dental implant through a middle meatal antrostomy. *The British journal of oral & maxillofacial surgery*, Vol.45, No.5, (July 2007), pp. 408-409, ISSN 0266-4356

Kitamura A. (2007). Removal of a migrated dental implant from a maxillary sinus by transnasal endoscopy. *The British journal of oral & maxillofacial surgery*, Vol.45, No.5, (July 2007), pp. 410-411, ISSN 0266-4356

Lamb, JF., Husein, OF. & Spiess, AC. (2009). Ectopic molar in the maxillary sinus precipitating a mucocele: a case report and literature review. *Ear, nose, & throat journal*, Vol.88, No.8, (August 2009), pp. E6-E11, ISSN 0145-5613

Lee, KC. & Lee, SJ. (2010). Clinical Features and Treatments of Odontogenic Sinusitis, *Yonsei Medical Journal*, Vol.51, No.6, (November 2010), pp. 932-937. ISSN 0513-5796

Leong, SC., Karkos, PD., Krajacevic, J., Islam, R. & Kent, SE. (2010). Ameloblastoma of the sinonasal tract: A case report. *Ear, nose, & throat journal*, Vol.89, No.2, (February 2010), pp. 70-71, ISSN 0145-5613

London, SD., Schlosser, RJ. & Gross, CW. (2002). Endoscopic management of benign sinonasal tumors: a decade of experience. *American journal of rhinology*, Vol.16, No.4, (July – August 2002), pp. 221-227, ISSN 1050-6586

Lopatin, AS. & Kapitanov, DN. (2005). Endonasal removal of a large ethmoidal cementoblastoma. *Rhinology*, Vol.43, No.2, (June 2005), pp. 156-158, ISSN 0300-0729

Lopatin, AS., Sysolyatin, SP., Sysolyatin, PG. & Melnikov, MN. (2002). Chronic maxillary sinusitis of dental origin: is external surgical approach mandatory? *Laryngoscope*, Vol.112, No.6, (June 2002), pp. 1056-1059, ISSN 0023-852X

Lubbe, DE., Aniruth, S., Peck, T. & Liebenberg, S. (2008). Endoscopic transnasal removal of migrated dental implants. *British dental journal*, Vol.204, No.8, (April 26th, 2008), pp. 435-436, ISSN 0007-0610

McMains, KC. (2008). Safety in endoscopic sinus surgery. *Current opinion in otolaryngology & head and neck surgery*, Vol.16, No.3, (June 2008), pp. 247-251. ISSN 1068-9508

Mehra, P. & Murad, H. (2004). Maxillary sinus disease of odontogenic origin. *Otolaryngologic clinics of North America*, Vol.37, No.2, (April 2004), pp. 347-364, ISSN 030-6665

Micozkadioglu, SD & Erkan, AN. (2007). Endoscopic removal of a maxillary dentigerous cyst. *B-ENT*, Vol.3, No.4, pp.213-216. ISSN 1781-782X

Nakamura, N., Mitsuyasu, T. & Ohishi, M. (2004). Endoscopic removal of a dental implant displaced into the maxillary sinus: technical note. *International journal of oral and maxillofacial surgery*, Vol.33, No.2, (March 2004), pp. 195-197, ISSN 0901-5027

Nemec, SF., Peloschek, P., Koelblinger, C., Mehrain, S., Krestan, CR. & Czerny, C. (2009). Sinonasal imaging after Caldwell-Luc surgery: MDCT findings of an abandoned procedure in times of functional endoscopic sinus surgery. *European Journal of Radiology*, Vol.70, No.1, (April 2009), pp. 31-34, ISSN 0720-048X

Nkenke, E., Schlegel, A., Schultze-Mosgau, S., Neukam, FW. & Wiltfang, J. (2002). The endoscopically controlled osteotome sinus floor elevation: a preliminary prospective study. *The International journal of oral & maxillofacial implants*, Vol.17, No.4, (July – August 2002), pp. 557-566, ISSN 0882-2786

Ramotar, H., Jaberoo, MC., Koo Ng, NK., Pulido, MA. & Saleh, HA. (2010). Image-guided, endoscopic removal of migrated titanium dental implants from maxillary sinus: two cases. *The Journal of laryngology and otology*, Vol.124, No.4, (April 2010), pp. 433-436, ISSN 0022-2151

Stammberger, H. (1986). Endoscopic endonasal surgery--concepts in treatment of recurring rhinosinusitis. Part II. Surgical technique. *Otolaryngology--head and neck surgery:*

official journal of American Academy of Otolaryngology-Head and Neck Surgery, Vol.94, No.2, (February 1986), pp. 147-156. ISSN 0194-5998

Ucer, TC. (2009). A modified transantral endoscopic technique for the removal of a displaced dental implant from the maxillary sinus followed by simultaneous sinus grafting. *The International journal of oral & maxillofacial implants*, Vol.24, No.5, (September – October 2009), pp. 947-951, ISSN 0882-2786

Varol, A., Türker, N., Göker, K. & Basa, S. (2006). Endoscopic retrieval of dental implants from the maxillary sinus. *The International journal of oral & maxillofacial implants*, Vol.21, No.5, (September – October 2006), pp. 801-804. ISSN 0882-2786

Yilmaz, T., Suslu, AE. & Gursel, B. (2003). Treatment of oroantral fistula: experience with 27 cases. *American journal of otolaryngology*, Vol.24, No.4, (July – August 2003), pp. 221-223. ISSN 0196-0709

Zimbler, MS., Lebowitz, RA., Glickman, R., Brecht, LE. & Jacobs, JB. (1998). Antral augmentation, osseointegration, and sinusitis: the otolaryngologist's perspective. *American journal of rhinology*, Vol.12, No.5, (September – October 1998) , pp. 311-316, ISSN 1050-6586

5

Sialendoscopy: Endoscopic Approach to Benign Salivary Gland Diseases

Meghan Wilson, Kyle McMullen
and Rohan R. Walvekar
Department of Otolaryngology Head & Neck Surgery,
Louisiana State, University Health Science Center,
New Orleans, Louisiana
USA

1. Introduction

Sialadenitis, or recurrent salivary gland infection associated with pain and swelling of the major salivary glands, is a common presentation to emergency rooms and outpatient clinics. One of the most frequent causes of sialadenitis is obstruction in the salivary ductal system. Salivary calculi affect 1.2% of the population and account for 60-70% of salivary duct obstruction (Nahlieli 2004; Kim 2007; Bomeli 2009; Nahlieli 2006). Additional causes of obstruction to salivary flow include strictures in 25-25%, inflammation (5-10%) and other rare pathologies such as foreign bodies (1%)

Conservative treatment is the first line of therapy that includes treatment with antibiotics, salivary stimulants or sialogogues, and anti-inflammatory agents. However, conservative therapy fails in up to 40% of people with sialadenitis; in which case the recommended treatment is excision of the involved salivary gland. There as several important nerves that are in close proximity to the major salivary glands. The facial nerve, motor to facial muscles, runs through the parotid glandular system. Similarly, the submandibular gland is associated with the lingual nerve that is 1sensory to the anterior two thirds of the oral tongue; marginal mandibular nerve that allows movement of the angle of the mouth; and the hypoglossal nerve, motor to the tongue. Surgical excision of the gland carries numerous risks include but are not limited to paresis or palsy of the facial nerve, lingual nerve, and hypoglossal nerve. Other complications include Frey syndrome (gustatory sweating), sialoceles, salivary fistula, xerostomia, numbness in the distribution of the greater auricular nerve, infection, and hemorrhage. Consequently, although surgical resection in experienced hands is safe, it's often not desired due to the associated surgical risk and external scar in the neck associated with it.

In 1988, salivary duct endoscopes were introduced. Since their introduction, sialendoscopes have undergone technical refinements that have been instrumental in permitting clear and high definition visualization and manipulation of the salivary ductal system. Today, salivary duct endoscopy or "Sialendoscopy" allows the minimally invasive endoscopic visualization of major salivary gland ductal system and endoscopic interventions to treat chronic sialadenitis with or without sialolithiasis.

As in many other surgical areas, the advent of sialendoscopy has added additional options to the diagnosis and management of non-neoplastic salivary pathology. Initially, sialendoscopy was created for diagnostic evaluation of the salivary glands and ductal system as well as treatment of obstruction through the removal of sialoliths or dilation of strictures. Nahlieli et al, in their study in 2004[1] described successful endoscopic treatment of recurrent parotitis and juvenile recurrent parotitis. The scope of sialendoscopy was further expanded to treat radioactive iodine sialadenitis (Kim 2007; Bomeli 2009; Nhlieli 2006) and sialadenitis induced by autoimmune diseseases (Schacham 2011). Today, sialendoscopy is regarded as an acceptable and often preferred diagnostic and treatment tool for chronic sialadenitis and non-neoplastic obstruction of the salivary ductal system.

2. Indications and contraindication

Current evidence has validated sialendoscopy for the treatment of non-neoplastic disorders of the salivary glands, including sialolithiasis. Sialolithiasis is one of the most common non-neoplastic disorders of the major salivary glands and a major cause of sialadenitis and unilateral diffuse swelling of the major salivary glands (Marchal F, Dulguerov P. 2003; Nahlieli O. 2006). In general, stones less than 4 mm in the submandibular gland and less than 3 mm in the parotid gland are amenable to endoscopic removal. Intermediate size stones between 5-7 mm may need further fragmentation either using a Holmium laser or lithotripsy prior to endoscopic extraction. In general stones larger than 8 mm require a combined approach technique for stone removal (Karavidas K, Nahlieli O, Fritsch N, et al. 2010). The combined approach technique is a technique that uses the sialendoscope for stone localization and either an intra-oral or an external approach for removal of large submandibular or parotid gland stones, respectively (Bodner L. 2002; Lustmann J, Regev E, Melamed Y. 1990; Marchal F. 2007; Raif J, Vardi M, Nahlieli O, et al. 2006; Seldin HM, Seldin SD, Rakower W. 1953; Walvekar RR, Bomeli SR, Carrau RL, et al. 2009).

Sialendoscopy indications include diagnostic evaluation of recurrent or chronic sialadenitis, including unexplained swelling of the major salivary glands associated with meals, ductal stenosis, and intra-ductal masses (Nahlieli O. 2006; Walvekar RR, Razfar A, Carrau RL, et al. 2008). The authors of limited series have also suggested benefit in patients with radioiodine-induced sialadenitis (Kim JW, Han GS, Lee SH et al. 2007; Bomeli SR, Schaitkin B, Carrau RL, et al. 2009; Nahlieli O and Nazarian Y. Sialadenitis 2006). Recent studies and the authors' experience suggest benefit in children with recurrent sialadenitis (Nahlieli O, Shacham R, Shlesinger M, et al. 2004; Jabbour N, Tibesar R, Lander T, et al. 2010; Martins-Carvalho C, Plouin-Gaudon I, Quenin S, et al. 2010; Faure F, Querin S, Dulguerov P, et al. 2007) and also in patients who have recurrent sialadenitis from autoimmune processes such as Sjogren's syndrome or Systemic Lupus Erythematosis (Shacham R, Puterman MB, Ohana N, et al. 2011).

The only absolute contraindication is acute sialadenitis. The use of the rigid dilator system and/or a semi-rigid endoscope during an acute episode increases the chance of ductal trauma and irrigation as well as ductal injury could increases the potential spread of infection in the head and neck soft tissues. Sialendoscopy can be challenging in patients with microstomia or trismus. These could be considered as relative contraindications for the procedure.

2.1 Sialendoscopy: Technique

Sialendoscopy may be performed in the clinic setting with local anesthesia or in the operating room with sedation or general anesthesia. The decision of where to perform the procedure is physician and/or patient preferences. The basic work up for sialendoscopy is summarized in **Table 1.**

History	Symptoms
	Number of infections
	Previous treatments
	History of external beam radiation therapy
	History of Radioactive iodine treatment
Physical Examination	Full Head and Neck examination
	Bimanual palpation of glands
	Examine and note location of papilla
	Note any anatomical limitations (trismus, small oral commissure, temporomandibular joint pathology, etc.)
Imaging	Computed Tomography Scan (CT)
	Ultrasound
	Magnetic Resonance Imaging Scan (MRI)

Table 1. Preoperative Evaluation

2.1.1 Basic workup

Workup of all salivary disorders begins with history of present disease. Important questions to ask include symptoms, number of infections, previous treatments, and previous testing or other studies. Questions regarding history of external beam radiation or radioactive iodine therapy are important as well to understand possible etiologies of salivary disease.

Examination should first include a complete head and neck exam. Bimanual palpation of the salivary gland should be performed to examine for any masses or palpable stones, noting any asymmetry. Examine the papilla and its location. Assess the patency and saliva flow and quality of the saliva from the papilla. It is important to make notes regarding the papilla in the chart to aid in identification when ready to perform sialendoscopy; pictorial illustrations are particularly helpful. In addition, the surgeon must evaluate access to the oral cavity by paying close attention to the size of the oral commissure (e.g., microstomia), size of tongue, ability to open the mouth (e.g., preoperative trismus), and pathology of temporomandibular joints

Laboratory and imaging studies ordered will depend on the patient's symptoms and physical exam findings. Frequently used imaging studies include ultrasonography, computed tomography (CT), and magnetic resonance imaging (MRI), (**Figures 1 and 2**). The authors' preference for diagnosis and surgical planning is CT scan with and without contrast.

2.1.2 Instrumentation

The basic instrumentation includes a specialized dilator system that permits gradual serial dilation of the salivary duct papilla from the lowest No.0000 dilator to a maximum of No.8,

(**Figure 3**). The sialendoscopes most frequently used are the "all-in-one" interventional sialendoscopes, which can range from 1.1.mm to 1.6 mm in diameter, (**Figure 4**). The sialendoscopes have an optic channel that transmits the image using fiberoptic channels, and an irrigation channel allows a continuous irrigation to be performed to maintain duct patency for endoscopic visualization of the salivary duct lumen and to allow working space for surgical intervention. A working channel is used to introduce instruments for intervention. The 1.1 and 1.3 mm sialendoscopes permit introduction of 0.4 mm stone wire baskets (**Figure 5 A-C**) and a hand-held micro burr to break stones. The 1.6 mm sialendoscope permits the use of 0.6 mm stone wire basket and a cup forceps in addition.

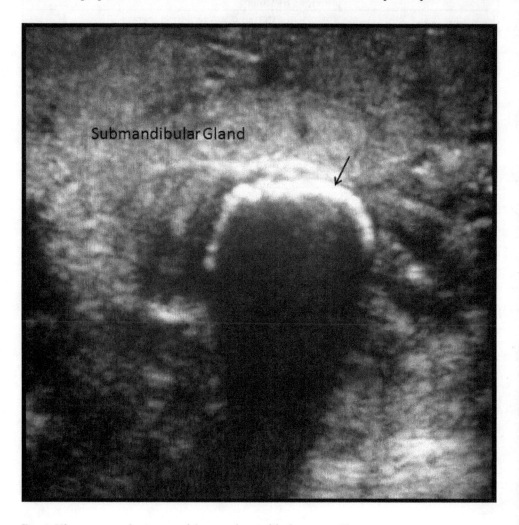

Fig. 1. Ultrasonography image of large submandibular stone. The stone appears as a hyperechoic rim while throwing a shadow that is a pathognomic finding of a salivary stone visualized via ultrasound, (black arrow points to the stone).

Holmium laser fibers can be used as well through the interventional channels for intra-ductal laser fragmentation of stones, (**Figure 6**). Another important tool for sialendoscopy is the conical dilator that permits gradual dilation of the duct and allows one to transition from a smaller dilator to the next size, (**Figure 7**).

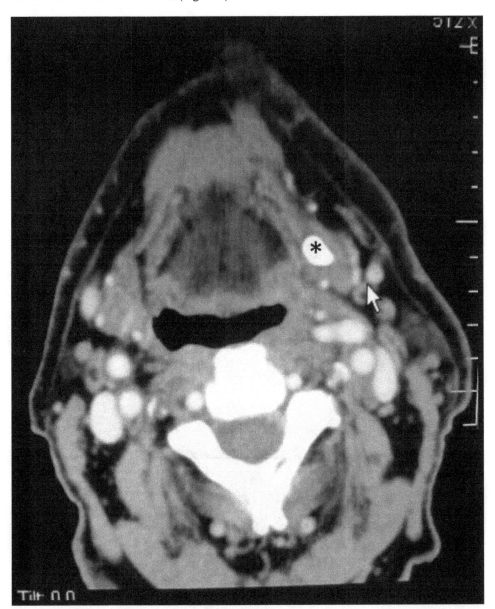

Fig. 2. An contrast enhanced axial CT scan showing a large irregular left submandibular stone in the hilum, (the asterix denotes the salivary stone).

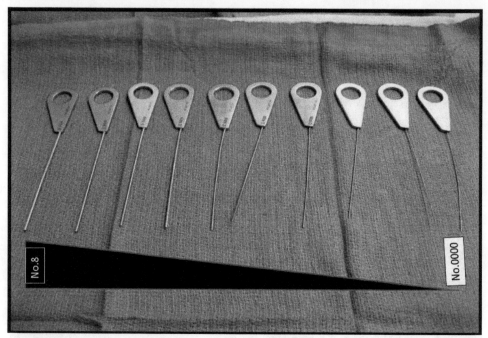

Fig. 3. Marchal Dilator System

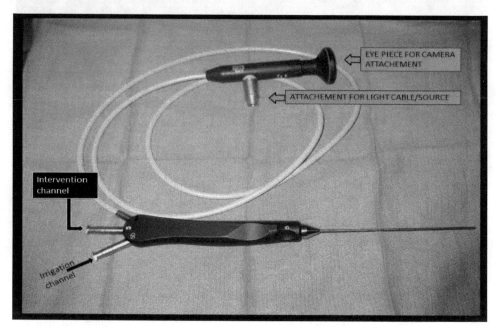

Fig. 4. 1.6 mm Erlangen "All-In-One" Sialendoscope

Salivary duct stents or cannulae can usually left in place following the procedure to decrease the risk of scarring and papilla stenosis, (**Figure 8**)

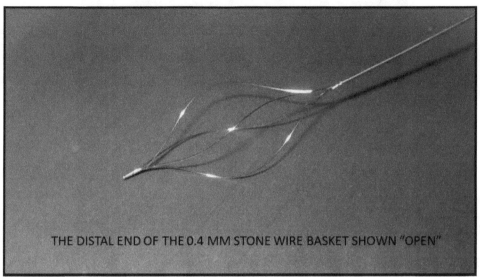

THE DISTAL END OF THE 0.4 MM STONE WIRE BASKET SHOWN "OPEN"

A)

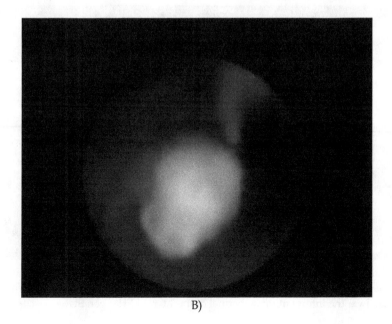

B)

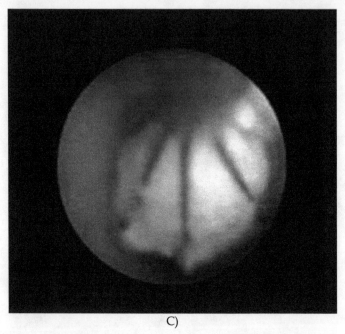

C)

Fig. 5. A) 0.4 mm stone wire basket. B) A free floating submandibular duct stone. C) The wire basket can be inserted through the interventional port of the sialendoscope and used for trapping the stone for endoscopic removal

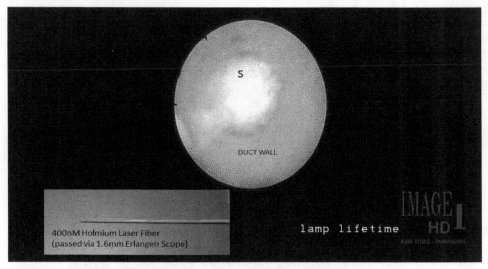

Fig. 6. A Holmium laser fiber being used for intra-ductal laser fulguration of an impacted 6mm submandibular stone (S). Inset shows the tip of the 400 nM Holmium laser fiber that can be passed via the interventional channel of the 1.6 mm Erlangen Sialendoscope.

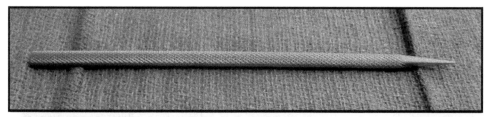

Fig. 7. Conical Dilator

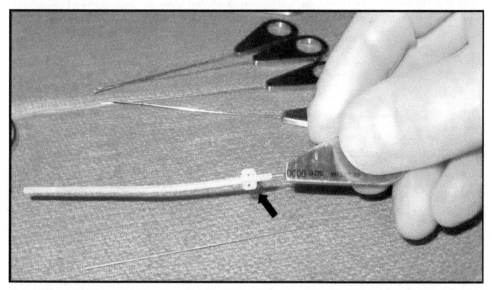

Fig. 8. The Schaitkin Salivary Canula (Hood Laboratories, Pembroke, MA) can be inserted over a No.0000 Marchal dilator to prevent subsequent stenosis of the duct or papilla. Black arrow points to distal end of stent that projects out of the papilla. Two holes on either side of the flange of the stent facilitate securing the stent to the floor of mouth or buccal mucosa via non-absorbable stitches.

2.1.3 Operative technique
Operative technique can be divided into two main components:
1.   Access to the salivary duct i.e. dilation of the papilla
2.   Endoscopy with or without intervention.
Management of papilla is the rate-limiting step of the procedure. Care must be taken to dilate the papilla. Poor handling of the papilla can lead to papillary stenosis in the future that can lead to obstructive sialadenitis. In addition, perforation of the duct (minor or major ductal tear) and creation of a false passage are potential complications of papilla dilation that add morbidity to the procedure and also are reasons for sialendoscopy failure.
Identification of the papilla can be aided by a using an operating microscope or surgical loupes. The author recommends the use of at least surgical loupes to identify and dilate the papilla. In office localization and documentation of the location of the papilla with imaging

is very helpful in intra-operative identification of the papilla. Massage of the gland may also assist in localizing the papilla by denoting the point of saliva flow. After identification of the papilla, serial dilation of the papilla is then performed using the Marchal dilator system, **(Figure 3)**. Injection of local anesthetic around the papilla often helps the process of serial dilation by making the ductal opening more prominent and by stiffening the surrounding tissues to facilitate serial cannulation of the duct. In this procedure, salivary probes of increasing diameter, beginning with the smallest (No. 0000), are sequentially introduced into the duct. Dilation up to No.3 or No.4 is adequate to allow introduction of a sialendoscope of 1.3mm diameter. For the introduction of larger endoscopes (1.6mm), dilation up to No.6 probe is necessary (Marchal F. 2003). Other techniques used to dilate the papilla or facilitate the identification of the papilla are the Seldinger's technique that uses a series of bougies of increasing diameter that are inserted over a guide wire that is placed in the salivary duct **(Figure 9)**, the placement of a papillotomy or an incision at the entry point of the salivary duct to facilitate entry into the it, and use of Methylene blue to identify the duct orifice (Marchal F. 2003; Geisthoff UW. 2009; Papadaki ME, Kaban L, Kwolek C, et al. 2007; Iwai T, Matsui Y, Yamagishi M, et al. 2009; Luers JC, Vent J, Beutner D. 2008).

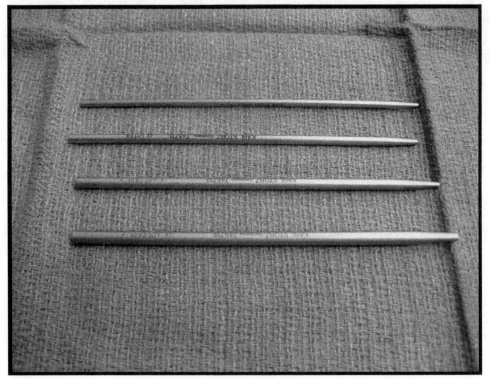

Fig. 9. Bougies of increasing diameter used in the Seldinger's technique of salivary duct dilation.

Nahlieli et al have suggested performing a papillotomy to allow introduction of the scope (Nahlieli O. 2006). However, in the authors' experience, a papillotomy prevents the creation of a mucosal seal around the endoscope, resulting in leakage of the irrigation, consequently preventing maximum dilation of the duct through hydraulic pressure. The authors reserve the use of a papillotomy for one of two scenarios: difficult cases in which standard dilation or the Seldinger's technique fails and if necessary for the delivery of larger stones at the conclusion of a procedure.

2.1.4 Endoscopy with or without intervention

Despite its apparent simplicity, sialendoscopy is a technically challenging procedure that requires organized and sequential learning(Marchal F. 2003). Once this is acquired, the success rates for diagnostic as well as interventional sialendoscopy can be more than 85% (Marchal F, Dulguerov P. 2003; Nahlieli O. 2006; Marchal F. 2003).

Sialendoscopy allows visualization of the entire ductal system with ability to navigate the scope into primary, secondary and at time tertiary branching systems, (**Figure 10**). With respect to diagnostic sialendoscopy, Marchal and Dulguerov reported a 98% success rate (Marchal F, Dulguerov P. 2003), whereas (Nahlieli O, Baruchin AM. 1999) reported a success rate of 96% in their case series. Though diagnostic sialendoscopy is possible in most patients, failure to pass the scope along the entire ductal system may result from ductal stenosis, inflammation, or because of the presence of an acute masseteric bend of the parotid duct, making navigation with the scope difficult.

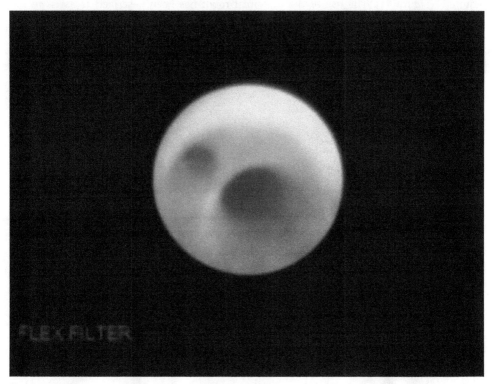

Fig. 10. Intraoperative view of the ductal lumen showing branching ductal system.

In the interventional setting, stone removal is the most common indication for sialendoscopy. Success rates for endoscopic stone removal without adjuvant lithotripsy with forceps or laser fragmentation range from 74-89% in several case series(Marchal F, Dulguerov P. 2003; Nahlieli O. 2006; Marchal F. 2007; Walvekar RR, Razfar A, Carrau RL, et al. 2008; Bowen MA, Tauzin M, Kluka, EA, et al. 2010; Nahlieli O, Nakar LH, Nazarian Y, et al. 2008; Walvekar RR, Carrau RL, Schaitkin B. 2009). Nahlieli et al reported a success rate of 86% and 89%, respectively, for endoscopic parotid and submandibular sialolithotomy in 736 cases of sialolithiasis (Nahlieli O. 2006). However, their success rate for endoscopic sialolithotomy was 80% in an earlier series of 3 years experience, during which they reported a total of 32 cases of sialolithiasis with 4 failures (Nahlieli O, Baruchin AM. 1999).

Stones larger than 3mm in the parotid gland and 4mm in the submandibular gland have a lower success rate for removal (Marchal F, Dulguerov P. 2003). Laser fragmentation and lithotripsy are useful for removal of intermediate-size stones (up to 6 or 7 mm). External lithotripsy can be performed prior to sialendoscopy to fragment the stones into smaller fragments that can be more readily removed with wire baskets or forceps. External lithotripsy for the management of salivary stone is not currently FDA approved in the United States. Consequently, the authors have not incorporated this into their practice. Laser stone fragmentation and intra-ductal lithotripsy have been described. The Holmium has been used for stone fragmentation(Papadaki ME, McCain JP, Kim K, et al. 2008). For larger stones or stones that cannot be accessed endoscopically, a combined approach technique is required, (**Figure 11**). The use of the da Vinici robot has been described to assist in the

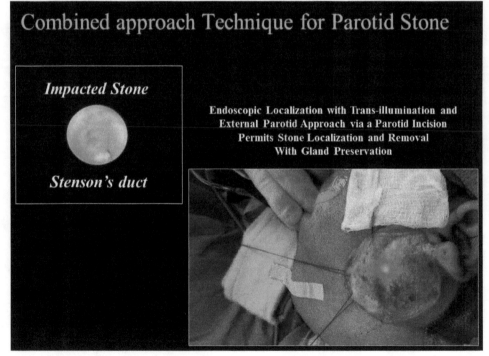

Fig. 11. Combined Approach Technique for Parotid Stones via an External Approach.

management of large hilar and intra-glandular submandibular salivary stones are traditionally difficult to access via a transoral route, (**Figure 12**)(Walvekar RR, Tyler PD, Tammareddi N, et al. 2011).

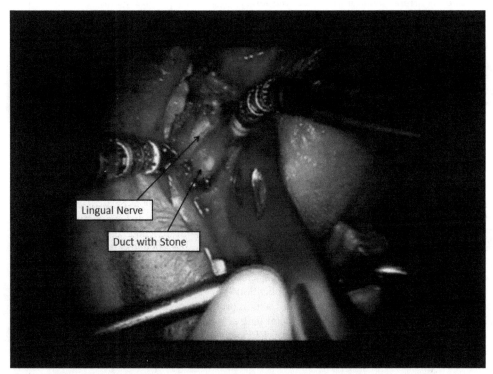

Fig. 12. Combined Approach Technique (Robot-Assisted) for Submandibular Stones via a Transoral Approach. Right submandibular stone is exposed with identification and dissection of the lingual nerve with excellent visualization via the da Vinci robotic system.

Radioactive iodine (RAI) treatment can induce sialadenitis with inflammation and consequently stenosis of the ductal system (Kim JW, Han GS, Lee SH et al. 2007; Bomeli SR, Schaitkin B, Carrau RL, et al. 2009; Nahlieli O and Nazarian Y. 2006). This occurs because the salivary glands in addition to the thyroid gland concentrate iodine. Up to 60% of patients treated with RAI can develop chronic sialadenitis (Kim JW, Han GS, Lee SH et al. 2007; Bomeli SR, Schaitkin B, Carrau RL, et al. 2009; Nahlieli O and Nazarian Y. 2006). Sialendoscopy has shown to be effective in the treatment of this disorder. Bomeli et al. (Bomeli SR, Schaitkin B, Carrau RL, et al. 2009) studied radioactive iodine induced sialadenitis in 12 patients. 37 glands were studied in these 12 patients. Mucous plugs were found in 44% of glands; strictures had developed in 30%. Therapeutic maneuvers involve flushing the gland to expel mucous plugs, dilation of stenotic areas with an endoscopic balloon dilator, or , intra-ductal instillation of steroids during the procedure. Sialendoscopy was able to be performed in 84% of patients and 75% of patients had resolution of symptoms following the procedure. Overall success rates for resolution of symptoms range between 50 and 100%. Failure is most commonly due to severe ductal stenosis(Kim JW, Han GS, Lee SH et al. 2007; Bomeli SR, Schaitkin B, Carrau RL, et al. 2009; Nahlieli O and Nazarian Y. 2006).

Juvenile recurrent sialadenitis most frequently affects the parotid gland. The etiology is unknown. Sialendoscopy can be used as both a diagnostic tool and treatment (Nahlieli O, Shacham R, Shlesinger M, et al. 2004; Jabbour N, Tibesar R, Lander T, et al. 2010; Martins-Carvalho C, Plouin-Gaudon I, Quenin S, et al. 2010; Faure F, Querin S, Dulguerov P, et al. 2007). Sialendoscopy with irrigation of the duct with or without injection steroids has been shown to be effective in treating this condition. Characteristic findings are seen on sialendoscopy originally include whitish appearance of the duct and lack of vascular markings seen on the ductal wall. Shacham et al. (Shacham R, Droma EB, London D, et al. 2009) studied 70 children with recurrent sialadenitis. In 56 of the children, symptoms were eliminated after one procedure; only 5 children required a repeat procedure.

3. Complications

Major complication rates are low with sialendoscopy. Gland swelling post-operatively is expected and usually resolves in approximately 24-48 hours. This is particularly important to consider in submandibular procedures, as swelling could cause airway compromise (Iwai T, Matsui Y, Yamagishi M, et al. 2009). Consequently, when performing bilateral submandibular gland procedures, it is important to examine the gland and oral cavity after completing one side and determine whether it is safe for the patient to proceed with the contralateral gland.

One of the more serious iatrogenic complications is avulsion of the duct. This complication can be prevented by avoiding excessive traction on the stone while it is engaged in the wire basket,. If duct avulsion or a major ductal tear occurs, subsequent gland excision could be necessary (Walvekar RR, Razfar A, Carrau RL, et al. 2008).

Lingual nerve paresthesias can occur in up to 15% of patients undergoing transoral combined procedures in the immediate post-operative period and resolves with time (Walvekar RR, Razfar A, Carrau RL, et al. 2008; Bowen MA, Tauzin M, Kluka, EA, et al. 2010; Nahlieli O. 2009). The development of a post-operative stricture has been reported (Bowen MA, Tauzin M, Kluka, EA, et al. 2010; Nahlieli O. 2009). Taking care not to cause trauma to the duct or papilla during the procedure minimizes the risk of this complication. In addition, in the event the duct is traumatized or a papillotomy is required, placement of a salivary stent for up to 2 weeks can help prevention of subsequent ductal or papillary stenosis. Salivary fistulas, sialoceles, minor ductal tears, development traumatic ranulas, minor bleeding, and infection have been reported (Nahlieli O. 2006; Walvekar RR, Razfar A, Carrau RL, et al. 2008; Bowen MA, Tauzin M, Kluka, EA, et al. 2010) (4,21,31). Other complications may include inability to retrieve the stone and failure of the procedure due to ductal stenosis or an acute masseteric bend (Nahlieli O. 2006; Walvekar RR, Razfar A, Carrau RL, et al. 2008; Bowen MA, Tauzin M, Kluka, EA, et al. 2010; Nahlieli O. 2009).

4. Future directions and conclusions

Diagnostic and interventional sialendoscopy are safe and effective options for treating non-neoplastic disorders of the major salivary glands. Sialendoscopy is technically challenging and requires sequential learning in which success rates appear to be proportional to the surgeon's level of experience Marchal F, Dulguerov P. (2003). The authors recommend that future sialendoscopist's should familiarize themselves with the anatomy and physiology of the salivary glands and floor of the mouth. They should be competent in taking care of any potential complication and should be comfortable with major salivary gland resections if required. Sialendoscopy training via hands-on courses and case observations should be pursued prior to initiating a sialendoscopy practice

5. Further resources for sialendoscopy-related information

1. www.salivaryendoscopy.net
2. http://emedicine.medscape.com/article/1520153-overview
3. Marchal F. Sialendoscopy. In: E Myers, Ed. Salivary Gland Disorders. Berlin, Germany: Springer; 2007:127-48.
4. Marchal F, Dulguerov P. Sialolithiasis management: the state of the art. Arch Otolaryngol Head Neck Surg. Sep 2003;129(9):951-6.
5. Marchal F. Sialendoscopy: The Endoscopic Approach to Salivary Gland Ductal Pathologies. Tuttlingen, Germany: Endo Publishing; 2003.
6. Koch M, Zenk J, Iro H. Algorithms for treatment of salivary gland obstructions. Otolaryngol Clin North Am. 2009.

6. References

[1] Nahlieli O, Shacham R, Shlesinger M, et al.(2004). Juvenile recurrent parotitis: a new method of diagnosis and treatment. *Pediatrics*; Vol. 144,No. 1, (Jul 2004),pp. 9-12.
[2] Kim JW, Han GS, Lee SH et al.(2007). Sialendoscopic treatment for radioiodine induced sialadenitis. *Laryngoscope* Vol. 117, No. 1, (Jan 2007), pp. 133-136.
[3] Bomeli SR, Schaitkin B, Carrau RL, et al. (2009), Interventional sialendoscopy for treatment of radioiodine-induced sialadenitis. *Laryngoscope, Vol 119, No.5* ,(May 2009), pp. 864-867.
[4] Nahlieli O and Nazarian Y. Sialadenitis following radioiodine therapy - a new diagnostic and treatment modality. *Oral Dis,* 2006;12:476-479.
[5] Shacham R, Puterman MB, Ohana N, et al. (2011) Endoscopic treatment of salivary glands affected by autoimmune diseases. *J Oral Maxillofac Surg,* Vol. 69, No. 2 (Feb 2011), pp.476-481.
[6] Marchal F, Dulguerov P. (2003) Sialolithiasis management: the state of the art. *Arch Otolaryngol Head Neck Surg,* Vol. 129, No. 9 (Sept 2003), pp. 951-956.
[7] Nahlieli O. (2006) Sialendoscopy: a new approach to salivary gland obstructive pathology. *J Am Dent Assoc,* Vol. 137, No. 10, (Oct 2006), pp. :1394-1400.
[8] Karavidas K, Nahlieli O, Fritsch N, et al.(2010) Minimal surgery for parotid stones: a 7-year endoscopic experience. *In J Oral Maxillofac Surg,* Vol. 39, No. 1, (Jan 2010), pp. 1-4.
[9] Bodner L. (2002) Giant salivary gland calculi: diagnostic imaging and surgical management. *Oral Surg Oral Med Oral Pathol Oral Radiol Endo,.* Vol. 94, No. 2, (Sep 2002), pp. 320-233.
[10] Lustmann J, Regev E, Melamed Y. (1990) Sialolithiasis. A survey on 245 patients and a review of the literature. *Int J Oral Maxillofac Surg,* Vol. 19, No. 3, (Jun 1990), pp. 135-138.
[11] Marchal F. (2007) A combined endoscopic and external approach for extraction of large stones with preservation of parotid and submandibular glands. *Laryngoscope,* Vol. 117, No. 2 (Feb 2007), pp. 373-377.
[12] Raif J, Vardi M, Nahlieli O, et al. (2006) An Er:YAG laser endoscopic fiber delivery system for lithotripsy of salivary stones. *Lasers Surg Med,* Jul 2006;38(6):580-587.

[13] Seldin HM, Seldin SD, Rakower W. (1953) Conservative surgery for the removal of salivary calculi. *Oral Surg Oral Med Oral Pathol*, Vol 6, No. 5, (May 1953), pp. 579-587.

[14] Walvekar RR, Bomeli SR, Carrau RL, et al. (2009) Combined approach technique for the management of large salivary stones. *Laryngoscope*. Vol. 119, No. 6, (Jun 2009), pp.1125-1129.

[15] Walvekar RR, Razfar A, Carrau RL, et al. (2008) Sialendoscopy and associated complications: a preliminary experience. *Laryngoscope*. Vol. 118, No. 5, (May 2008), pp. 776-779.

[16] Jabbour N, Tibesar R, Lander T, et al. (2010) Sialendoscopy in Children. *Int J Pediatr Otorhinolaryngol*, Vol 74, No. 4, (Apr. 2010), pp. 347-350.

[17] Martins-Carvalho C, Plouin-Gaudon I, Quenin S, et al. (2010) Pediatric Sialendoscopy: a 5-year experience at a single institution. *Arch Otolaryngol Head Neck Surg*, Vol 136, No. 1, (Jan 2010)pp. 33-36.

[18] Faure F, Querin S, Dulguerov P, et al. (2007) Pediatric salivary gland obstructive swelling: sialendoscopic approach. *Laryngoscope*, Vol 117, No. 8 (Aug 2007), pp. 1363-1367.

[19] Marchal F. Sialendoscopy: The *Endoscopic Approach to Salivary Gland Ductal Pathologies*. Tuttlingen, Germany: Endo-Publishing; 2003.

[20] Geisthoff UW. (2009) Technology of sialendoscopy. *Otolaryngol Clin North Am* Vol. 42, No. 6, (Dec 2009), pp. 1001-1028.

[21] Papadaki ME, Kaban L, Kwolek C, et al. (2007) Arterial stents for access and protection of the parotid and submandibular ducts during sialoendoscopy. *J Oral Maxillofac Surg* Vol 65, No. 9 (Sept 2007), pp. 1865-1868.

[22] Iwai T, Matsui Y, Yamagishi M, et al. (2009) Simple technique for dilatation of the papilla in sialoendoscopy. *J Oral Maxillofac Surg*, Vol. 67, No. 3, (Mar 2009) pp. 681-2.

[23] Luers JC, Vent J, Beutner D. (2008) Methylene blue for easy and safe detection of salivary duct papilla in sialendoscopy. *Otolaryngol Head Neck Surg* Vol. 139, No. 3 (Sept 2008), pp. 466-467.

[24] Nahlieli O, Baruchin AM. (1999) Endoscopic technique for the diagnosis and treatment of obstructive salivary gland diseases. J Oral Maxillofac Surg. Vol. 25, No. 12, (Dec 1999), pp. 1394-401; discussion 1401-1402.

[25] Bowen MA, Tauzin M, Kluka, EA, et al. (2010) Diagnostic and interventional sialendoscopy: a preliminary experience. *Laryngoscope*, Vol. 121, No. 2 (Feb 2010), pp. 299-303.

[26] Nahlieli O, Nakar LH, Nazarian Y, et al. (2008) Sialoendoscopy: a new approach to salivary gland obstructive pathology. *J Am Dent Assoc*, Vol. 137, No. 10, (Oct 2008), pp. 1394-1400.

[27] Walvekar RR, Carrau RL, Schaitkin B. (2009) Sialendoscopy: Minimally invasive approach to the salivary ductal system. *Operative Techniques in Otolaryngology*. Vol. 20, No. 2, (Jun 2009), pp. 131-135.

[28] Papadaki ME, McCain JP, Kim K, et al. Interventional sialoendoscopoy: Early Clinical Results. *J Oral Maxillofac Surg*, Vol. 66, No. 5, (May 2008), pp. 954-962.

[29] Walvekar RR, Tyler PD, Tammareddi N, et al. (2011) Robotic-assisted Transoral removal of a submandibular Megalith. *Laryngoscope* Vol. 131, No. 3, (Mar 2011), pp. 534-7.

[30] Shacham R, Droma EB, London D, et al. Long-term experience with endoscopic diagnosis and treatment of juvenile recurrent parotitis. *J Oral Maxillofac Surg*, Vol. 67, No. 1, (Jan 2009), pp. 162-167.

[31] Nahlieli O. Advanced Sialoendosocpy Techniques, Rare Findings and Complications. *Otolaryngol Clinc North Am*. Vol. 42, No. 6, (Dec 2009), pp. 1053-1072.

6

Virtual Endoscopy of the Nasal Cavity and the Paranasal Sinuses

Sumeet Anand, Rickul Varshney and Saul Frenkiel
McGill University, Department of Otolaryngology – Head & Neck Surgery
Canada

1. Introduction

The ideal approach to sinus surgery has been a mystery that many Otolaryngologists have attempted to discover throughout their career. The intricate and complex anatomy of the nasal cavity and paranasal sinuses has challenged many in terms of adequate exposure during surgery, as well as proper relief of patient symptoms. From the days of Hirschmann, who used a modified cystoscope to examine the sinuses in 1901 (Draf, 1983, as cited in Rice & Schaefer, 2004), to the work of Messerklinger and Wigand in establishing operative techniques later in that century (Rice & Schaefer, 2004), surgeons have appreciated the obscurity and complexity of endoscopic sinus surgery for decades.

Traditionally, pre-operative planning has consisted of imaging modalities, namely x-rays and computed tomography (CT) scans, as well as flexible or rigid endoscopy in the clinic. With the advent of helical CT in the late 1980s, pre-operative imaging has improved dramatically. It is faster than the conventional CT scanner and provides more details (Wood & Razavi, 2002). In fact, helical CT has provided physicians with the ability to attain reconstruction of axial images into coronal and sagittal views with resolution quality equivalent to the original axial cuts. Imaging for the paranasal sinuses is ideally viewed in coronal slices as Otolaryngologists enter the nasal cavity in an anterior-posterior direction rather than the cephalocaudal direction represented by axial slices. Furthermore, the coronal view allows the examination of critical relationships such as the osteomeatal complex, not provided by axial imaging. The use of MRI for better soft tissue examination and less artifacts has also improved imaging of the head and neck (Kettenbach et al., 2008). The dependence of Otolaryngologists on proper pre-operative imaging highlights the strong relationship between radiologists and otolaryngologists in endoscopic sinus surgery in order to precisely locate numerous vital structures, such as the orbits and the internal carotid arteries, surrounding the nasal cavity and the paranasal sinuses and to identify benign and pathologic anomalies.

Recently, virtual endoscopy (VE) through reconstruction of CT images has interested Otolaryngologists that perform endoscopic sinus surgery. This contemporary technology facilitates the difficult task of mentally conceptualizing complex and intricate anatomy in a three-dimensional model from two-dimensional CT images, a task that requires years of experience to truly master. VE utilizes the technique of surface or volumetric rendering to process data provided by CT images to allow three-dimensional visualization of tubular anatomical structures (Rubin et al., 1996). This modality has been used in the past for imaging of the colon (Pineau et al., 2003) and more recently in imaging of the tracheobronchial tree (Vining et al., 1996), urinary tract, vessels, the middle ear and the paranasal sinuses (Han et al., 2000; Ossoff & Reinisch, 1994; Rogalla et al., 1998). This chapter explores the use of VE in the imaging of the nasal cavity and the paranasal sinuses. The technical aspects of VE, the uses in Otolaryngology and Radiology, the benefits for pre-operative and intra-operative planning, the roles in endoscopic sinus surgery training, as well as future directions will be discussed.

2. Technical aspects of Virtual Endoscopy

In essence, VE is a reformation of axial CT images into a 3D model using sophisticated software. In the present age where the medical system is influenced by a paucity of resources and increasing waiting times for diagnostic tests, VE provides a useful diagnostic adjunct for the surgeon, without the need of additional tests. There are no required particular CT specifications over the standard scanner and thus, any patient who can undergo a CT sinus can have a three-dimensional model created.

The process begins with a low-dose spiral CT scan, as routinely performed for sinus imaging. Axial slices of 2.5mm thickness are acquired at an interval of 1.25 mm, therefore providing an overlap of collected information. No intravenous contrast is used for the scan. The images are then reconstructed into thinner 0.625 mm slices at an increment of 0.625 mm using a standard algorithm. Thereafter, these images are processed through rendering into a three-dimensional model using software provided with a 64-multislice General Electrics (GE) LightSpeed scanner (Milwaukee, WI). VE software is accessed on a GE workstation in our radiology department, which was provided with the scanner without an additional fee. There are two main methods for post-processing, namely surface rendering and volume rendering. We use volume rendering at our institution for reasons that will be explained later in this chapter. Although the process of post-processing is complex, we present a brief overview of the two methods.

In order to understand the process of reformatting, it is useful to appreciate the significance of a voxel. The latter is defined as a volume element (Rogalla et al., 2000) or the smallest distinguishable volume part of a 3D space. These individual voxels merge to create the three-dimensional model, analogous to a two-dimensional image formed by pixels (Gilani et al., 1997).

2.1 Surface rendering

Surface rendering works by defining a certain threshold as to determine which pixels will be included in the model and which ones will not (Rogalla et al., 2000). Surface rendering then creates a 3D model by linking the contours of selected objects from one slice of a CT with the adjacent slices (Wood & Razavi, 2002). Segmentation, as an intermediate step, is done to transform the volume into a mesh of polygons (Kettenbach et al, 2008; Rogalla et al., 2000). The polygons are then formed into a 3D model using specialized software often provided with the CT scan machine. Authors have suggested threshold ranges from -520 to -200 Hounsfield units (HU) in order to remove voxels denser than -500 HU. They recommend that thresholds of -250 and -400 HU be used to optimally view the nasal anatomy in healthy patients or those with sinonasal disease (Kettenbach et al, 2008). Although it is faster than volume rendering, surface rendering has poorer definition (Wood & Razavi., 2002), as there is data loss about the inner aspects of the polygons and artifacts. Furthermore, the axial images can be manipulated to show the surface structures modified by shading techniques, a process entitled surface shaded display. Surface shading can be done based on distance of the surface from the observer or the orientation of the surface in question. This differential shading pattern allows the surgeon to appreciate the position of one structure relative to another (Rogalla et al., 2000).

2.2 Volume rendering

Volume rendering consists of creating images by casting rays from an observation point from two possible locations, either outside the volume being visualized or from within it. The difference between surface and volume rendering is that it does not focus solely on the surface features, but also displays the structures as though they are partially transparent by modifying the percentage of light ray within a voxel (Kettenbach et al, 2008). In volume rendering, the volume data itself is analysed without the surface representation step of surface rendering.. (Rogalla et al., 2000) Also, all the pixels are kept in memory, as oppose to surface rendering which has a set threshold (Rogalla et al., 2000). This allows the acquisition of more information and increased detail with an expense, however, of increased need of data processing and time consumption. The quality of the processed three-dimensional model can be improved with increased quality of the original axial images, namely through thinner slices and greater pixel formatting (Kettenbach et al., 2008).

2.3 Flight path

The three-dimensional model provides the surgeons the ability to navigate through the created structure. VE software displays an optical electronic apparatus to dynamically navigate an organ lumen – the virtual endoscope. The navigation tool allows the operator to "fly through" or "sail through" the three-dimensional anatomy, traveling in any direction or any position in the nasal cavity and paranasal sinuses. The virtual endoscope is shown here (Figure 1) simultaneously traveling in the axial, sagittal and coronal planes. Orientation to the virtual endoscope is made easier to follow by these corresponding reference planes. Images are initially presented in a greyscale, though functions of the software allow subjective colour assignments to represent anticipated anatomic tissue hues.

The "flight path" is the route of flight as determined by the operator. This course can be set to emulate a course similar to conventional fiberoptic endoscopy or can be set to explore areas and obtain perspectives not available by routine fiberoptic exam. Pre-operatively, this has the potential to allow adequate planning and mapping of the operative approach in a safe manner, while localizing delicate and vital structures. Also, the surgeon can correlate the 3D images with the endoscopic view as to understand the limitations and imperfections of surface and volume rendering of the CT images, as there is a certain learning curve as with most novel technologies.

3. Virtual Endoscopy in otolaryngology and radiology

In the past two decades, multiplanar reformatting in coronal and sagittal planes of cross-sectional axial imaging has offered a capability to visualize with detail complex bony and

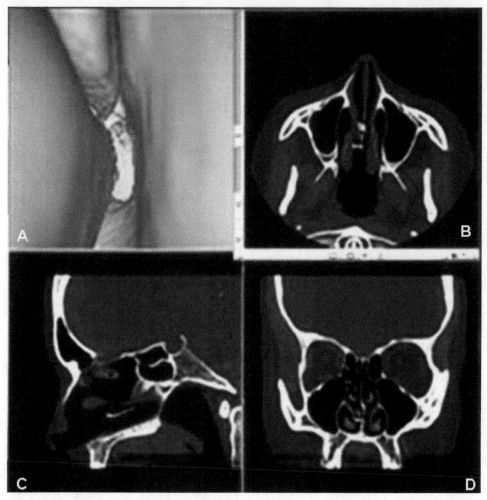

Fig. 1. Virtual Endoscopy
Virtual endoscope traveling in the right nasal cavity towards the nasopharynx (A),
simultaneously being pursued in the axial (B), sagittal (C), and coronal planes (D); original
figure.

soft tissue nasal structures. The otolaryngologist and radiologist, however, must routinely
undertake a practice of mentally unifying two-dimensional images to accurately envision
three-dimensional anatomy. VE offers a unique advantage of noninvasively carrying out
this mental practice for the user to pictorially display the true anatomical site. Used in
complement with high resolution thin-slice CT, VE significantly advances a users level of
visualization of the paranasal sinuses, providing great utility to the clinical practice of
both the otolaryngologist and radiologist. Many of the applications described here are
relevant to the practice of both specialties, emphasizing the multidisciplinary utility of
this technology.

3.1 Clinical applications

In direct patient care, VE offers numerous advantages that can complement office-based rhinoscopy. Foremost, VE has the ability to surmount the anatomical boundaries of the sinuses, visualizing areas and obtaining perspectives that are not achievable with conventional fiberoptic rhinoscopy. The virtual endoscope can in effect be directed in an innumerable array of flight paths, limited only by the creativity of the operator. A user can instantly traverse across bony and soft tissue landmarks such as the medial maxillary wall or the curvature of the turbinates to visualize an adjacent structure. Systematically, the user can follow pathways of mucociliary clearance from the originating sinus, via the narrow ostia, to ultimately the area of natural drainage. For instance, drainage of the maxillary sinus can be followed from within the cavity, through the narrow maxillary sinus ostia to the ethmoid infundibulum and ultimately the maxillary sinus meatus at the semilunar hiatus (see figure 2A). Distinctively, VE allows the user to reach anatomically arduous to reach landmarks not amenable via conventional endoscopy such as the frontal and sphenoid sinus cavities or ostia (see figure 2B).

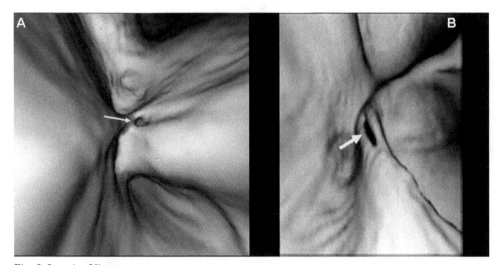

Fig. 2. Interior Views
En face three-dimensional view of a non-diseased right maxillary sinus ostium (A; thin arrow) and right sphenoethmoidal recess (B; thick arrow); original figure.

Unique perspectives, such as a retrograde evaluation of the nasal choanae via the nasopharynx or looking medially towards a maxillary sinus ostia from within the maxillary sinus, can be appreciated. VE also permits access to narrow and painful areas as small as 1-2 mm in diameter including the inferior meatus and stenotic pathology such as an obstructed osteomeatal complex or choanal atresia (Han et al., 2000). In each of these instances, VE affords superior visualization than fiberoptic rhinoscopy.

We have previously reported that VE has great utility in visualizing anatomical landmarks of the sinonasal tract (Anand et al., 2009). Similar to CT, in the presence of an air-tissue or air-fluid interface, VE has equivocal utility in recognizing sinonasal pathology (Figures 3 and 4). Visualization is strongly dependent on this interface to delineate the surface anatomy of a structure as viewed en face by the virtual endoscope. In instances of soft tissue obliteration, like CT, VE finds difficulty in distinguishing mucinous secretions from soft-tissue anatomy.

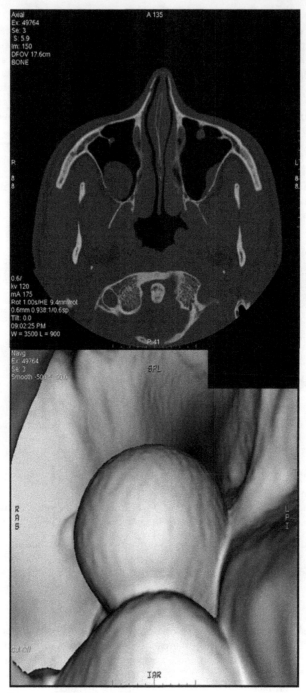

Fig. 3. Right maxillary sinus cyst; original figure.

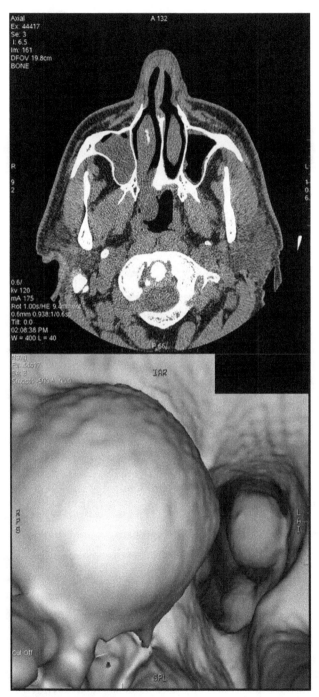

Fig. 4. Right choanal polyp; original figure.

VE remains an imaging technology and unlike conventional rhinoscopy there is no opportunity for the otolaryngologist to simultaneously culture, lavage or biopsy pathology (Greess et al., 2000). Table 1 outlines the advantages and disadvantages of VE. Overall, the advanced visualization inherent in VE makes it an excellent complement to flexible or rigid clinic endoscopy.

Advantages	Disadvantages
Visualize areas inaccessible by nasal endoscopy (ostia, paranasal cavities)	Cannot appreciate quality of the mucosa
Antro- and retro-grade views, 360° analysis	Learning curve
Traverse painful stenotic areas	No density measurements
No additional morbidity (no special CT, no IV contrast/aerolized medication/local trauma/discomfort or complications)	Cannot culture, lavage or biopsy pathology

Table 1. Advantages and Disadvantages of virtual endoscopy

Unlike fiber-optic rhinoscopy, there is no additional morbidity with VE beyond that associated with a routine non-contrast CT. No particular CT specifications are required and any patient that can undergo a CT sinus can have VE completed using the same image dataset. For the Radiologist, VE can offer the unique advantages of superior visualization described above without additional imaging of the patient or a considerable amount of additional image processing. For communication amongst colleagues, VE can serve as an additional tool to CT for subjects on whom the Otolaryngologist has not performed rhinoscopy. If care is being provided in a remote area where there is limited or no access to fiberoptic rhinoscopy or for discussing a patient case across two or more centers, VE can increase communication amongst treating physicians.

There are limitations to the use of VE in both Otolaryngology and Radiology. As with other advances in medical technology there is a learning curve with the introduction of a new modality (Chin et al., 2007). Once the user is familiar with VE software, however, navigation of the virtual endoscope is instantaneous. Specific limitations of VE arise in evaluating mucosal surfaces and secretions. For the Otolaryngologist, it is difficult to appreciate the quality and colour of the mucosal lining, prohibiting a differentiation of erythema or leukoplakia. Radiologically, mucous in the nasal cavity can be mistaken for a false soft tissue density; however, this is a similar pitfall in conventional two-dimensional CT (Anand et al., 2009).

3.2 Pre-operative and intra-operative planning

As a preoperative tool in surgical planning VE holds widespread potential. Prior to undertaking either open or endoscopic sinus surgery, the operative approach can be mapped out with the virtual endoscope. The influence of removing or partially altering surgical landmarks can be evaluated from the direction of anticipated view during surgery, as well as from several perspectives adjacent to the anatomic landmark to evaluate the functional impact of the intended surgical step. This could assist in making both endoscopic and open nasal surgery even safer and minimally invasive by assisting in preservation of vital functional structures. A step-by-step anatomic prosection can be formulated with VE for each individual case, allowing the surgeon to plan out an entire procedure in the preoperative setting. This is a great assist for both active surgeons and in simulation-based teaching for trainees; the latter is an advantage that will be explored in detail later in this chapter. Several institutions have already begun using VE as a preoperative tool, and its use has been described in combination with multiplanar imaging, to preoperatively decide safe surgical entrance points for paranasal sinus mucoceles (Nakasato et al, 2000). The advantage of being able to traverse stenotic segments inaccessible by conventional rhinoscopy increases the utility of VE in advanced skull base surgery. Visualization and thorough preoperative localization of critical structures such as the carotid and optic canal within the sphenoid, frontal sinus recess, anterior and posterior ethmoid arteries, fovea ethmoidalis and cribriform plate at the skull base increases operative safety in endoscopic and open skull base approaches. Intra-operatively, VE can be used as a navigational aid with image-guided applications to identify complex anatomy. The surgeon can herein use VE in real-time for intraoperative decision making to help direct the surgery, increase efficiency, localize detailed landmarks and importantly reduce the complication rate of advanced sinonasal surgery.

3.3 Anatomical correlation

To date several reports have evaluated the capability of VE to identify nasal cavity and paranasal sinus landmarks and a high level of agreement has been seen between volume rendering virtual three-dimensional imaging methods and conventional fiber-optic rhinoscopy (Di Rienzo et al., 2003; Han et al., 2000). Reports also demonstrate considerable agreement among VE and intra-operative findings in the vast majority of patients (Bisdas et al., 2004). We completed a preliminary evaluation of our VE interpretation experience and compared this to operative identification of landmarks in yet unpublished data. In a retrospective series, VE of 25 patients undergoing CT imaging of the paranasal sinuses for chronic nasal symptoms was compared to operative fiberoptic endoscopy findings. None of the patients were given aerosolized nasal decongestant prior to their CT imaging. Nineteen anatomic landmarks relevant in the mucociliary clearance of paranasal sinus secretions were objectively evaluated to be either not, partially or very well identified and scored with a 0, 1, or 2 out of 2 respectively (Table 2).

VE outperformed operative findings in visualizing hard to access areas such as the superior turbinate, superior meatus, choanae, nasopharynx, sphenoid and sphenoethomoidal recess. VE also identified more clearly structures of the osteomeatal complex, namely the maxillary sinus ostium, uncinate process, and infundibulum, where most often pathology is localized in chronic sinonasal disease. Operative endoscopy better identified the middle and inferior meati and turbinates, as similarly described by Han et al. (2003). Surgeons are able to dissect away diseased mucosa or suction secretions to gain entry into a meatus, a feat not feasible with VE. Operative endoscopy also better visualized the ethmoid air cells, frontoethmoidal recess and frontal sinus, areas routinely addressed in dissection during endoscopic sinus surgery.

	VE			FOE		
	0	1	2	0	1	2
Septum	0	0	25(100%)	0	1	25(96.2%)
Nasal cavity	1(4.0%)	2(8.0%)	22(88.0%)	3(12.0%)	3(12.0%)	19(76.0%)
Infer Turbinate*	0	2(8.3%)	22(91.7%)	0	1(4.2%)	23(95.8%)
Mid Turbinate*	6(25.0%)	2(8.3%)	16(66.7%)	1(4.8%)	2(9.5%)	18(85.7%)
Super Turbinate	13(52.0%)	0	12(48.0%)	25(100%)	0	0
Infer Meatus*	1(4.2%)	2(8.3%)	21(87.5%)	0	1(4.2%)	23(95.8%)
Mid Meatus*	4(16.7%)	3(12.5%)	17(70.8%)	1(4.8%)	1(4.8%)	19(90.4%)
Super Meatus	10(40.0%)	0	15(60.0%)	25(100%)	0	0
Choanae	2(8.0%)	1(4.0%)	22(88.0%)	2(8.0%)	2(8.0%)	21(84.0%)
Nasopharynx	1(4.0%)	0	24(96.0%)	3(12.0%)	3(12.0%)	19(76.0%)
Uncinate process	9(37.5%)	7(29.2%)	8(33.3%)	0	20(83.3%)	4(16.7%)
Infundibulum	9(37.5%)	10(41.7%)	5(20.8%)	0	20(83.3%)	4(16.7%)
Max sinus ostium	8(32.0%)	4(16.0%)	12(48.0%)	0	21(84.0%)	4(16.0%)
Maxillary Sinus	3(12.0%)	6(23.1%)	17(68.0%)	0	19(76.0%)	6(24.0%)
Frontal Sinus*	8(32.0%)	6(24.0%)	11(44.0%)	2(8.0%)	10(40.0%)	13(52.0%)
Sphenoid Sinus	7(28.0%)	6(24.0%)	12(48.0%)	1(4.0%)	16(64.0%)	8(32.0%)
Ethmoid cells*	6(24.0%)	9(36.0%)	10(40.0%)	0	13(52.0%)	12(48.0%)
FER*	8(32.0%)	6(24.0%)	11(44.0%)	2(8.0%)	10(40.0%)	13(52.0%)
SER	8(32.0%)	5(20.0%)	12(48.0%)	1(4.0%)	16(64.0%)	8(32.0%)

*FER: frontoethmoidal recess; SER: sphenoidoethmoidal recess; *Only 24 were observed as opposed to 25 as these structures were surgically removed in the past.*

Table 2. Total number and percentages of scores for each anatomical landmark observed by virtual endoscopy (VE) and by fiberoptic operative endoscopy (FOE).

4. Virtual Endoscopy in resident and trainee education

Apart from clinical uses for the Otolaryngologist, virtual endoscopy also has potential applications in resident training. In the past, resident education in most surgical disciplines has been heavily based on the apprenticeship model, where trainees learned various procedures through clinical encounters. This fact is particularly still prevalent in endoscopic sinus surgery, where technical expertise is gained mainly from practice on real patients. However, the intricate anatomy of the nasal cavity and paranasal sinuses, as well as the numerous surrounding vital structures, create the potential for significant morbidity of endoscopic sinus surgery in inexperienced hands.

In the past decade, there has been an emergence of novel teaching modalities, such as simulation training and virtual reality. Numerous authors in the past have reported improved resident performance after simulation and virtual reality training (Grantcharov et al., 2005; Seymour et al., 2002). More recently, VE has become an innovative educational method for training residents. In terms of Gastroenterology, improvement in technical accuracy and time needed to reach technical competency has been shown for colonoscopies after virtual endoscopy training (Ferlitsch et al., 2010). Improved trainee performance with surgical simulation training in endoscopic sinus surgery has been demonstrated, although there is a lack of data with virtual endoscopy. Edmond published his work with an endoscopic sinus surgical simulator as a training device for Otolaryngology residents and suggested a positive impact in performance in certain procedures such as anterior ethmoidectomies and also increased surgical confidence (Edmond, 2002). Similar response to simulation in endoscopic sinus surgery was demonstrated by Glaser with his work with medical students, who praised the ability for simulation training to help with 3D visualization and understanding of nasal anatomy (Glaser et al., 2006). There is a lack of data on the use of the virtual endoscope in Otolaryngology training, which we hope will be addressed as VE becomes more popular amongst endoscopic sinus surgeons.

In our institution, similar to many programs, endoscopic sinus surgery is typically performed by senior residents, starting in the upper years of residency. The use of VE would allow exposure for younger junior residents to explore and properly understand the anatomy early in their training, potentially improving their ultimate performance and safety on real patients. It is common knowledge within the discipline of Otolaryngology, furthermore, that the anatomy of the paranasal sinuses is a challenge to truly comprehend. A realistic virtual portrayal of the anatomy can strengthen the comprehension of natural pathways of mucociliary clearance as well as rhinoscopy and operative assessment. As mentioned previously, users are not restricted to spaces defined by mucosal surfaces in the nasal cavity as they are during real endoscopy. They are able to permeate through mucosal and bony structures and therefore learn the complex anatomical relationships. The literature has shown on numerous occasions that an operator can better appreciate spatial relationships in a three-dimensional model than in a series of two-dimensional images (Greess et al., 2000; Remy-Jardin et al., 1998).

VE provides many advantages over surgical experience for early training. It is non-invasive, thus there is no compromise in patient care. The same approaches and technical exercises can be performed multiple times or variant approaches can be designed and practiced. A resident can thus attempt to discover numerous pathways to a certain anatomical structure, such as a specific meatus or the maxillary, sphenoid or frontal sinus ostia. VE also provides crucial information to the location of surrounding anatomical structures. This will provide teaching faculty with pre-operative knowledge of what procedures are safe to be performed by resident trainees at varying levels of experience, thus objectifying procedure delegation.

5. Future directions

Three-dimensional rendering of helical CT images has modified the way Otolaryngologists and Radiologists approach the investigation of tubular anatomical structures. It is evident that VE of the paranasal sinuses provides surgeons with a new tool for both pre-operative and intra-operative planning, as well as a teaching modality for residents. The limitations of VE are in its ability to assess mucosal surfaces and secretions. In particular, current VE processing does not allow adequate differentiation of color and density, thus mucus or other secretions can be mistaken for a false soft tissue density. The differentiation between erythema and leukoplakia also can not be addressed by VE as opposed to direct visualization of color by conventional rhinoscopy. Moreover, VE is currently not able to identify tissue densities with imaging. Ultimately understanding from density measurements the nature of individual structures will allow improved identification of critical landmarks and pathologic anomalies possibly without conventional invasive rhinoscopy. Further research and innovation of VE technology will likely address this issue in the future. Finally, prospective trials in its use in training can objectively explore the role of this innovation in resident education.

6. Conclusion

As we enter a new decade, we are fortunate to constantly being challenged by novel diagnostic and therapeutic modalities to enhance patient care. VE has the potential to improve pre-operative diagnosis of pathologies, intra-operative patient management, post-operative follow-up, as well as trainee education. In this chapter, we have explored this relatively new technology, with an overview of its numerous utilities in clinical practice and residency training. VE has already been implemented routinely in certain centers for imaging of the colon and bronchial tree. It is our belief that VE will continue to progress as a technology and will certainly be an essential armamentarium of Otolaryngologists in the near future.

7. References

Anand SM, Frenkiel S, Le BQH, Glikstein R. Virtual Endoscopy: Our Next Major Investigative Modality? J Otolaryngol Head Neck Surg. 2009 Dec;38(6): 642-5.

Bisdas S, Verink M, Burmeister HP, et al. Three-dimensional visualization of the nasal cavity and paranasal sinuses: clinical results of a standardized approach using multislice helical computed tomography. J Comput Assist Tomogr 2004; 28(5):661-669.

Chin JL, Luke PP, Pautler SE. Initial experience with robotic-assisted laparoscopic radical prostatectomy in the Canadian health care system. Can Urol Assoc J 2007; 1(2):97-101.

Di Rienzo L, Coen Tirelli G, Turchio P, et al. Comparison of virtual and conventional endoscopy of nose and paranasal sinuses. Ann Otol Rhinol Laryngol 2003; 112:139-142.

Edmond, C. V. Impact of the Endoscopic Sinus Surgical Simulator on Operating Room Performance. The Laryngoscope 2002;112:1148–1158.

Ferlitsch A, Schoefl R, Puespoek A, Miehsler W, Schoeniger-Hekele M, Hofer H, Gangl A, Homoncik M. Effect of virtual endoscopy simulator training on performance of upper gastrointestinal endoscopy in patients: a randomized controlled trial. Endoscopy 2010;42(12):1049-56.

Gilani S, Norbash AM, Ringl H, et al. Virtual endoscopy of the paranasal sinuses using perspective volume rendered helical sinus computed tomography. Laryngoscope 1997;107:25–9

Glaser AY, Hall CB, Uribe S JI, Fried MP. Medical students' attitudes toward the use of an endoscopic sinus surgery simulator as a training tool. Am J Rhinol 2006;2:177-9.

Grantcharov, TP, Kristiansen, VB, Bendix, J, Bardram, L, Rosenberg, J, Funch-Jensen, P. Randomized clinical trial of virtual reality simulation for laparoscopic skills training. Br J Surg 2005;91(2): 146-150.

Greess H, Nomayr A, Tomandl B, et al. 2D and 3D visualization of head and neck tumours from spiral-CT data. European Journal of Radiology 2000; 33:170-177.

Han P, Pirsig W, Ilgen F, et al. Virtual endoscopy of the nasal cavity in comparison with fiberoptic endoscopy. Eur Arch Otolaryngol 2000; 257:578-583.

Kettenbach, J., Birkfellner, W., Rogalla, P. (2008). Virtual Endoscopy of the Paranasal Sinuses, In: *Image Processing in Radiology*, Neri, E., Caramella, D., Bartolozzi, C., (151-171), Springer Berlin Heidelberg, 978-3-540-49830-8, Berlin Heidelberg.

Nakasato T, Katoh K, Ehara S, et al. Virtual CT Endoscopy in Determining Safe Surgical Entrance Points in Paranasal mucoceles. J Comput Assist Tomogr 2000; 24(3):486-492.

Ossoff RH, Reinisch L. Computer-assisted surgical techniques: a vision for the future of otolaryngology, head and neck surgery. J Otolaryngol 1994; 23(5):354-359.

Pineau BC, Paskett ED, Chen GJ, et al. Virtual colonoscopy using oral contrast compared with colonoscopy for the detection of patients with colorectal polyps. Gastroenterology 2003; 125(2):304-10.

Remy-Jardin M, Artaud D, Fribourg M, et al. Volume rendering of the tracheobroncial tree: clinical evaluation of bronchographic images. Radiology 1998;208:761–70.

Rice, DH, Schaefer, SD. (2004). Introduction, In: *Endoscopic paranasal sinus surgery*, Rice, DH, Schaefer, SD. (XV), Lippincott Williams & Wilkins, 0-7817-4077-0, Philadelphia.

Rogalla P, Nischwitz A, Gottschalk S,et al. Virtual endoscopy of the nose and paranasal sinuses. Eur Radiol 1998; 8(6): 946-950.

Rogalla, P. (2000). Virtual Endoscopy of the Nose and Paranasal Sinuses, In: *Virtual endoscopy and related 3D techniques*, Rogalla, P., Terwisscha van Scheltinga, J., Hamm, B., (17-38), Springer, 3-540-65157-8, Berlin Heidelberg New York.

Rubin GD, Beaulieu CF, Argiro V, et al. Perspective volume rendering of CT and MR images: applications for endoscopic imaging. Radiology 1996; 199(2):321-330.

Seymour, NE, Gallagher, AG, Roman, SA, O'Brien, MK, Bansal, VK, Andersen, DK, Satava, RM. Virtual Reality Training Improves Operating Room Performance. Results of a Randomized, Double-Blinded Study. Ann Surg 2002; 236(4):458-464.

Vining DJ, Liu K, Choplin RH, et al. Virtual bronchoscopy: Relationships of virtual reality endobronchial simulations to actual bronchoscopic findings. Chest 1996; 109(2):549–553.

Wood BJ, Razavi P. Virtual Endoscopy: A Promising New Technology. Am Fam Physician 2002;66:107-12.

7

Endoscopically Guided Balloon Dilatation of Recurrent Choanal Stenosis

B.J. Folz and C.-G. Konnerth
Department of Otorhinolaryngology,
Karl Hansen Medical Center, Bad Lippspringe
Germany

1. Introduction

Balloon Sinuplasty is a treatment modality, which has gained much attention since its introduction in 2005. Nasal and paranasal sinus disease can be treated with this new method in a less traumatic way than by Functional Endoscopic Sinus Surgery (FESS) or conventional sinus surgery. One of the advantages of Balloon Sinuplasty is the preservation of anatomical structures within the nose. Also there is no loss of mucosal lining, i.e. ciliated nasal epithelium normally remains intact. The basic principle is to place a balloon catheter (Fig. 1) via a guidewire into a sinus ostium, to inflate the balloon and thus to dilate the sinus ostium. Improved ventilation and drainage of the sinus via the dilated ostium ensures healing of the diseased cavity. Dilatation catheters, which are now being used in Rhinology derive from vascular medicine, where these devices are used to open occluded or partially occluded arteries. In this field dilatation catheters have led to significant reduction of operative trauma compared to conventional vascular surgery.

FESS currently is the gold standard in the treatment of recurrent sinusitis, if conservative therapy fails to achieve a permanent relief. It provides good results with acceptable discomfort for the patient. In most cases postoperative packing is necessary after FESS to stop nasal bleeding. Packing is uncomfortable for the patient and thus there are ongoing endeavours to develop even less traumatic methods to treat nasal diseases than FESS. Balloon dilatation is supposed to have the following benefits compared to FESS: less bleeding, more tissue preservation, less trauma to surrounding tissue, less complications, faster patient recovery and less postoperative care.

Initially all Balloon Sinuplasty procedures were performed under fluoroscopy. This fact was bound to technical prerequisites, which not every ENT-Department was able to provide. In addition exposure of patients and surgeons to X-rays during the procedure was a matter of continuous debate, especially in paediatric patients. This problem was overcome, when the LUMA™ technology was developed and catheters could be placed into the respective sinuses under endoscopic and diaphanoscopic control. We decided to use this technique for the restoration of the nasal airway passage in a child with recurrent choanal atresia. At the explicit wish of the parents no conventional surgery or FESS procedure was carried out. The parents reported, that the first operation had severely traumatized the child, therefore the parents asked for the least traumatic method, which was likely to give the child relief of his complaints.

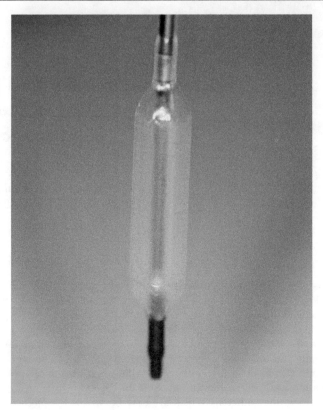

Fig. 1. Inflated Sinus Balloon. The size of the respective Balloon catheter was 7 mm x 16 mm in diameter.

2. Case report

A 4 year-old boy had been operated on a right-sided choanal atresia via a transnasal approach at the age of two years. A silicone stent had been inserted for a period of three months postoperatively. Initially nasal breathing had been restored successfully, however within two years symptoms recurred. The child again suffered from persistent anterior rhinorrhoea, recurrent airway infections and snoring. Examination by flexible endoscopy and CT scanning revealed recurrent stenosis, which was partially bony and partially membranous (Fig.2). Repeated surgery was recommended, but the parents specifically asked for a less invasive treatment. The parents reported, that the child had suffered a lot after the initial operation and during the postoperative period, when the stent had to be kept in place for many months. The balloon method was explained to the parents and the interventional procedure was offered. Simultaneously it was pointed out that the balloon method was a treatment attempt and no standard therapy, as there were only few accounts in literature reporting that this method had already been used to open a choanal atresia. After weighing the potential advantages of the balloon dilatation method against their past experiences with endoscopic sinus surgery the parents explicitly asked for the balloon method.

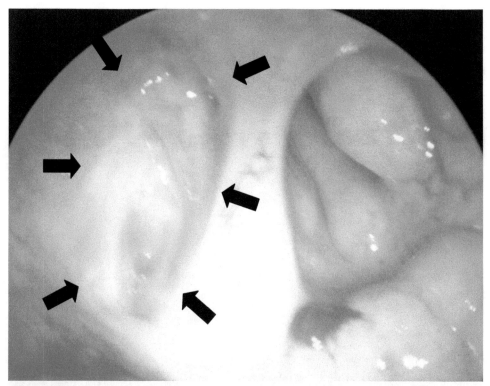

Fig. 2. Intraoperative view into the nasopharynx with a rigid 90° angled endoscope (transoral view). The left-sided choana shows a normal appearance. The posterior ends of the inferior and middle turbinate can be identified. The right-sided choana is occluded by a membranous plate (→) and a bony stenosis .

3. Method

A balloon catheter was placed in the nasal cavity under control with a 0°-degree rigid endoscope (Karl Storz Company, Tuttlingen) while the child was under general anaesthesia (Fig. 3). After decongestion of the nasal mucosa with cottonoids soaked in decongestant nose drops, a pinpoint-sized lumen within the atretic plate could be identified. Under simultaneous transoral endoscopy of the nasopharynx with a rigid 90°-angled endoscope (Karl Storz Company, Tuttlingen) (Fig 4.) a light source catheter was placed in the small choanal opening (Acclarent Company, Relieva LumaTM Sinus Illumination System, 7 mm diameter) (Fig. 5). The light source catheter was subsequently advanced into the nasopharynx. The sinuplasty balloon catheter was then gently rotated into the residual lumen, with the light source catheter as guide wire. The balloon was inflated with normal saline solution until a pressure of 8 atm. was reached (Fig. 6). The balloon remained inflated for 5 minutes and was then deflated. The residual lumen was thus enlarged to a diameter of 7 mm without any signs of hemorrhage or swelling (Fig.7). No packing was necessary and no postoperative bleeding occurred. After some

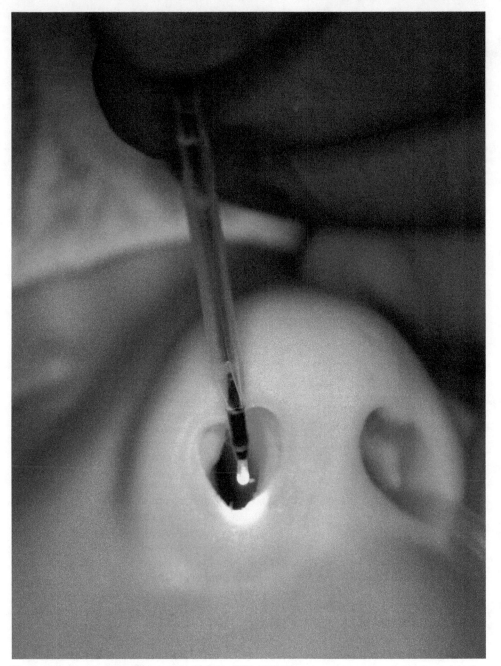

Fig. 3. The flexible light-fibre of the Relieva LUMA™ illumination system (straight tip) is the guide wire for the balloon catheter. The guide wire and the balloon catheter are inserted into the right nose and advanced to the stenosis.

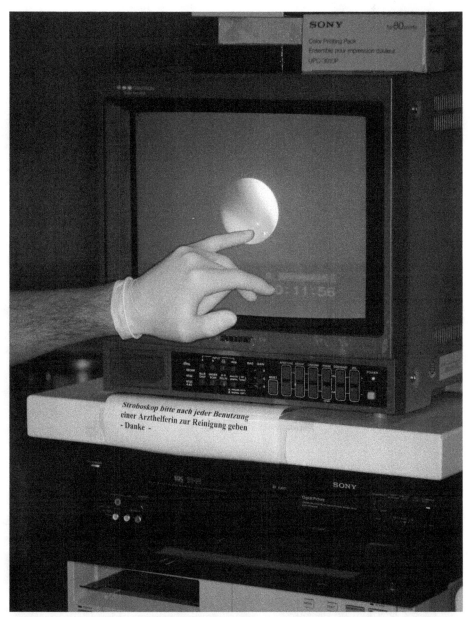

Fig. 4. Simultaneously the nasopharynx is controlled transorally with a 90° endoscope coupled with a digital camera. The position of the catheter can be controlled on a monitor. The position of the catheter is correct, if the choana lightens up on diaphanoscopy. By transnasal endoscopy the residual lumen of the choana was identified and the catheter was placed into the lumen.

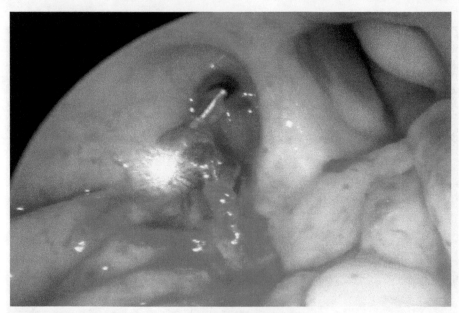

Fig. 5. The LUMA™ catheter is advanced into the nasopharynx (endoscopic image with a 90°-angled endoscope).

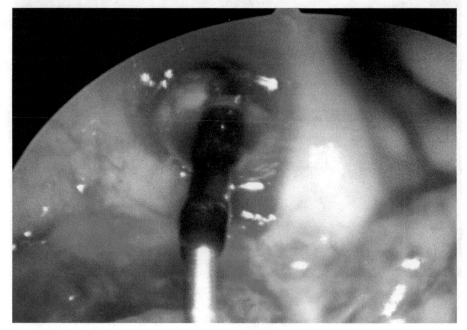

Fig. 6. Once the balloon catheter is in the correct position it is inflated with normal saline solution to a pressure of 8 atmospheres. The catheter stays in situ for 5 minutes.

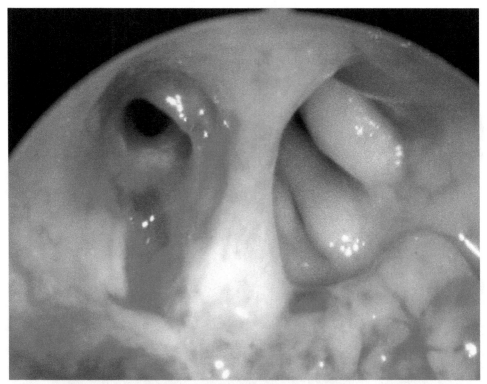

Fig. 7. After the removal of the catheter a circular dilatation of the atretic membrane is evident. The diameter of the choana is approximately 7 mm. Stenting of the choana was not necessary.

uneventful hours in the recovery area the patient was discharged home. Normal saline solution for nasal rinsing and nasal antiseptic cream were prescribed two times daily for the treatment of possible crusting.

4. Result

Intraoperatively the procedure was performed as planned, no adverse events occured. The pressure in the balloon was successively increased at paces of 2 atms at each step until a target pressure of 8 atmospheres was reached. As shown in the respective image (Fig. 7), there was hardly any bleeding. The child had a normal recovery and did not complain about any pain or discomfort. There was no need for any specific postoperative therapy other than lubricating ointments, decongestive nose drops and rinsing the nose with normal saline. No antibiotics were administred. The child was under observation as an inpatient for 24 hours postoperatively. The boy was discharged on the following day. Postoperative packing or stenting was not necessary. On controls 6, 12, 18 and 24 months postoperatively the enlarged choanal lumen remained stable. Nasal breathing was restored successfully as could be shown by the mirror test (Fig. 8). There were no signs of rhinorrhoea, snoring or recurrent stenosis. The patient and his parents were extremely happy with the result and the fact that the operation and postoperative phase was considerably less traumatizing than the initial operation. No specific therapy other than the above mentioned topical treatments were prescribed. The child is currently observed at 6 month intervals in our outpatient department.

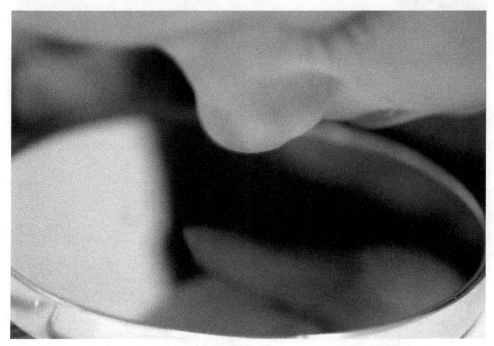

Fig. 8. The patient at 6 months postop. The mirror test proves patency of the nasal airway. During an observation period of >24 months the child has been free of complaints.

5. Discussion

Balloon catheter dilatation started in February 1974, when Andreas Grüntzig of Zürich/Switzerland used this method for the first time to dilate a vascular stenosis. Grüntzig had designed, constructed and produced the Balloon catheters all by himself. In September 1974 he used a catheter of an advanced design to dilate an occluded coronary artery for the first time in medical history. Today the method which has been developed by Grüntzig is the standard treatment for occluded vessels in interventional cardiology and vascular medicine. Since Grüntzig's invention, balloon catheters have become a well established technique in modern medicine (Schlupf, 2004). This applies not only to Cardiology and Angiology, but also to many other medical specialities including Otorhinolaryngology. Most frequently balloon dilatations are performed in Rhinology in so-called Balloon Sinuplasty procedures. The principle idea of this technique is to dilate intranasal or sinusoidal bottle-necks without any classical surgical intervention, like incisions, tissue removal, suturing or coagulation. Balloon Sinuplasty also allows to perform interventions in areas of the nose and sinuses, which are difficult to access by conventional endonasal techniques, like Functional Endoscopic Sinus Surgery (FESS). Based on these thoughts the idea of dilating a recurrent, predominantely membranous stenosis seemed to be promising. According to Meyer and Riemann stenoses and atresias of the choanae may be congenital, iatrogenic, post inflammatory or a result of radiation therapies for e.g. nasopharyngeal carcinoma (Meyer & Riemann, 2010). The incidence of a congenital choanal atresia is estimated to occur in 1:8000 children, girls are twice as often affected than boys (Jacob, 2001). In up to 2/3 of the cases choanal atresias may be combined with further congenital defects. The CHARGE syndrome (Coloboma of the eye, Heart disease, Atresia of choanae, Retarded growth and development and/or CNS anomalies, Genital hypoplasia, and Ear anomalies and/or deafness) may be an example for this observation (Pagon et al, 1981). Bilateral choanal atresia becomes evident in newborns immediately after birth. The healthy newborn usually breathes through the nose at rest. Nasal breathing is crucial for newborns especially while being fed. Newborns with bilateral choanal atresia show the clinical sign of „paradox cyanosis," while being fed, i.e. first they become cyanotic, then they stop swallowing and start to cry. At this point cyanosis resolves because the newborns can breathe orally again. In newborns with bilateral choanal atresia immediate action is therefore required. Unilateral choanal atresia on the other hand often is not recognized immediately. This defect usually becomes evident at a later point of time in life, when parents recognize permanent or recurrent unilateral rhinorrhoea. Therapy of unilateral choanal atresia mostly is surgical, either via the transnasal route or via the palatal route. Sometimes even a combined transnasal – transoral approach can be helpful. Although surgery nowadays is minimally invasive, large wounds and tissue defects may occur, necessitating intensive postoperative care and in some cases stenting. Despite all measures like excellent postoperative care, stenting or Mitomycin-C applications, the rate of secondary stenoses is high. Aside from the fact of a surgical intervention, insertion of a stent, which is supposed to keep the widend stenosis open, is often uncomfortable for the patient. Patients complain of foreign body sensation, rhinorrhaea and pain. Inflammation due to mucosal abrasions or foreign body reactions may occur. Many surgeons believe that only the reduction of trauma to surrounding tissue is likely to reduce the rate of recurrent stenoses. In 2006 Brown and Bolger described a new method for the dilation of sinus ostia for the treatment of recurrent nasal and paranasal sinusitis. One of the advantages of this new method was minimal trauma to surrounding tissues (Brown & Bolger, 2006, Siow et al., 2009). When performing Balloon Sinuplasty the surgeon can generally choose between two different techniques. The correct position of the guide wire can be controlled by fluoroscopy in a similar fashion like in interventional cardiology or interventional radiology. However, in the head and neck region this leads to a considerable radiation exposure, first of all for the patient and secondly for the surgeon. Due to the fact that the hands of the surgeon manipulate in close proximity to the nose, they are regularly exposed to radiation during fluoroscopy, which is needed to control the position of the guide wire and the balloon. Patient´s eyes and the lenses are exposed to the radiation beam and it is not uncommon that patients, who are frequently exposed to radiation may develop cataract. The estimated radiation dose during Balloon Sinuplasty accounts to approximately 730 mrem (Bolger et al., 2007). In comparison the radiation dose of a CT scan of the head accounts to only 200 mrem, CT scan of the chest sums up to approximately 800 mrem. Angioplasty on the other hand exposes the patient to radiation between 750 and 5,700 mrem (Siow et al. 2008).

Due to the problem of unwanted radiation exposure and due to the fact that not every hospital offers the technical requirements, which are needed for Balloon Sinuplasty under fluoroscopy a novel technique was developed. The presented patient was also treated with the new technique, which is known under the acronym LUMA technology. The principle of LUMA technology is that the position of the guide wire and the balloon is not controlled by fluoroscopy, but by endoscopy and diaphanoscopy. In this variation of Balloon Sinuplasty the guide wire contains a flexible light fiber, which can be coupled to a cold light source, which is usually present in every ENT operating room. The tip of the guide wire is extremely soft and emits light in an intensity, that it illuminates the frontal and maxillary sinus perfectly. Thus the position of the guide wire can be controlled from the outside by diaphanoscopy and from the inside by routine endoscopy with rigid endoscopes. Correct placement of the balloons in the frontal recess or in the maxillary ostium is thus possible without any radiation. The advantages of the LUMA technology rendered the treatment of our presented patient, who was four years old at the time of treatment. We feel that this technique allows minimally invasive dilatations in paediatric patients or even in pregnant women. The risk of perforating the orbit or the skull base is low, due to the flexibility of the guide wire/light fiber. Complications or undesired side effects are unlikely to occur. This method seemed ideal for the presented case and a thorough analysis of the medical literature showed that balloon dilatation had already been tried in a similar case. Goettman and coworkers were probably the first, who had treated recurrent choanal atresia by balloon dilatation. They used repeated balloon dilatations in a 16-year-old girl, which had presented herself with a restenosis 3 weeks after conventional and laser surgical therapy of a choanal atresia. In their publication from the year 2000 the authors reported about good results during a follow-up period of 2 years (Goettman et al., 2000). We could show similar results with only one dilatation. In addition, our method had the advantage that all manipulations were carried out under endoscopic control with the LUMA™ technique, i.e. no X-ray control was needed to position or control the balloon. Thus exposure of the patient or the surgeons to radiation was not necessary. The presented technique may be especially suited for membranous recurrent stenosis. A comparison between Balloon Sinuplasty for dilatation of a choanal stenosis with conventional transnasal, transoral or combined operations show that the Balloon technique requires more resources in disposable material (Fig. 9), the time for the actual intervention however is considerably shorter than operation time in conventional surgery. It seems to be recommendable to increase the pressure in the balloon stepwise. An increase of pressure of 2 atmospheres during each step is sufficient to build up adequate pressure in the balloon, as Brehmer recommended (Brehmer D., 2008). There are no uniform recommendations about the ideal pressure or the duration of the actual dilatation process in literature. We chose to build up a pressure of 8 atmospheres within 5 minutes to dilate the atresia. Meyer und Riemann reported on dilatation of a choanal atresia in an oncologic patient with 12 atmospheres within 12 seconds (Meyer and Riemann, 2010) , Brown und Bolger used pressures between 10-16 atmospheres (mean maximum pressure 13 atm) for about 5 seconds, with an inflation/deflation interval of 10 seconds each (Brown & Bolger, 2006). Other authors like Brehmer estimate that the required pressure may be considerably lower, i.e. 8 atmospheres (Brehmer D., 2008).

Since it´s initial description dilatation procedures in the nose have become more and more accepted in Otorhinolaryngology. The procedure are regarded to be safe, with hardly any side-effects. Bolger and coworkers could prove the safety and efficacy of Balloon Sinuplasty in a prospective multicentric trial with 115 patients. Patients were followed up for a period

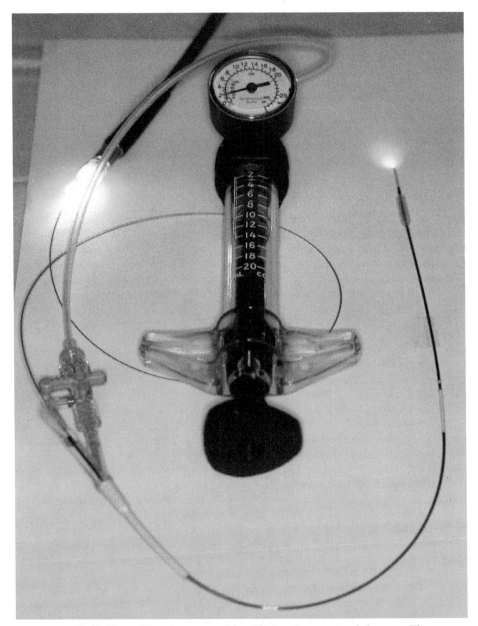

Fig. 9. System for Balloon dilatation as used for dilating the atresia of choanae. The guidewire is connected to a bright external light source with a detachable connector. Intraoperative the distal tip with the light fiber provides a direct visual confirmation via diaphanoscopic illumination. With the attached syringe-like Relieva® Sinus Balloon Inflation Device the balloon was inflated with normal saline solution until a pressure of 8 atm. was reached.

of 24 weeks and postinterventional endoscopies were performed. The trial showed a successful and persistent dilatation of sinus ostia in 80,5% of the patients. In 1,6% of the cases a persitent ostium could not be seen on endoscopy, in 17,9% of the cases the interior nose could not be assessed adequately by endoscopy (Bolger et al, 2007). Nine patients had developed bacterial sinusitis, which could be treated successfully by oral antibiotic therapy. Major complications had not occurred. In our case of a child with recurrent choanal atresia the results are similarily positive. Neither were there any undesired events during the intervention nor in the postinterventional period. No secondary hemorrhage or infection was observed. The good result encourages us to report this procedure as a possible alternative to conventional surgery in selected cases.

6. Conclusion

There is preliminary evidence that dilatation of membranous choanal atresia is feasible with balloon catheters. It is less invasive than FESS and requires only little postoperative care. Postoperatively no stents have to be inserted. This is of importance for patient´s quality of life aspects. The patients does not have to endure any foreign bodies in his nasal airway. Additionally a second surgical procedure for removal of the stent is not necessary. Thus it seems to be of great value especially in the treatment of paediatric patients.

7. References

Brown CL, Bolger WE. Safety and feasibility of balloon catheter dilation of paranasal sinus ostia: a preliminary investigation. *Ann Otol Rhinol Laryngol* 2006; 115:293-299

Bolger WE, Brown CL, Church CA, Goldberg AN, Karanfilov B, Kuhn FA, Levine HL, Sillers MJ, Vaughan WC, Weiss RL. Safety and outcomes of balloon catheter sinustomy: a multicenter 24-week analysis in 115 patients. *Otolaryngol Head Neck Surg* 2007; 137:10-20

Brehmer D. Cathter-based balloon dilatation of the frontal, maxillary und sphenoid ostia: a new procedure in sinus surgery. *HNO* 2008; 56:65-70

Goettman D, Strohm M, Strecker EP. Treatment of a recurrent choanal atresia by balloon dilatation. *Cardiovasc Intervent Radiol* 2000; 23:480-481

Meyer HJ, Riemann R. Behandlung erworbener Choanalstenosen durch Ballon-Dilatation. *Laryngorhinootologie* 2010; 89:289-10

Siow JK, Al Kadah B, Werner JA. Balloon sinuplasty: a current hot topic in rhinology. *Eur Arch Otorhinolaryngol.* 2008; 265:509-11

Schlupf M. 30 Jahre Ballonkatheter: Andreas Grüntzig, ein Pionier in Zürich. *Schweizerische Ärztezeitung,* 2004; 85, 7: 346-351

Jacob R. 2001. Erkrankungen der Nase und des Pharynx: Pharynx. In: *Praxis der HNO-Hielkunde, Kopf- u. Halschirurgie,* J.Strutz & W.Mann. p 396, Thieme-Verlag Stuttgart, New York; ISBN: 3-13-116971-0

Pagon RA, Graham JM Jr, Zonana J, Yong SL: *Coloboma,* congenital heart disease, and choanal atresia with multiple anomalies: CHARGE association. *JPediatr.*1981; 2:223-7.

8

Evolution of the Adenoidectomy in the Endoscopic Era

Fabio Pagella, Alessandro Pusateri,
Georgios Giourgos and Elina Matti
Foundation IRCCS Policlinico San Matteo
and University of Pavia
Italy

1. Introduction

During the last 20 years, we have observed an increasing recognition of the high prevalence of sleep-disordered breathing (SDB) in children. Adenotonsillar enlargement, leading to a partial or a complete obstruction of the nasopharynx (or epipharynx, or rhinopharynx) and/or of the oropharynx, accounts for the vast majority of cases. Consequently, the number of adenoidectomies performed in children for SDB has increased significantly. An adenoidectomy can be performed as an isolated procedure or as part of an adenotonsillectomy operation. As a matter of fact, adenoidectomy with or without tonsillectomy is one of the most common surgical procedures performed by Otolaryngologists in the paediatric population. Historically, tonsil and adenoid surgery increasingly began to be carried out together in the early 20th century, as the popular "focus on infection" theory attributed various systemic disorders to diseased tonsils and adenoids; thus, tonsillectomy plus adenoidectomy were recommended as a standard treatment for several different conditions as anorexia, mental retardation and enuresis, or simply as a general measure to promote good health (Hays, 1924; Kaiser, 1932). In certain communities the surgical procedure was performed widely in the entire population of scholars in public school buildings (Baker, 1953). Over the years, things have changed, and precise indications were proposed for tonsillectomy and adenoidectomy. Adenoid hypertrophy can lead to obstructive sleep apnea, otitis media with effusion, recurrent otitis media and nasal obstruction, and nowadays these remain the most common indications for adenoidectomy.

Techniques and instruments have considerably evolved from the first techniques described by Cornelius Celsus in the first century A.D. (Thornval, 1969) and Paul of Aegina in 625 A.D. (Paul of Aegina, 1847) to the later contributions of surgeons such as Wilhelm Meyer of Copenhagen and Samuel J. Crowe in the last centuries (Curtin, 1987; Meyer, 1870; Wiatrak & Wooley, 2005; Younis & Lazar, 2002). Pioneers of tonsillectomy and adenoidectomy have developed novel techniques and instruments in order to increase the speed of the procedure, especially in the pre-anesthesia era, and to decrease the intra-operative complications and postoperative morbidity.

The classic surgical technique performed with an adenoid curette or an adenotome has recently evolved by the introduction of the endoscopic sinus surgery (ESS) instrumentation, with an improved patients' outcome and a better satisfaction of the surgeon (Havas & Lowinger, 2002; Rodriguez et al., 2002; Stanislaw et al., 2000). The standard adenoidectomy technique is to remove the nasopharyngeal lymphatic tissue with an adenoid curette or an adenotome (Figure 1 – 3), under general anaesthesia via oro-tracheal intubation, with the patient placed in the Rose position, and a mouth gag inserted (Kornblut, 1987; Paradise 1996).

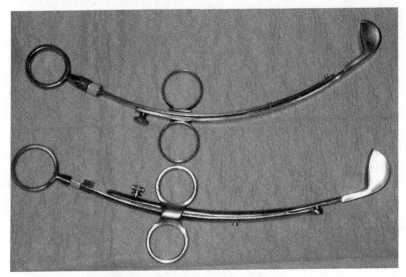

Fig. 1. Two, different sized, standard Shambaugh adenotomes.

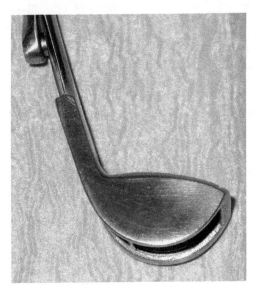

Fig. 2. Distal end of the Shambaugh adenotome.

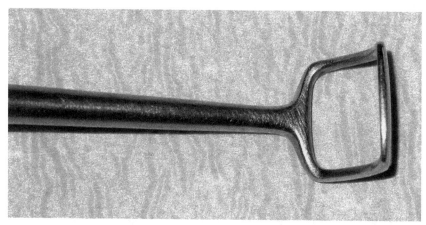

Fig. 3. Distal end of an adenoid curette.

The surgeon is placed at the head of the patient (Figure 4). The curette is transorally applied to the nasopharynx thus, by-passing the soft palate and the main bulk of the adenoids is removed, with a single or repeated passes. The majority of surgeons perform the procedure blindly, without a direct visualization of the nasopharynx (Figure 5). In some cases a partial visualization of the adenoid pad can be achieved by retracting the soft palate with rubber catheters or by using a laryngeal or a dental mirror. Bleeding is controlled by compression, through the placement of a gauze pack in the nasopharynx for several minutes.

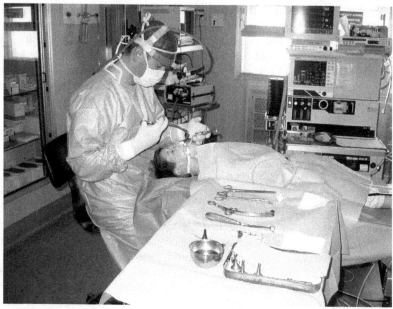

Fig. 4. Surgical position during a traditional adenoidectomy.

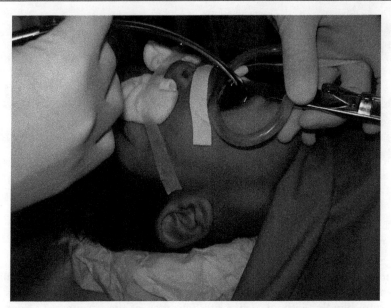

Fig. 5. External view of a traditional adenoidectomy performed with a Shambaugh adenotome; as underlined, the procedure is conducted without the visualization of the nasopharynx.

The visualization of the operative field is particularly useful in avoiding damages to important structures located nearby the adenoid tissue, such as the Eustachian tube and/or the pharyngeal muscles. Postoperative complications such as velopharyngeal insufficiency, tubaric stenosis and nasopharyngeal stenosis are rare but difficult to resolve when occurred. Several investigations prove that in up to one-third of children with clinically significant adenoid hypertrophy, conventional curettage adenoidectomy does not achieve an adequate removal of obstructive adenoid tissue, especially when there is an intranasal extension of the tissue, or a bulky mass of adenoids superiorly in the nasopharynx and in the peritubaric region (Buchinsky et al., 2000; Elluru et al, 2002; Havas & Lowinger, 2002; Stanislaw et al., 2000).

To possibly reduce the morbidity linked to the adenoid tissue persistence and to prevent recurrences, total excision of the adenoids is the most important goal of this operation. Initially, the surgical clearance was confirmed by a digital palpation of the rhinopharynx and this procedure is still performed by some Otolaryngologists (Buchinsky et al., 2000). Subsequently, the use of an angled mirror or an endoscope during the adenoidectomy provided adequate visualization of the field, and these techniques are currently preferred by most surgeons (Brodsky, 1996; Cannon et al., 1999; Discolo et al., 2001). A recent study published by Ark et al. showed that in order to achieve a complete adenoid tissue removal, a direct/indirect visual assistance is necessary. The authors considered a group of patients that underwent a conventional adenoidectomy (surgical efficacy confirmed by digital palpation at the end of the procedure); subsequently, the surgical field was inspected through an indirect laryngeal mirror visualization. Their finding was that only one-fifth of the patients had no residual adenoid tissue. Instead, in the 81% of the patients a residue of lymphatic tissue was still present on the pharyngeal roof nearby the choanal opening; also, 11.4% of the patients had a residue along the torus tubarius on either side of the nasopharynx and in 6.3% the residual tissue was located at both cited sites (Ark et al., 2010).

The recurrence of adenoid hypertrophy after the surgical procedure is under debate in the literature, but several reports do not offer comparable results. According to Lundgren, the recurrence rate is 4 – 8%, in Hill's series instead it is 23.7 – 50% and Crowe states a recurrence rate of over 75% (Tolczynski, 1955). More recent studies cite a significantly lower recurrency rate till a 0.5% (Joshua et al., 2006; Monroy et al., 2008), and this success could be attributed to the evolution of the techniques. Historically, Tolczynski (Tolczynski, 1955) considered various situations to be responsible for the recurrence of adenoid hypertrophy, summarized in:

- Anatomical difficulties.
- Adenoidectomy is often performed in a hurry, and sometimes the inadequate anaesthesia could be responsible for an insufficient relaxation of the palato-pharyngeal muscles, whose contracture interferes with the manipulations of the adenoid pad.
- In many cases it is a "Surgical operation in the dark", without a visualization of the operatory field.

A recent paper in a cohort of over 300 patients reports that, when an endoscopic examination was performed at the end of the adenoidectomy, in the 14.5% of the cases some residual adenoid tissue that required additional removal was found; during the follow-up of these patients only 0.85% needed a revision adenoidectomy in the next 2 years. In contrast, when that endoscopic examination was not performed, there was a 6.7% persistence of the initial symptoms and a 5.6% of the patients required a revision adenoidectomy. By comparing such results, it becomes evident that the endoscopic examination at the end of the procedure, significantly reduces the incidence of recurrence and thus the need for a revision surgery (Ezzat, 2010).

In the last years, several surgical techniques have been proposed to ensure a finer removal of the adenoid mass, as well as to achieve a better control of intraoperative bleeding.

Suction diathermy was initially introduced for haemorrhage control following conventional curettage of the adenoid pad (Kwok & Hawke, 1987). Subsequently, the whole procedure was performed with this technique, always along a transoral approach and an indirect visualization by a laryngeal or dental mirror (Owens et al., 2005; Sherman, 1982; Skilbeck et al., 2007). As an evolution, in the following years suction diathermy was performed via a transnasal approach and under a transnasal endoscopic control, in the older paediatric population (Shin, 2003).

The introduction of powered instrumentation for sinus surgery prompted the use of a shaver system with an overbent cannula for a, power-assisted, total or partial adenoidectomy; however, the approach still was a transoral one, along with an indirect visualization through a laryngeal mirror (Heras et al., 1998; Koltai et al., 1997, 2002; Stanislaw et al. 2000).

In a recent article Walner et al presented a survey between 300 members of the American Society of Pediatric Otolaryngology, which examined the equipment used in adenotonsillectomy along the last 15 years in order to assess the surgical trends in instrument usage for paediatric adenotonsillectomy. About the adenoidectomy, there has been less consistency in the choice of an instrument over the years than for tonsillectomy.

The most promising instrument 15 years ago was a monopolar electrocautery curette, the use of which instead declined over the years against the simple curette adenoidectomy. One other instrument with a decreasing usage over the years is the adenotome. On the other hand, three adenoidectomy instruments faced an increasing success over the last 15 years. Firstly, a monopolar electrocautery's usage passed from a 7.1%, 15 years ago to a current 25.9%. This upgrade is, most likely, due to the increased speed of the procedure, the better control of the blood loss and the lower cost of the instrument. Secondly, although the use of a simple debrider showed a modest rise in popularity, instead its model enriched with a monopolar electrocautery went from a 0% to a current 19.8% in the surgeon's preferences during the last 15 years. According to the present study, when combining the data from debrider alone and debrider with monopolar electrocautery, the instrument is currently used more commonly than curette with monopolar electrocautery touch-up and is second only to monopolar electrocautery in total usage for adenoidectomy. A major advantage of the microdebrider is the possibility to use the angled blades to within the nasopharynx, the anatomy of which is problematic for some instruments, such as the curette or the adenotome. In addition, debrider's usage showed a low incidence of complications. One study evidenced no long-term complications, including significant blood loss, in over 1000 procedures carried out with the power-assisted instrument (Rodriguez et al., 2002). Finally, coblation adenoidectomy gained significant popularity over the years. When combining the current data from pure coblation adenoidectomy and adenoidectomy with monopolar electrocautery coblation procedures, the instrument is used by the 8.6% of the surgeons in over 50% of their cases (Walner et al, 2007). We must recognize that the cited survey was conducted in a restricted national cohort (U.S.A.), and this may not reflect the international trend on the surgical equipment for the adenoidectomy.

In the '90s, the advent of ESS popularized the use of intranasal scopes and the endoscopic adenoidectomy became the natural evolution of the conventional adenoidectomy, permitting a direct visualization throughout the procedure (Becker et al., 1992; Cannon et al., 1999). By using this technique the adenoid remnants along the superior portion of the nasopharynx, the choanae and the peritubal region, can be clearly visualized and, thus, removed; moreover, the likelihood of damage of the Eustachian tube and/or of the pharyngeal muscles is reduced, and the haemorrhage may be effectively controlled by a direct identification of the bleeding point. In addition to the endoscopic-assisted adenoid curettage, residual adenoid tissue can be removed piece by piece using, transnasally, either a straight or a 45° Blakesley forceps, always under an endoscopic view (Huang et al., 1998). In the following years, a power-assisted adenoidectomy conducted completely through a transnasal approach and under an endoscopic guidance was suggested by Parson in 1996 (Parson, 1996) and firstly reported by Yanagisawa in 1997 (Yanagisawa, 1997).

As reported in the literature, the usual approaches to the adenoid tissue with power-assisted instruments are: pure transnasal (Al-Mazrou et al., 2009; Havas & Lowinger, 2002; Pagella et al., 2009), transorally inserted curved debrider under a transoral control (with laryngeal mirrors or with 45° or 70° scopes) (Koltai et al., 2002; Rodriguez et al., 2002; Stanislaw et al., 2000) or transorally inserted curved microdebrider combined with a transnasal endoscopic control (Pagella et al., 2010).

In this chapter we expose the evolution of the adenoidectomy during the last decades, from the traditional procedures to the modern endoscopic-assisted methods, with a description of each surgical technique.

2. Preoperative evaluation

All children underwent a preoperative flexible fiberoptic nasal endoscopy; we used a paediatric flexible endoscope, diameter 3.6 mm. Before the exam, nasal secretions were removed either by nasal-blowing or by a gentle aspiration through a small flexible rubber tube. No topical intranasal decongestant was used to avoid a misdiagnosis of an inferior turbinate hypertrophy or generalized nasal mucosa congestion; moreover, the National guidelines proposed by the Italian Drugs Agency, permit the use of intranasal vasoconstrictor drugs in children over 12 years of age. No local or general anesthesia was used. We preferred the presence of the parents in the examination room, for a better compliance of the patient. Most children fully collaborated during the nasal endoscopy; if necessary, the head of the patient was gently immobilized by the assistant/nurse during the performance. The entire procedure could be followed on the video screen and taped, which facilitated review and discussion of the disease along with the parents.

The procedure enables the visualization of the entire nasal fossae and, in particular, key-areas as the inferior and middle turbinates, the septum, the Osteo-Meatal Complex (OMC), the fontanella area, the Spheno-Ethmoidal Recess (SER) and the nasopharynx. The child is laid supine on an examination bed with his head bent by about 30° - 45°. The endoscopic evaluation can be divided into three main phases. At first, the endoscope is introduced along the nasal floor (between the inferior turbinate and the septum) so as to evaluate the inferior turbinate volume, the inferior meatus and the septum's morphology; then, the scope proceeds towards the nasopharynx to evaluate the presence of lymphatic tissue (adenoids), oedema, pathologic drainages and the condition of the Eustachian orifices. As a second step, the scope is gently retracted thus, permitting the investigation of the SER and the lateral nasal wall along with the fontanella area and the OMC. In this area, evidence of pathological drainage is crucial. Purulent secretions at the level of the OMC and of the posterior fontanella zone are an endoscopic sign of an anterior compartment rhinosinusitis (maxillary, anterior ethmoid and frontal sinuses), whereas secretions within the SER mean rhinosinusitis of the posterior compartment (posterior ethmoid and sphenoid sinuses). As a final step, if requested, an endoscopic visualization of the oropharynx and of the hypopharynx/larynx can be obtained by passing through the nasopharynx. During this step particular importance should be given to the posterior extension of the palatine tonsils within the oropharynx, as long as both the laryngeal morphology and motility. The entire procedure lasts about 30 sec – 1 min.

The degree of obstruction by the adenoid tissue over the posterior choanae was estimated using the grading system proposed by Parikh et al. (Figure 6): grade 1 for adenoid tissue not in contact with adjacent structures; grade 2 for adenoid tissue in contact with torus tubarius, grade 3 for adenoid tissue in contact with vomer, and grade 4 for adenoid tissue in contact with soft palate (at rest) (Parikh et al., 2006). Other diseases usually noted during the examination, include inferior turbinate hypertrophy, septal deviation, choanal stenosis or atresia, mucosal infections and polypoid formations.

A clinical examination of the ear and the oropharynx is, usually, obtained in all children. Further exams as pure-tone audiometry (in children over 4 years-old) and timpanometry, are suggested in cases of referred hearing impairment or middle otitis.

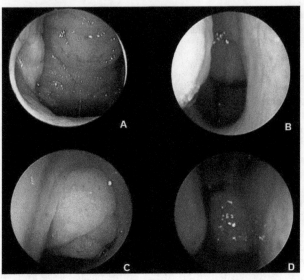

Fig. 6. Adenoid hypertrophy grading system proposed by Parikh et al. (Parikh et al., 2006): grade 1 (A), grade 2 (B), grade 3 (C) and grade 4 (D).

3. Evolution of surgical techniques

3.1 Adenoidectomy in the pre – endoscopic era
3.1.1 Traditional adenoidectomy

This is the "standard" surgical procedure of an adenoidectomy. As an initial step, the hard palate is inspected and palpated for the detection of an eventual submucous cleft (bifid uvula, zona pellucida, notching of the posterior hard palate). The palate's length should also be inspected. In the present procedure, the whole procedure is conducted without visualization of the nasopharynx. A complete set of three adenotomes (Shambaugh or LaForce) – small, medium and large size – is prepared, and an adenoid curette is chosen based on the dimension of the child's oropharynx and should fit between the tori (Figure 7).

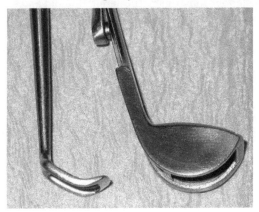

Fig. 7. An Adenoid curette (left) and a Shambaugh adenotome (right).

The large-sized adenotome is inserted in the oral cavity by-passing the oropharynx in order to reach the nasopharynx and the adenoid pad; when the target is reached the adenotome is applied in order to remove the lymphatic nasopharyngeal tissue (Figure 8). The procedure is, then, repeated with both the medium and small sized adenotomes. After this passage, the curette is transorally inserted in the superior nasopharynx and in contact with the vomer; then is swept inferiorly with a side-to-side rocking motion to completely remove all the remaining adenoids. Care is taken to avoid injury to the deep muscular and vertebral plane, to the torus region or to the choanal area. A smaller curette can consequently be used to remove any retained tissue. After several saline solution irrigations, hemostasis is obtained by placing a tonsillar pack in the nasopharynx for some minutes. Complete removal of the adenoid tissue is confirmed by digital palpation.

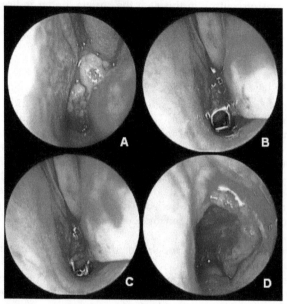

Fig. 8. Intraoperative steps of a traditional adenoidectomy with an adenotome. The procedure is showed under endoscopic view (transnasal 0° endoscope) only for didactic purposes because, as mentioned, the procedure is usually performed blindly. In A the adenoid pad is visualized from the left nasal fossa in the nasopharynx. In B and C the adenotome is transorally inserted to reach the adenoid tissue, opened (B), and then closed (C) in order to remove the lymphatic tissue. In D the surgical field at the end of the adenoidectomy.

The main limitations of the traditional technique include: less precise removal and potentially less effective treatment, possible increased bleeding, risk of neck pain and velopharyngeal insufficiency, and lack of surgical visualization. As known, this procedure does not always remove completely the adenoid tissue (Cannon et al., 1999).

This method showed an efficacy of tissue removal only in 30% of cases (Bross-Soriano et al., 2004). The superior and the peritubaric portions of the adenoid that obstruct the nasopharynx and the orifice of the Eustachian tube should be considered as zones of potential adenoid remnants. Moreover, excessive removal of adenoid tissue by curettage may provoke damage to the pharyngeal muscles, to the posterior choana, to the Eustachian tubes, or to other structures. As a result, several complications might result from an excessive traditional adenoidectomy, including velopharyngeal insufficiency and persistence of obstructive symptoms (Gelder, 1974).

3.1.2 Laryngeal-mirror assisted adenoidectomy
In all these surgical techniques the surgical field is controlled through a transorally placed laryngeal (or dental) mirror, in order to achieve an adequate view of the nasopharynx.

3.1.2.1 Traditional adenoidectomy with transoral laryngeal-mirror control

The already described traditional adenoidectomy may also been conducted under a transoral laryngeal mirror control; in this case the curette, under indirect visualization, is passed through the oral cavity in order to reach the adenoid tissue, and adenoidectomy is performed. Hemostasis can also be obtained with an electrocautery under the mirror control.

3.1.2.2 Power assisted adenoidectomy with transoral laryngeal-mirror control (Koltai et al., 2002; Rodriguez et al., 2002; Stanislaw et al., 2000)

This technique consists in performing the adenoidectomy with a debrider under an indirect visualization, through a laryngeal mirror. The shaver cannula is usually curved (mainly 45° or 60°). The cannula is, transorally, introduced into the nasopharynx under indirect transoral mirror visualization, and the oscillating blade is then switched on. The adenoidectomy starts high in the nasopharynx, near the choanal sill. The resection is performed in a side-to-side manner, progressing on an even level until the inferior edge of the adenoid pad is reached. The depth of adenoid resection, as well as the resection around the choana and torus, is precisely controlled. The tip of the oscillating cannula is always under visual control via the laryngeal mirror. Electrocautery can be used in order to obtain an adequate hemostasis.

A complete adenoidectomy with a microdebrider was shown to be faster than, and as safe as, a traditional curettage adenoidectomy. A recent review evidenced that operative time was significantly less when applying the debrider and that blood loss, recovery time, and complications were comparable between those two techniques. Moreover, the main advantage of debrider adenoidectomy resides in its precision.

3.1.2.3 Suction diathermy (Elluru et al., 2002;Walker, 2001)

This technique is usually performed with an indirect visualization of the nasopharynx through a laryngeal mirror (but it can also be conducted under endoscopic control), as already seen. Diathermy ablation of the adenoid pad is accomplished by using an insulated, curved Frazier-type suction system or, more commonly, a disposable, malleable 10 French size, hand-switching suction coagulator (E2610–6, ValleyLab, Boulder, CO). When the Frazier-type system is used, a monopolar diathermy is applied. Typically, a setting of 30 to 45 W (depending on the patient's weight) is used to ablate the adenoid tissue.

The suction electrocautery device is applied to the adenoid pad, beginning at the most superior part of it (within the central bulk of the adenoid tissue, and not superficially). As the pad is cauterized, it shrinks and the suction device helps in evacuating the smoke. Thus, the obstructive adenoid tissue is ablated with care taken not to traumatize the soft palate, the opening of the Eustachian tube, or other adjacent pharyngeal structures. Surgery is completed when the choanae are clearly visible and the nasopharynx presents a smooth level contour. There should be no heat damages on the vomer, nasal turbinates, soft palate, or lateral nasopharyngeal walls. In the literature, this method is defined as precise, easy to perform, fast, bloodless and relatively inexpensive.

In a recent prospective study published by Jonas et al., a comparison between suction-diathermy ablation and curettage adenoidectomy was performed. The majority of patients experienced symptom improvement after 6 months, regardless of the method used. Both techniques were very effective in controlling the symptoms of the adenoidal hypertrophy. As referred, suction diathermy technique was superior in reducing adenoidal regrowth at 6 months. Although this result was statistically significant, it is uncertain whether it is of a true clinical significance, as the symptom improvement for both groups were in excess of 95% (Jonas et al., 2007).

3.2 Adenoidectomy in the endoscopic era
3.2.1 The pure endoscopic approaches

3.2.1.1 Nasal endoscopic-guided curettage transoral adenoidectomy (EGA) (Wan et al., 2005)

The nasal cavities and nasopharynx are examined through a 0° nasal scope. A throat pack is then inserted to prevent blood from entering the trachea. A Boyle- Davis mouth gag is used to open the mouth widely as during the classic adenoidectomy. A suitably sized Beckmann adenoid curette is transorally placed into the nasopharynx. Under nasal endoscopic guidance, the blade of the adenoid curette is placed just above the superior border of the adenoid. The lateral ends of the blade should just be away from the Eustachian tube area on both sides. The nasal endoscope is then taken out from the nose and the curette is used as in conventional curettage.

Transoral packing gauze is used for some minutes to control bleeding, which usually stops spontaneously without need for cauterization. Nasal endoscopy, simply, allows an assessment of the adenoid size and extension and improves the accuracy of the adenoidectomy with the curette. This method is particularly useful in younger patients with a small oral cavity; in fact, adenoid palpation, mirror examination and consequent laryngeal mirror-adenoidectomy is challenging in patients with narrow passages. These problems can be addressed by the rigid nasal endoscope, which allows accurate and safe placement of the curette at the superior border of the tissue. Thus, we obtain a complete removal of the main bulk of the adenoid without the need for nasal grasping forceps or a debrider. Moreover, teaching is much easier when combined with the real-time video presentation. Last but not least, as sophisticated instruments are not required, the cost-effectiveness of such method remains highly acceptable.

In all cases, the EGA curettage method is sufficient to remove the main bulk of the adenoids in one attempt. In contrast, the adenoid tissue is removed piece by piece during the classic curette adenoidectomy. In conclusion, the EGA allows a more complete and precise removal of the adenoid compared with the conventional method.

3.2.1.2 Transoral endoscopic adenoidectomy with adenoid curette and St. Claire Thomson forceps (El-Badrawy & Abdel-Aziz, 2009)

Under general oro-tracheal anesthesia, a Boyle-Davis mouth gag is used. The soft palate is retracted with rubber catheters passed from the nose to the mouth. The 4 mm-70° rigid nasal scope is introduced through the mouth, and the nasopharyngeal adenoid mass is identified. Curettage of the main adenoid mass is carried out using an adequate size adenoid curette; removal of any residual tissue is performed by a St. Claire Thomson forceps while suction is used to clear the field. At the end, a pack of gauze is inserted into the nasopharynx for some minutes.

According to the authors, the advantage of this method is the direct visualization of the operative field that would decrease the incidence of post-op adenoidal remnants, the reduced possibility of injury to the Eustachian tube with a consequent long-term fibrosis and the finer control of possible haemorrhage sites. Moreover, the procedure does not need any expensive equipment and it needs just a few minutes more than the conventional mirror-adenoidectomy method. However, the transoral endoscopic approach demands some experience in endoscopic surgery through curved scopes.

3.2.1.3 Transoral adenoid ablation by suction diathermy under a 45° scope vision (Lo & Rowe- Jones, 2006)

The procedure is undertaken under general anaesthesia. The patient is positioned and prepared as described in the latter technique. The surgeon stands on the right side of the patient's head. A 45° rigid scope is introduced through the oral cavity to the oropharynx with the lens pointing towards the nasopharynx. The suction coagulator device is introduced alongside the endoscope. Using a setting of 30 W of monopolar coagulation combined with suction, the adenoidectomy is performed under direct endoscopic vision.

The known limitations of the traditional indirect mirror adenoidectomy are mainly associated to the poor visualization and manoeuvrability. Thus, the endoscopic transoral approach overwhelms those limitations. More specifically, by the 30° endoscope and in particular in patients with small mouth opening, visualization of the nasopharynx, although better, could be limited. With a 90° endoscope, although the whole nasopharynx could be effectively visualised, however a closer look into the nasopharynx would be very difficult, and the endoscope and suction coagulator would be oriented at different axis, thus limiting manoeuvrability.

By using a 45° endoscope the entire nasopharynx can be easily visualised. In addition, the axis of introduction in both, scope and suction-coagulator, is the same so, bimanual co-ordination is easily achieved. As referred, with this technique and in patients with submucous cleft palate, adenoid tissue may be excised under direct vision preserving, however, a small pad inferiorly to avoid velopharyngeal insufficiency. In conclusion, this technique is both effective and presents a short learning curve.

3.2.1.4 Transnasal power assisted adenoidectomy with transnasal endoscopic control (Al-Mazrou et al., 2009; Havas & Lowinger, 2002)

The shaver blade used is the XPS Xomed Power System with the lightweight magnum-scaled handpiece and a 2.9-mm Tricut blade with straight-through suction irrigation (Medtronic Xomed Surgical Products, Jacksonville, Fl). The theater setup and positioning is as for a standard functional endoscopic sinus surgery. Using the 0°, 2.7-mm rigid telescope (4 mm scope is used in older children with larger nasal cavities), the posterior choanae and nasopharynx are assessed. Under endoscopic vision the shaver cannula is passed into the nose with the suction switched off to allow passage to the adenoids without traumatizing the turbinates or the septum. The suction is then turned on and the obstructive tissue is removed under constant endoscopic vision with care not to lacerate the torus tubarius. The cutting and aspirating action of the shaver removes both adenoid tissue and blood, providing a clear view. Tissue is removed at the site of the oscillating blade only, and the blade is kept under vision all the time using the telescope. Working from proximal to distal, intranasal adenoid and hypertrophic nasopharyngeal adenoid are removed until the surgeon is satisfied with the clearance. A small inferior rim of adenoid tissue can be left intact intentionally to preserve the velopharyngeal sphincter. With this technique a finer peritubal and perichoanal tissue clearance is possible, and a better control on the depth of the tissue resection is achieved. Careful tissue removal is carried out with the concomitant visual-protection of important nearby structures like Eustachian tubes, torus tubarius and the posterior pharyngeal wall. Moreover, this technique is reported to be faster and bloodless than the traditional curette adenoidectomy. A possible disadvantage, is the cost of the disposable blade of the shaver.

3.2.1.5 Transoral power assisted adenoidectomy with transoral 70° endoscopic control (Costantini et al., 2008)

A general orotracheal anaesthesia is performed for the surgery. The patient is placed in a supine position with the neck slightly extended and the surgeon placed to the right of the patient. A mouth gag, the same as for tonsillectomy, is positioned; two rubber catheters are introduced through the nasal fossae to apply light upward traction to the soft palate, thereby increasing the forward-back diameter of the passage. The slight stretching of the palate achieved with this manoeuvre can also help to detect a possible soft palate cleft.

A 70° endoscope with a video attachment is introduced through the mouth to visualize the nasopharynx, and consequently a 40° curved blade microdebrider is introduced through the mouth (Figure 9).

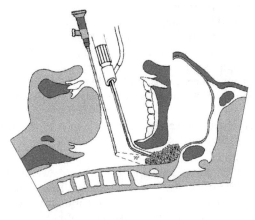

Fig. 9. Schematic representation of the transoral power assisted adenoidectomy with transoral 70° endoscopic control

The instrument is connected to an aspirator, and set a rotational speed of 1200 rpm. Removal of the adenoid tissue starts from the choanal extension, and proceeds backwards along the vault towards the posterior wall of the nasopharynx. The smooth tip of the microdebrider can be introduced into the recess between the side vegetations and the tubaric ostium so that the tissue can be completely removed without damaging the mucosa covering the torus tubarius.

The resection is interrupted at the passage from the regular adenoid vegetations to the chaotic aspect of the lymphatic tissue in this zone (Passavant ridge). From a functional point of view, the removal can be considered complete at this point. In doing so, such procedure prevents transitory velo-pharyngeal insufficiency and avoids excessive intraoperative bleeding.

At the end of the resection, a gauze packing could be placed and is maintained for some minutes. The packing is then removed and the cavity is checked for possible remnants and for the absence of bleeding. In the uneventful case of persistent bleeding, hemostasis can be established using a curved suction-coagulator, always under an endoscopic transoral control.

Several authors have described the high percentage of residual tissue remnant after traditional (adenotome or curette) adenoidectomy, especially in the choanal and the peritubaric region. A blindly performed surgical procedure is no longer satisfactory. A clear vision of the operating field is essential and this can be obtained, with excellent illumination and focus, with a transorally inserted 70° endoscope. Compared to the image obtained by a laryngeal or dental mirror, the quality of the image is unquestionably better.

In some cases, introduction of the catheters for suspending the soft palate can be rather difficult (especially in the presence of an important choanal obstruction), but, according to these authors, they do offer considerable advantages. The safety and precision of the transoral curved microdebrider for adenoidectomy is well documented by the Rodriguez et al. (Rodriguez et al., 2002), Koltai et al. (Koltai et al., 2002), and Murray et al. (Murray et al., 2002). This method can be effective to remove the lateral (peritubaric) adenoidal tissue with a precision that is difficult to achieve with any other instrument, thereby minimizing the risk of damaging the surrounding structures. If a partial adenoidectomy is appropriate, it is also possible to perform very selective removal of the adenoid tissue. Moreover, the continuous suction generated by the microdebrider maintains a bloodless field.

Although the technique described may appear, at a first view, more difficult than those traditionally used, it is easier to learn, particularly for the surgeon who is, somewhat, familiar with the endoscopic nasal surgery. Moreover, it is easy to teach using the video images. The duration of the procedure is slightly longer than a standard adenoidectomy. The organization and preparation times are also longer, while ablation and haemostasis times are substantially the same. However, the slightly longer duration is more than compensated by the greater precision and confidence gained by the surgeon.

3.2.2 The combined methods

A recent report (Saxby et al., 2009) comments on the incidence of residual adenoid tissue after 425 consecutive traditional curette adenoidectomies. This residual tissue can lead to a combination of potential problems, including peritubaric obstruction, bacterial reservoirs and hyperplasia of the remnants with the persistence of obstructive symptoms; all these aspects highlight the importance of addressing a complete removal of the adenoid tissue. In this report, the majority (73%) of patients who underwent to a traditional curettage adenoidectomy had some endoscopic evidence of residual adenoids, 26% of which presented also symptoms of nasal obstruction (grade 2 or 3 adenoid hypertrophy).

The incidence of residual adenoid tissue found in this study agrees with previously published results. (Havas & Lowinger, 2002; Cannon et al., 1999). Residual tissue revealed by the endoscopic control of the nasopharynx, occurred in a significant proportion of cases and would have been missed by palpation alone; this fact highlights the advantage of endoscopically inspecting the nasopharynx after the curettage. However, it is still not clear whether lesser grades of residual tissue warrant further resection. In this study, and also according to our experience, all the residual lymphatic tissue should be removed. Some authors argue that grade 1 (up to one-third of choanal occlusion) is not clinically significant, but it appears interesting that this occurs in most cases. Herein, we report some of the different combined methods described in the literature.

3.2.2.1 Conventional curettage adenoidectomy with transnasal endoscopic forceps' residual asportation (Huang et al., 1998)

In this procedure, the patient is placed supine in Rose position with the head extended. The mouth is opened with a Dingmann mouth gag. Disinfection of the face and oral cavity is performed to avoid contamination. The soft palate is retracted with a Hurd tonsil retractor. After this passage, an adenoid curette is transorally applied to the nasopharynx and the main bulk of adenoid is removed. Care is required during this process in order to avoid injury to the choana and to the pharyngeal muscles, which could result in a massive bleeding.

Subsequently, a 4-mm or 2.7-mm, 0° or 30° endoscope is inserted transnasally till the nasopharynx. Residual adenoid tissue at the superior portion of the rhinopharynx and at the orifice of the Eustachian tube, is usually detected at this time. Under endoscopic guidance, the adenoidectomy is completed by removing the residual tissue piece by piece using either a straight or a 45° Blakesley forceps. The nasopharynx and the orifice of the Eustachian tube can be inspected by a direct endoscopic visualization without damage to other structures. Adjunctively, control of the hemostasis can be performed through a direct endoscopic view.

The use of endoscopic equipment allows a piece by piece adenoid removal. However, in patients with important tissue volume, such approach requires more time than conventional surgery, which prolongs the anesthesia times and increase the peri-operative risks. In such cases, conventional surgical methods (curette and adenotome) may remove the main bulk of the adenoid mass. On the other hand, direct endoscopic visualization reduces the likelihood of damage to other structures by excessive excision and hemorrhage due to residual adenoid tissue. Direct visualization allows direct identification and treatment of the source of bleeding, thus sparing unaffected structures and is therefore highly suitable for children. If necessary, suction cautery or other hemostatic methods can be locally used under endoscopic control.

A similar method was proposed also by Cannon et al. in 1999 (Cannon et al., 1999) and called "Endoscopic-assisted adenoidectomy (EAA)"; according to this technique, at the end of a conventional adenoidectomy, both the nasal cavities and the rhinopharynx were inspected with a 4-mm 0° rigid telescope. Adenoid remnants in the rhinopharynx were removed under direct visualization by paediatric straight forceps or pituitary forceps.

3.2.2.2 Endoscopic-assisted combined curettage adenoidectomy (Regmi et al., 2011)

This is a simple but effective technique, as confirmed in our personal experience too. Surgery is conducted under general oro-tracheal anaesthesia, with the child placed in the Rose's position, and a mouth gag inserted to expose the oropharynx. A rubber catheter may be inserted through the mouth to obtain an adequate palatal retraction. As a first step a traditional curettage and / or adenotome adenoidectomy without a direct visualization of the nasopharynx is performed. Subsequently, the nasal cavities and nasopharynx are endoscopically examined with a rigid endoscope. If adenoid remnants are observed, those are removed under transnasal endoscopic control through the transoral adenoid curette.

By this method, the main disadvantages of the traditional technique such as the damage to the torus tubarius or the pharyngeal muscles and the persistence of adenoid remnants could be avoided.

3.2.2.3 Endoscopic suction diathermy following traditional curettage adenoidectomy (Saxby et al., 2009)

All the adenoidectomies are performed under general anaesthesia with the patient appropriately positioned and draped. A Boyle–Davis mouth gag is used in order to hold the mouth open. Digital palpation of the palate is performed to assess adenoidal size, and to identify any eventual submucosal cleft. The first part of the surgical procedure consists in the removal of the adenoid tissue with sweeping movements of an appropriately sized adenoid curette. Haemostasis is achieved with a moist gauze swab left in place for several minutes. After removal, any eventual residual adenoid tissue is transnasally assessed using a 0° scope. A Y-suction catheter is used to clear the field and allow assessment of the epipharynx. Ablation of residual tissue by electrocautery is achieved using a suction diathermy coagulator (Valleylab, Tyco Healthcare Group, Boulder, Colorado, USA) placed transorally under a transnasal endoscopic visualization. The suction diathermy is bent 90°, 2.5 cm from the distal end to get to the epipharynx through the mouth. Care should be taken to avoid a Eustachian injury by the diathermy tip. Thus, the removal of the residual adenoid tissue should proceed medially from anterior to posterior.

3.2.2.4 Traditional curette and transnasal endoscopic adenoidectomy (transnasal straight microdebriders and transnasal endoscopic view) (Pagella et al., 2009)

With the child under general anaesthesia via an orotracheal tube, a Crowe-Davis mouth gag is inserted; the patient is placed supine in the Rose position, then a conventional adenoidectomy with a Shambaugh adenotome and Shambaugh curette is performed. A catheter is passed through the nose to assure cessation of bleeding and removal of any clot, and the nasopharynx is inspected using a 0°, 2.7 mm rigid fibre-optic endoscope with a video attachment.

In the presence of residual adenoid tissue still causing a significant obstruction of the nasopharynx, the patients undergo completion of adenoidectomy using a powered shaver. The shaver used is the XPS (Xomed Powered System by Medtronic, Jacksonville, FL) with a 2.9 mm Tricut straight blade and straight-through suction irrigation (Figure 10).

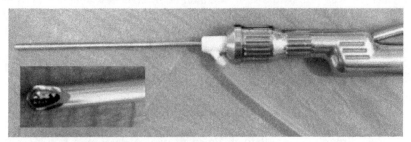

Fig. 10. The straight XPS shaver, as described above in the text.

The device should be set at 500 rpm in the oscillating mode, with concomitant irrigation. Under constant endoscopic view the shaver cannula is passed through the nose with the suction switched off, so as to allow passage to the nasopharynx without traumatizing the nasal mucosa. The suction is then switched on and residual adenoid tissue is removed under endoscopic vision with care not to damage the torus tubarius (Figure 11 – 14). The cutting and aspirating action of the shaver removes both adenoid tissue and blood, providing a clear surgical field and keeping the oscillating cannula always under visual control. Once haemostasis is achieved by several saline solution irrigations, the equipment is removed and the child is then handed back to the anaesthetists for awakening and extubation.

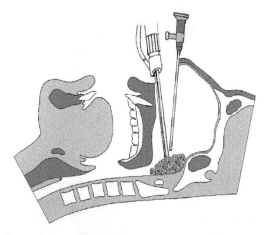

Fig. 11. Schematic representation of the traditional curette and transnasal endoscopic adenoidectomy.

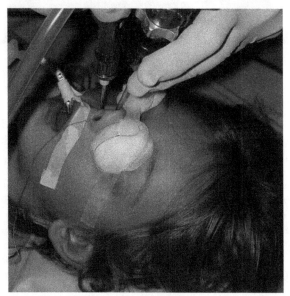

Fig. 12. External view of the microdebrider and the endoscope, both placed in the nasal cavity.

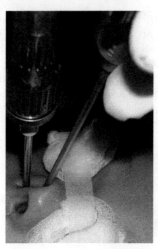

Fig. 13. Closed-detail of the relative placement of the two instruments into the right nostril.

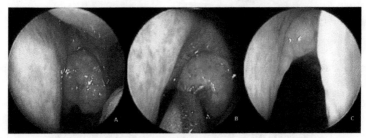

Fig. 14. Intraoperative sequential steps of the removal of adenoid remants after a traditional adenoidectomy. The scope is introduced in the left nasal fossa to permit a safe control of the entire surgical act. Lymphatic tissue still obstructing the nasopharynx (A); removal of the latter tissue with the straight shaver (B); the surgical field at the end of the procedure (C).

The value of a transnasal endoscopic view for assessing the complete adenoid removal at the end of a traditional adenoidectomy has been repeatedly underlined; this counts especially for the tissue placed superiorly in the nasopharynx and around the choanal sill but is effective as well for the control of active bleeding areas. (Buchinsky et al., 2000; Elluru et al., 2002; Havas & Lowinger, 2002; Shin & Hartnick, 2003; Stanislaw et al., 2000)
The use of the transnasal microdebrider assures a complete adenoidectomy and, in particular, a better control over the extent of the resection, especially around the choanal sill, the posterior nose and the torus tubarius. On the other hand, and in the presence of bulky/obstructing adenoids, a pure microdebrider adenoidectomy is time-consuming procedure; moreover, sometimes results as a difficult act because of the limited manoeuvrability of the instruments in the inferior nasopharynx. In our experience, in case of children with large adenoids, a conventional curettage and/or the usage of the adenotome removes rapidly the main tissue bulk. Then, the transnasally controlled power-assisted endonasal approach, permits an accurate residual tissue exeresis, a correct evaluation and

effective treatment of active bleeding points, and a decreased traumatism of the region. By performing the combined adenoidectomy approach, there is an obvious increase in operative time when both curette and power-assisted techniques are used. However, in experienced hands, this increase is limited to some minutes. According to Koltai et al. (Koltai et al., 2002), initially it may appear that the power-assisted adenoidectomy is a more hemorrhagic operation than the traditional operation; this happens because the microdebrider removes small pieces of tissue with each oscillation, leaving a raw surface that bleeds during the rest of the procedure. However, when continuous suction is used, the blood is evacuated along with the excised tissue, leaving a clear and unobstructed view of the operating field. In our experience, there was no increased primary or secondary bleeding related to the use of the microdebrider. By contrast, we were certain that we had achieved a complete clearance of the rhinopharynx in every single patient.

3.2.2.5 Transoral Endonasal-Controlled Combined Adenoidectomy (TECCA) (Pagella et al., 2010)

As a first step a traditional transoral adenoidectomy is performed with a Shambaugh adenotome and Shambaugh curette. Secondarily, a 0°, 2.7-mm, rigid fiber optic endoscope with a video attachment is introduced through the nostrils to inspect the nasopharynx and ensure a complete removal of the adenoid tissue. In the presence of residual adenoid tissue still obstructing the nasopharynx, the patient undergoes a completion of the adenoidectomy with the curved microdebrider. We use the 60° curved, 4-mm Tricut blade and straight-through suction irrigation microdebrider by XPS (Xomed Powered System by Medtronic, Jacksonville, FL). The device is set at 500 rpm in the oscillating mode. Under endoscopic transnasal view the curved microdebrider, with the suction switched off to avoid oropharyngeal damages during the introduction, is advanced through the oral cavity and reaches the nasopharynx. The suction is then switched on and the residual adenoid tissue is removed under transnasal endoscopic vision, with care not to damage the torus tubarius or the pharyngeal muscles (Figure 15 – 17). The constant aspiration of the power-assisted instrument permits a complete removal of the adenoid tissue and a bloodless surgical area. Once haemostasis is achieved, and abundant irrigation of the field with saline solution is performed, the equipment is removed.

This new technique seems to be as safe and effective as the previous described one (transnasal microdebrider and transnasal endoscopic control). Moreover by performing the TECCA technique, some problems encountered during the latter procedure (Traditional curette and transnasal endoscopic adenoidectomy), as the contact between the scope and the debrider if both are passed transnasally, seem to be addressed; to us, the efficacy and safety of both procedures are similar. As stated before, we underline that we would rather not perform the entire procedure with the debrider so as not to significantly extend the total operative time; this is why we propose to perform the first step with standard adenoidectomy instruments. One possible limitation of this technique might be the higher price of the curved blades, as usually happens with the new equipment.

In conclusion, TECCA appears to be efficient in removing adenoid tissue that still obstructs the nasopharynx, in particular, when such remnants are situated in the superior part of the nasopharynx and/or the peritubaric region. Apparently, such procedure carries no additional risk compared to other techniques. Indeed, it permits a better maneuverability of the instruments in cases of narrow nasal spaces for a complete clearance of the nasopharyngeal area.

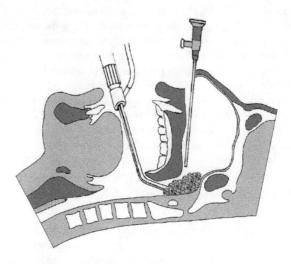

Fig. 15. Schematic representation of the second surgical step of the TECCA, as described in the text.

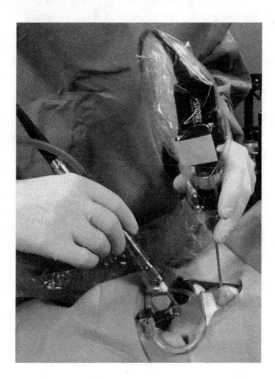

Fig. 16. External view of the second surgical step of a TECCA procedure.

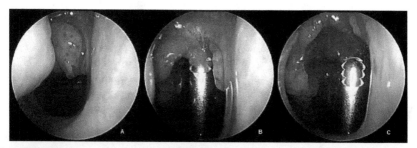

Fig. 17. Intraoperative sequential steps of residual adenoid removal by the TECCA technique. The scope is placed transnasally between the septum and the right inferior turbinate in order to control the transoral adenoidal clearance by the curved microdebrider. In A adenoid remnants at the end of a traditional adenoidectomy. In B and C remnant's exeresis through the transorally placed power-assisted instrument.

4. Conclusion

Since many years, adenoidectomy is one of the most common surgical procedures performed by Otolaryngologists in children. Historically, in the pre-endoscopic era, this procedure was performed blindly, without a direct visualization of the surgical field. Conventional "blind" adenoidectomy (adenotome or curette) may achieve the desired results in many patients; however, as many authors state, it frequently fails to obtain a complete tissue removal and, thus is less effective than direct/indirect visualization techniques. The indirect, mirror-controlled adenoidectomy was the first attempt to obtain a view of the nasopharynx during the operation. More recently, in the endoscopic era, the use of the endoscopes and other modern surgical equipment (p.e. microdebriders, suction-diathermy) permitted the development of several endoscopic-assisted approaches; these innovative techniques offered the surgeon a clear, direct view of the rhinopharynx, enabling a complete and fine removal of the adenoid tissue, thus, avoiding an excessive and unnecessary trauma to the surrounding structures.

5. References

Al-Mazrou, KA; Al-Qahtani, A & Al-Fayez AI. (2009). Effectiveness of transnasal endoscopic powered adenoidectomy in patients with choanal adenoids. *International Journal of Pediatric Otorhinolaryngology*, Vol.73, No.12, pp. 1650-1652.

Ark, N; Kurtaran, H; Ugur, KS; Yilmaz, T; Ozboduroglu, AA & Mutlu, C. (2010). Comparison of adenoidectomy methods: examining with digital palpation vs. visualizing the placement of the curette. *International Journal of Pediatric Otorhinolaryngology*, Vol.74, No.6, pp. 649-651.

Baker, S. (1939). *Fighting for life*, pp. 140-141. The Macmillan Company. New York, NY.

Becker, SP; Roberts, N & Coglianese, D. (1992). Endoscopic adenoidectomy or relief of serous otitis media. *Laryngoscope*, Vol.102, No.12 Pt 1, pp./1379-1384.

Brodsky, L. (1996). Adenoidectomy, In: *Atlas of Head & Neck Surgery-Otolaryngology*, Bailey, BJ; Calhoun, KH; Coffey, AR & Neely, JG, pp. 816–817, Lippincott-Raven, Philadelphia, PA.

Bross-Soriano, D; Schimelmitz-Idl, J & Arrieta-Gomez, JR. (2004), Endoscopic adenoidectomy: use or abuse of technology? *Cirugia y Cirujianos*, Vol.72, No.1, pp. 15-19, 21-22.

Buchinsky, FJ; Lowry, MA & Isaacson, G. (2000). Do adenoids regrow after excision? *Otolaryngology-Head and Neck Surgery*, Vol.123, No.5, pp. 576-581.

Cannon, CR; Replogle, WH & Schenk, MP. (1999). Endoscopic-assisted adenoidectomy. *Otolaryngology-Head and Neck Surgery*, Vol.121, No.6, pp.740-744.

Costantini, F; Salamanca, F; Amaina, T & Zibordi, F. (2008). Videoendoscopic adenoidectomy with microdebrider. *ACTA Otorhinolaryngologica Italica*, Vol.28, No.1, pp.26-29.

Curtin, JM. (1987). The history of tonsil and adenoid surgery. *Otolaryngologic Clinics of North America*, Vol.20, No.2, pp. 415-419.

Discolo, CM; Younes, AA; Koltai, PJ. (2001). Current techniques of adenoidectomy. *Operative Techniques in Otolaryngology-Head and Neck Surgery*, Vol.12, No.4, pp. 199-203.

El-Badrawy, A & Abdel-Aziz, M. (2009). Transoral Endoscopic Adenoidectomy. *International Journal of Otolaryngology*, 949315. Epub 2009 Jul 28.

Elluru, RG; Johnson, L; Myer, CM. (2002). Electrocautery adenoidectomy compared with curettage and power-assisted methods. *Laryngoscope*, Vol.112, No.8 Pt. 2 Suppl.100, pp. 23-25.

Ezzat, WF. (2010). Role of endoscopic nasal examination in reduction of nasopharyngeal adenoid recurrence rates. *International Journal of Pediatric Otorhinolaryngology*, Vol.74, No.4, pp. 404-406.

Havas, T & Lowinger, D. (2002). Obstructive adenoid tissue: an indication for powered-shaver adenoidectomy. *Archives of Otolaryngology-Head and Neck Surgery*, Vol.128, No.7, pp. 789-791.

Hays, HM. (1924). Diseases of pharynx, nasopharynx and hypopharynx, In: *Pediatrics*, Abt IA, (3rd Ed.), pp. 217-218, Saunders WB, Philadelphia, PA.

Heras, HA & Koltai, PJ. (1998). Safety of powered instrumentation for adenoidectomy. *International Journal of Pediatric Otorhinolaryngology*, Vol.44, No.2, pp. 149-153.

Huang, HM; Chao, MC; Chen, YL & Hsiao, HR. (1998). A combined method of conventional and endoscopic adenoidectomy. *Laryngoscope*, Vol.108, No.7, pp. 1104-1106.

Jonas, NE; Sayed, R & Prescott, CA. (2007). Prospective, randomized, single-blind, controlled study to compare two methods of performing adenoidectomy. *International Journal of Pediatric Otorhinolaryngology*, Vol.71, No.10, pp. 1555-1562.

Joshua, B; Bahar, G; Sulkes, J; Shpitzer, T & Raveh, E. (2006). Adenoidectomy: long-term follow-up. *Otolaryngology-Head and Neck Surgery*, Vol.135, No.4, pp. 576-580.

Kaiser, AD. (1932). *Children's tonsils in or out?* pp. 2, 3, 8-10. JB Lippincott. Philadelphia, PA.

Koltai, PJ; Kalathia, AS; Stanislaw, P & Heras, HA. (1997). Power-assisted adenoidectomy. *Archives of Otolaryngology-Head and Neck Surgery*, Vol.123, No.7, pp. 685-688.

Koltai, PJ; Chan, J &Younes, A. (2002). Power-assisted adenoidectomy: total and partial resection. *Laryngoscope*, Vol.112, No.8 Pt.2 Suppl.100, pp. 29-31.

Kornblut, AD. (1987). A traditional approach to surgery of the tonsil and adenoids. *Otolaryngologic Clinics of North America*, Vol.20, No.2, pp. 349-363.

Kwok, P & Hawke, M. (1987). The use of suction cautery in adenoidectomy. *The Journal of Otolaryngology*, Vol.16, No.1, pp. 49-50.

Lo, S & Rowe- Jones, J. (2006). How we do it: Transoral suction diathermy adenoid ablation under direct vision using a 45 degree endoscope. *Clinical Otolaryngology*, Vol.31, No.5, pp. 436–455.

Meyer, W. (1870). On adenoid vegetations in the nasopharyngeal cavity: their pathology, diagnosis and tretament. *Medico-chirurgical Trans (London)*, Vol.53, pp. 191-216.

Monroy, A; Behar, P & Brodsky, L. (2008). Revision adenoidectomy – a retrospective study, *International Journal of Pediatric Otorhinolaryngology*, Vol.72, No.5, pp. 565-570.

Owens, D; Jaramillo, M & Saunders, M. (2005). Suction diathermy adenoid ablation. *The Journal of Laryngology and Otology*, Vol.119, No.1, pp. 34-35.

Pagella, F; Matti, E; Colombo, A; Giourgos, G & Mira, E. (2009). How we do it: a combined method of traditional curette and power-assisted endoscopic adenoidectomy. *Acta Otolaryngologica*. Vol.129, No.5, pp. 556-559.

Pagella, F; Pusateri, A; Matti, E & Giourgos, G. (2010). Transoral Endonasal-Controlled Combined Adenoidectomy (TECCA). *Laryngoscope*, Vol.120, No.10, pp. 2008-2010.

Paradise, JL. (1996). Tonsillectomy and adenoidectomy, In: *Pediatric Otolaryngology*, Blueston, CD; Stool SE; Kenna MA, (3rd Ed.), pp. 1054-1065, WB Saunders, Philadelphia, PA.

Parikh, SR; Coronel, M; Lee, JJ & Brown, SM. (2006). Validation of a new grading system for endoscopic examination of adenoid hypertrophy. *Otolaryngology-Head and Neck Surgery*, Vol.135, No.5, pp. 684-687.

Parson, SP. (1996). Rhinologic uses of powered instrumentation in children beyond sinus surgery. *Otolaryngologic Clinics of North America*, Vol.29, No.1, pp. 105-114.

Paul of Aegina (A.D. 625-690). *The seven books of Paulus Aegineta*. (1847). Translated from the Greek by Francis Adams, Sydenham Society Instituted, London.

Regmi, D; Mathur, NN & Bhattarai, M. (2011). Rigid endoscopic evaluation of conventional curettage adenoidectomy. *The Journal of Laryngology and Otology*, Vol.125, No.1, pp. 53-58.

Rodriguez, K; Murray, N & Guarisco, JL. (2002). Power-assisted partial adenoidectomy. *Laryngoscope*, Vol.112, No.8 Pt.2 Suppl.100, pp. 26-28.

Saxby, AJ & Chappel, CA. (2009). Residual adenoid tissue post-curettage: role of nasopharyngoscopy in adenoidectomy. *ANZ Journal of Surgery*, Vol.79, No.11, pp. 809-811.

Sherman, G. (1982). "How I do it"-head and neck and plastic surgery. A targeted problem and its solution. Innovative surgical procedure for adenoidectomy. *Laryngoscope*, Vol.92, No. 6 Pt. 1, pp. 700-701.

Shin, JJ & Hartnick, CJ. (2003). Pediatric endoscopic transnasal adenoid ablation. *The Annals of Otology, Rhinology, and Laryngology*. Vol.112, No.6, pp. 511-514.

Skilbeck, CJ; Tweedie, DJ; Lloyd-Thomas, AR & Albert, DM. (2007). Suction diathermy for adenoidectomy: complications and risk of recurrence. *International Journal of Pediatric Otorhinolaryngology*. Vol.71, No.6, pp. 917-920.

Stanislaw, P; Koltai, PJ & Feustel, PJ. (2000). Comparison of power-assisted adenoidectomy vs adenoid curette adenoidectomy. *Archives of Otolaryngology-Head and Neck Surgery*. Vol.126, No.7, pp. 845–849.

Thornval, A. (1969). Wilhelm Meyer and the adenoids. *Archives of Otolaryngology*, Vol.90, No.3, pp. 383-386.

Tolczynski, B. (1955). The recurrence of adenoids. *Canadian Medical Association Journal*, Vol.72, No.9, pp. 672-673.

Van Gelder, L. (1974). Open nasal speech following adenoidectomy and tonsillectomy. *Journal of Communication Disorders*, Vol.7, No.3, pp. 263–267.

Walker, P. (2001). Pediatric Adenoidectomy Under Vision Using Suction-Diathermy Ablation. *Laryngoscope*, Vol.111, No.12, pp. 2173–2177.

Walner, DL; Parker, NP & Miller, RP. (2007). Past and present instrument use in pediatric adenotonsillectomy. *Otolaryngology-Head and Neck Surgery* , Vol.137, No.1, pp. 49-53.

Wan, YM; Wong, KC & Ma, KH. (2005). Endoscopic-guided adenoidectomy using a classic adenoid curette: a simple way to improve adenoidectomy. *Hong Kong Medical Journal*, Vol.11, No.1, pp. 42-44.

Wiatrak, BJ & Wooley, AL. (2005). Pharyngitis and adeno tonsillar disease, In: *Otolaryngology-head and neck surgery*, Cummings, CW; Flint, PW; Harker, LA, et al., pp. 4150–4165, Mosby Inc., Philadelphia, PA.

Yanagisawa, E & Weaver, E. (1997). Endoscopic adenoidectomy with the microdebrider. *Ear Nose and Throat Journal*, Vol.76, No.2, pp. 72-74.

Younis, RT & Lazar, RH. (2002). History and current practice of tonsillectomy. *Laryngoscope*, Vol.112, No.8 Pt.2 Suppl.100, pp. 3–5.

Part 2

Endoscopy of the Central Nervous System

9

Technical and Clinical Evolution of Modern Neuroendoscopy

P. Grunert and J. Oertel
Johannes Gutenberg University
Germany

1. Introduction

Endoscopy plays an important part in the present minimally invasive neurosurgery. The concept, the indications and the technical development have a long history. We can distinguish an early period at the end of 19th and beginning of 20th century and an advanced period toward the end of the 20th century. Each of these periods can be further divided in a time of an obvious medical problem and first idea of possible solution, further in the next step a time of intensive technical improvements and finally the clinal application of endoscopes during surgical interventions. This historical development of endoscopy is true for all branches of surgical application. In this chapter it will described in the field of neurosurgery.

2. History of neuroendoscopy

2.1 Early endoscopic period in the 19th and beginning 20th century
2.1.1 The problem and the first technical solution by Philipp Bozzini

Originally the direct visual inspection of organs such as bladder, female genital organs or digestive tract through natural orifices was restricted to few centimetres with a speculum. To see deeper into the human cavities and to improve the visual quality, a better illumination was necessary.

The physician Philipp Bozzini constructed at the beginning of the 19th century an optical device which enabled to look deeper into the human cavities. Bozzini was born in Mainz Germany 1773 as a son of Italian immigrants (Doglietto et al 2005; Netzhat 2005; Shah 2002). He studied medicine in Mainz and Jena. After obtaining his decree he settled as a physician in Mainz and later in Frankfurt. He constructed a device equipped with a speculum and two chambers one for light conduction and a second for direct visual inspection. Candle light was used for the illumination of the cavity. The isolation between these two chambers was necessary to be not blinded during the inspection. Bozzini called this device "Lichtleiter" (illuminating conduction) (Fig. 1).

First experiments with this "Lichtleiter" were demonstrated in Vienna 1806/1807 in the Josephinum, a foundation of the emperor Joseph II as a college for training of surgeons for the Habsburg army. Bozzini performed there with his optical instrument experiments on cadavers in different orifices of the body. However the medical academy of the Josephinum had not recognized the diagnostic potential of his invention. They estimated the device as a mere curiosity and called the instrument laterna magica in corpore humano (magic lamp in human body). Unfortunately Bozzini died 1809 on typhus and his invention fell for long time into oblivion.

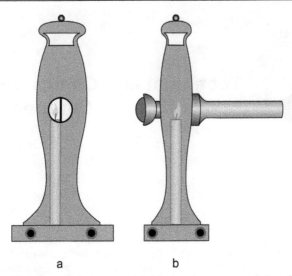

a   b

Fig. 1. Bozzini's "Lichtleiter". Front view(a). Notice the separated chambers for illumination and for observation. The black holes at the bottom are connected with the chamber and provide oxigen for the candle light.The opening on the top schould protect against overheating. Side view(b) with an attached speculum.

2.1.2 Technical development of endoscopes

50 years after the death of Bozzini his idea of illumination was again picked up. The French physician Antoine Jean Dèsormeaux constructed around 1853 a technically improved version of Bozzinis "Lichtleiter". He called this instrument an endoscope (Shah 2002). As the instrument of Bozzini the device was without optical lenses. The innovation in comparison to Bozzinis "Lichtleiter" consisted in the use of a single optical canal without separation of canals for light conductance and for observation. Additionally the candle light of the "Lichtleiter" was replaced by an external light source using gas oil, the light of which was reflected by means of a mirror from a side arm into the optic canal. 1865 he reported about the first clinical applications of this endoscope in the urethra and the bladder (Dèsormeau 1865). In the second half of the 19th century the endoscopes became increasingly important in urology and gynaecology.

Although having precursors in the second half of the 19th century such as Joseph Grünfeld in Vienna and Gustave Trouve in Paris, the development of the modern endoscopes is ascribed to Maximilian Nitze (1848–1912). Nitze organized partly in Berlin, partly in Dresden and partly in Vienna the development of each module of the endoscope the illumination, the optical system and the mechanical system. Under his surveillance the modules were set together to a functioning clinically applicable device. Therefore it is correct to speak of Nitze as the inventor of the modern endoscopy.

Nitze was born in Berlin 1848 (Doglietto et al 2005; Netzhat 2005; Verger-Kuhnke 2007). He studied medicine at different German universities and obtained his medical degree 1874. In 1875 he worked in the state hospital of Dresden. There in the department of gynaecology he saw the necessity to develop an optical device allowing better inspection of the female genital organs. The main idea of Nitze was to transfer the illumination source into the tip of the instrument and to use a system of lenses in imitation of a microscope. The optical problem solved by an order of Nitze Louis Charles Bénèche (Schultheiss & Moll 2009). Bénèche was borne in Berlin as a son of reformed Hugenotts. He was specialized in construction of microscopes. Regarding endoscopes he was confronted with the problem of a long shaft in relation to a very small diameter and thus a very restricted and small view. His ingenious basic solution was to construct a lens system based on the principle of a Kepler telescope (Fig. 2b). In front of the lens system at the very tip was placed wide-angle lens to increase the viewing angle and to bundle the rays inside the shaft. The first lens of the optic system at the tip with a short focus distance f1 produced a real image inside the shaft close to the tip in an upside down position. This image was zoomed by a second lens positioned at the middle of the shaft with a focus distance f2 measuring half of the shaft length. By this optical construction at the proximal end of the endoscope a zoomed and virtual image in upside down position was created (Fig. 2). The mechanical realisation was difficult to be performed in Dresden and Nitze was referred to the Viennes instrument maker Joseph Leiter. For this reason Nitze quit in Dresden and moved to Vienna where he started to work in the surgical department of Leopold knight of Dittel, who was professor of surgery at the university of Vienna and highly interested in urology and endoscopy. There Nitze found the best presuppositions for his scientific work. Already 1879 he presented with Leiter the first cystoscope. Leiter published the prototype 1880 with the title "electro-

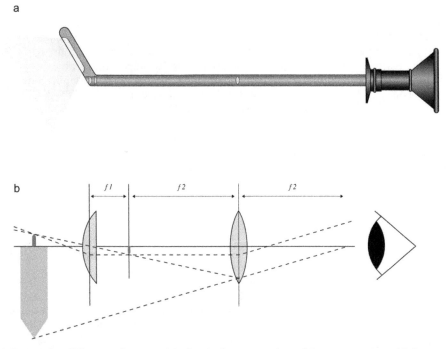

Fig. 2. Principle of Nitze endoscope. Mechanical construction of the cystoscope with lenses within the shaft and the illumination at the tip of the endoscope(a). Optic principle of Nitze endoscope constructed as a "Keppler" telescope producing an imaginary zoomed image in upside down position(b).

endoscopic instruments description and instruction by M. Nitze and J Leiter". Using platinium wire as distal illumination source this prototype had to be equipped with an expensive cooling system to prevent burning (Leiter 1880). After invention of the incandescent electric light bulb 1878 by Thomas Alva Edison the platinium wire was replaced in the endoscope by an electric lamp, which needed no additional cooling system. This endoscope became known as "von Dittel-Leiter cystoscope". The experiences with endoscopic diagnosis and treatment of the bladder published Nitze 1889 as a text book "Lehrbuch der Kystoskopie. Technik und klinische Bedeutung"(text book of cystoscopy: Technique and clinical relevance) (Nitze 1889). The handling of the Nitze endoscopes needed experience and practice because the images were originally upside down. Only 1907 the Swiss Zeiss company developed a prism for the endoscope which reversed the picture again into the upside position.

2.1.3 First clinical applications of endoscopy in neurosurgery

Although the basic development of endoscopes was associated with Germany and Austria, the serial production at the beginning of 20th century shifted to US where Reinhold Wappler (Shah 2002) a manufacturer for medical instruments who emigrated 1890 from Germany to the United States founded the American Cystoscope Makers Incorporation (ACMI). Thus at the beginning of the 20th century endoscopes mostly in form of Nitze type cystoscopes were available in the medical centres in the most American universities. Neurosurgery was in that time a new surgical field with great potential of innovation and technical improvement. Additionally at this time in the US neurosurgery much earlier than in Europe started to separate from the general surgery and was becoming an independent discipline with own development of instruments, new operative approaches and own medical training. This gave an additional push for neurosurgeons to apply new technologies in this promising surgical field. It is therefore not surprising that first endoscopic procedures in the brain started nearly simultaneously at different universities just in the United States in the 20s of the 20th century.

The first neuroendoscopic procedure was performed 1910 in the department of neurological surgery at the Northwest University, Chicago by the urologist Victor Darwin Lespinasse and the neurosurgeon Allen Buckner Kanavel, an innovative neurosurgeon who described also 1909 the infranasal transphenoidal approach to the sella turcica (Northwestern University, Dept. of History). With a cystoscope they coagualated the plexus chorioideus in two children with hydrocephalus. They had not continued with this type of procedure because one child died just after the operation and the other survived only 5 years.

Walter Edward Dandy is also associated with early neuroendoscopy (Hsu et al. 2009). Dandy was in the first half of 20th century one of the most innovative neurosgeons making substantial contributions to all fields of neurosurgery. Dandy was a son of British immigrants. He attended the medical school at John Hopkins University in Baltimore, Maryland and passed the examinations 1910. From 1910-1911 he worked in Cushings Hunterian laboratory at the John Hopkins University. Among many other topics, Dandy studied there experimental hydrocephalus produced in dogs by obstructions of the aqueduct with a cotton piece introduce from the posterior fossa through the IV. ventricle (Aschoff 1999, Dandy & Blackfan 1913, 1914). He published these results together with Blackfan 1913 as a short communication in JAMA (Dandy & Blackfan 1913) and 1914 as a comprehensive basic work in A. J. dis. Child (Dandy & Blackfan 1914). As consequence of their experimental study they distinguished between an obstructive and a communicating hydrocephalus. Based on the experimental work Dandy tried also to explain the so called "idiopathic" hydrocephalus of adults which corresponds mostly to the low pressure hydrocephalus in our present terminology (Dandy 1921). Due to their theoretical results on hydrocephalus the logical therapeutic approach for communicating hydrocephalus consisted in reduction of the CSF production by extirpation or coagulation the choroid plexus in the lateral ventricle (Dandy 1918) and for obstructive hydrocephalus in producing an artificial bypass from the ventricles into the subarachnoidal space. This was achieved anatomically by means of an open ventriculostomy perforating the lamina terminalis from a temporopolar approach (Aschoff et al 1999; King 2003). The disadvantage of this method consisted besides of the occasional necessity to sacrifice the optic nerve also in the frequent occurrence of hygromas (King 2003). To overcome this problem Dandy preferred since 1933 a more posterior extradural subtemporal approach (Aschoff et al 1999, Dandy 1933, King 2003). It is reported that Dandy performed also 2 endoscopic inspections in children with hydrocephalus. However he was not able to complete the operation endoscopically and he had to change to the open approach. Dandy called this endoscope due to the application in the human ventricles from this time on a "ventriculoscope". It is further reported that Dandy published the results of these two endoscopic operations in Johns Hopkins Hospital Bulletin 1922 in two papers "Cerebral ventriculoscopy" and "An operative procedure for hydrocephalus". These citations although often cited remain however dubious because a closer inspection of all publications of Dandy in John Hopkins Hosp. Bull shows, that in this journal were no publications concerning his neuroendoscopic work. Nevertheless the very thorough evaluation of Dandy's correspondence by Hsu (Hsu et al 2009) speaks in favour that Dandy was initially interested in the application of endoscopes in the ventricles and probably he performed also few endoscopic procedures in children with hydrocephalus but gave up very early this technique without publishing his experience on this topic.

Temple Fay and Francis Grant were other two neurosurgeons who tried endoscopically to treat hydrocephalus in children. Temple Fay born in Seattle worked as neurosurgeon at the Temple University Philadelphia. 1923 he published an endoscopic operation of a child with the title "Ventriculoscopy and intraventricular photography in internal hydrocephalus" (Fay & Grant 1923) he treated one year ago together with Francis Grant, the later chairman of the neurosurgery at the Temple University. They described the operation and discussed the potential and the limitations of this method. However their endoscopic operation was not successful.

The most successful pioneer of neuroendoscopy was William Jason Mixter.

Mixter graduated at the Havard medical school and worked as surgeon in the Massachusetts general hospital. There he worked together with his father Samuel Jason Mixter, a recognized surgeon, who described the spinal dorsal stabilisation at the level C1/C2 as early as 1910. With his father William Mixter had 2 beds for treating also neurosurgical patients. Their neurosurgical results were so good, that a neurosurgical unit was established. From 1933–1946 William Mixter was there the chief of the department of neurosurgery. He is well known to the neurosurgery by describing 1934 a disc herniation as reason for sciatica. 1923 William Mixter published the first successful endoscopic ventriculocisternostomy, performed with an cystoscope by transventricular approach through the foramen of Monroe by perforating the floor of the third ventricle (Mixter 1923). Exactly this technique was the example for later endoscopic ventriculostomies in the modern advanced neuroendoscopy.

The only neurosurgeon who continued with neuroendoscopy in the treatment of hydrocephalus till the development of shunt systems was John E. Scarff.

Scarff, finished his study at John Hopkins University 1924 and worked in the Hunterian laboratory at John Hopkins University between 1925-1927. He operated there also with

Dandy. Later working at the Columbia University in New York he continued with the neurosurgeon Byron Stookey to treat hydrocephalus as developed in the 20s (Scarff 1936, 1951, Scarff & Stookey 1936) perforating the lamina terminalis and the floor of the third ventricle in patients with obstructive hydrocephalus.

2.2 Advanced period of neuroendoscopy at the end of 20th century
2.2.1 Idea and motivation

Although the shunt operations were very successful in the treatment of hydrocephalus of any origin, they had typical complications due to implanted material such as shunt infections and shunt obstructions. This draw back made necessary in the life of the patient often repeated operative revisions. One of the starting ideas of the modern neuroendoscopy was therefore to reintroduce the endoscopic methods instead of shunt implantations in the treatment of obstructive hydrocephalus with technically advanced instrumensts. The endoscopic procedure in form of the ventriculocysternostomy had the advantage of being a single procedure and being more physiological regarding the CSF circulation than the shunt systems using a valve with constant flow. Other motivation to apply endoscopy in neurosurgery was the general trend in the operative disciplines in the late 80th toward a minimally invasive surgery.

2.2.2 Technical development

Present neuroendoscopy would not be possible without substantial improvements in image quality and endoscope flexibility. The major breakthrough in the endoscope technology and optical quality goes back to the work of Harold Horaz Hopkins (1918–1994), a professor of physics at the university of Reading, United Kingdom (Mc Combie & Smith 1998). He have probably remained only a recognized physicist, if he had not been approached 1951 at a dinner party by a physician who complained about the poor image quality and rigidity of the endoscopes. Encouraged by the subsequent discussion Hopkins developed the idea of using glass fibres for image transmission. 1951 he assembled a bundle of glass fibres with a higher refractory index of the core than of the cladded coat to improve light transmission over a longer distance by total reflexion (Fig. 3).

1953 he and his fellow researcher produced a bundle of fibres with precisely the same order at the proximal and distal ends, leading to a coherent image. They published their results in Nature 1954 (Hopkins & Kapany 1954). In the following years there was no interest from the industry in the technique and Hopkins could not continue his research. He sent letters about his invention and obtained a positive response only from Basil Hirschowitz, a gastroenterologist in Ann Arbor, US. He visited Hopkins and discussed the details of his work. After his return to US Hirschowitz continued the work of Hopkins. He improved the technique using a better permanent coating of the fibres. The prototype of this flexible fiberscope was presented for the first time at a meeting of gastroenterologists in Colorado Springs in 1957 (Hirschowitz et al 1958, McCombie & Smith 1998). To improve the image quality the number of glass fibres increased up to 200 000. For this amount of fibres the preservation of the topological fibre arrangement at both ends of the fibre bundle was essential. 1975 Max Eppstein, a German scientist developed a system of isolation which preserved the alignment of the fibers and thus guaranteed an undistorted image during twisting of the endoscope (Eppstein 1975, 1980). The development of the flexible fiberscope was completed by implementation of an external cold light source and an adjustable tip of the endoscope.

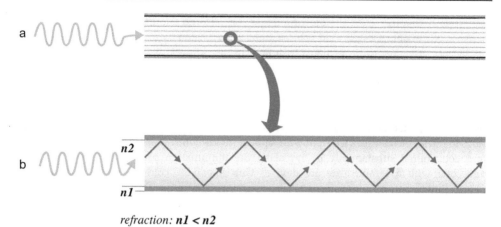

refraction: n1 < n2

Fig. 3. Principle of Hopkins flexible glass fiberscope. Complete fibre bundle (a). Single fibre showing the propagation of the image over long distance inside the endoscope(b). This works by total reflection based on the lower refraction of the coating n1 in comparison to the glass fibre n2.

In his theoretical work as physicist Hopkins made substantial contributions to mathematical calculations of relay lenses aberrations and its possible compensation (Hopkins 1950, Hopkins & Tiziani 1966). This theoretical knowledge was the presupposition for his main endoscopic invention the improvement of the image quality of the rigid endoscopes. His main idea was to replace the relay of lenses with long interspaces of air by rod glass lenses with small air gaps between the appropriate cut rod edges. This reversed the proportion of air and glass inside the shaft. The higher refractive index of glass in comparison with air improved the light transmission by a factor of 9 (Fig. 4).

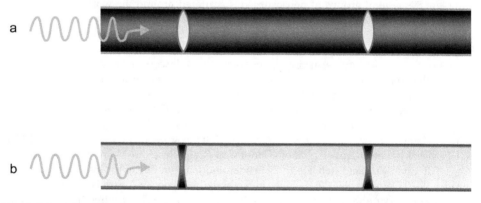

Fig. 4. Principle of rigid rod lens endoscope. Nitze optics with small lenses and long air interspaces between the lenses (a). Hopkins rigid rod lens endoscope (b) with reversed portion of glass to air in comparison to Nitze optic improving the optical quality and illumination by a factor of 9.

Additionally this increased the viewing angle and allowed simultaneously to decrease the diameter of the optics. Supported was the light transmission by an anti-reflection coating of the lenses. All this improvements resulted in an approximately 80 fold increase of illumination in comparison to the available standard rigid endoscopes of that time. The invention was made 1960 and the first prototype was presented 1961 during an urological meeting in Brazil (McCombie & Smith 1998). It followed the same silence and ignorance. In 1964 Hopkins presented the same invention again during a lecture in Düsseldorf. This time, however, the potential of his invention was immediately recognized by the attending Karl Storz, the head of the Storz Company for optical instruments. A fruitful cooperation began. Storz contributed substantially by replacing the illumination source from the tip of the endoscope with a remote external device. This so-called "cold light" was originally a halogen light that was transported via separate glass fibres through the shaft of the endoscope to its tip. 1967 the first commercial product was introduced to the market. Today xenon light sources are used instead halogen, whose effective power was restricted to 250 W and caused a yellow image quality.

The technical development of rigid rod-lens endoscopes was completed by the introduction of video cameras for imaging to replace direct observation by surgeon looking through the endoscope. For this purpose light, miniature electronic cameras equipped with charge-coupled (CCDs) transforming the light into a digital signal contributed essentially to the miniaturization of the cameras, which could be directly connected to the endoscope oculars with a sterile cover. This set up originally assembled for urology, minimally invasive abdominal surgery and arthroscopy was commercially available at the end of the 1980s.

For optical reasons the application of endoscopy is restricted to cavities of the human body. In the intracranial space this are the ventricles and the epiarachnoid space. Therefore pathologies in the ventricles constituted also the first applications of this minimally invasive endoscopic technique.

2.2.3 Clinical application

In the late 80s several groups of neurosurgeons scattered around the world such as Patric Kelly (Kelly et al 1986), Kim Manwaring and Allan Cohen in US, Jaques Caemaert in Belgium (Caemeaert 1992), (Jones et al 1996). Christiane Sainte-Rose in France (Sainte-Rose 1992) and Nigel Jones and Charles Teo in Australia made positive experience with the ETV technique. Strong activity regarding the systematic endoscope related basic anatomical research, the adaptation of endoscopic instruments to neurosurgical requirements and the indications, applications and standards in the neuroendoscopy are associated with 5 centres on the European continent. Activity at these centres started nearly simultaneously and independently of each other around 1990. Notable neurosurgical centres were in Germany Dieter Hellwig and Bernhard Bauer in Marburg (Hellwig & Bauer 1992, Hellwig et al 1997), Axel Perneczky, Peter Grunert, Nikolai Hopf and Klaus Resch in Mainz (Perneczky et al 1994, 1998) and Michael Gaab, Henry Schröder and Joachim Oertel in Greifswald (Gaab & Schröder 1998, Oertel et al 2009). Further in Netherland Nijmegen Andre Grotenhuis a close friend of Perneczky and in Belgium Ghent Jaques Caemaert. This centres had a common endoscopic concept and a synchronous development regarding neuroendoscopic technical innovations and an increase in clinical experience with a similar number of surgical patients. Despite some different opinions on details, the activity of these centres can be summarized due to their lasting effect abroad as a common "continental" development of modern contemporary neuroendoscopy. Their knowledge on endoscopy spread over the world due to many practical international courses organized in each centre every year.

The first practical experience in neuroendoscopy was gathered during intraventricular third ventriculostomies for the treatment of obstructive hydrocephalus. This was also in the 90s the most frequent type of neuroendopic operations.

Most of the centres performed initially the endoscopic third ventriculostomies (ETV) by frame based stereotactic technique. This enabled the planning of a precise trajectory through the foramen of Monro to the floor of the third ventricle. Additionally for the long nose-heavy cystoscopes the stereotactic frame provided in that time an excellent stable holding of the endoscope and made possible for the surgeon to work with both hands simultaneously. A disadvantage of framebased endoscopy consisted in the restricted mechanical flexibility to change the position of the endoscope under visual endoscopic view. This was partially overcome by construction of a guiding block with a ball joint which allowed under 0° a straight precise introduction of the endoscope and simultaneously after unlocking the endoscope in the block to have a free play in every direction under visual endoscopic view of 15° (Fig. 5).

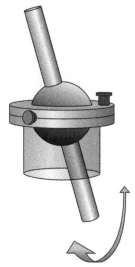

Fig. 5. Guiding block with ball joint. The ball joint allowed movement of the endoscope in any direction in a range of 15°. The upper metallic disc with the screws at the guiding block provided a fixation of the endoscope.

The stereotactic endoscopic third ventriculostomy was performed using CT images. With the CT adapted localisation frame the coordinates of two target points were calculated one at the level of the foramen of Monro and a second few slices below at the level of the floor of the third ventricle. Since in transversal CT slices the floor of the third ventricle was in general not visible the slice at the upper level of dorsum sellae was chosen for calculation. To protect the important surrounding anatomical structures the optimal target point was in the midline immediately behind the dorsum sellae and in front of the tip of the basilar artery (Fig. 6).

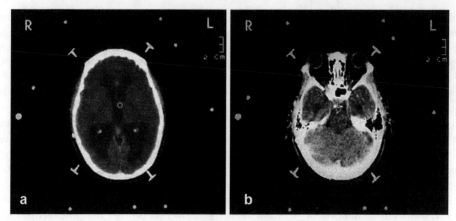

Fig. 6. CT-based stereotactic calculation of two target points for the ventriculostomy. Calculation of the foramen of Monro visualized by a circle (a) and the target at the floor of the third ventricle between the dorsum sellae and the basilar artery in the midline (b).

This CT –based calculation constituted the planed area for perforation. The final area for perforation was decided during the endoscopic procedure respecting the directly visible anatomical structures at the floor of the third ventricle. These two calculated target points one at the level of the foramen Monro and the second behind the dorsum sellae defined geometrically a line in the space which corresponded to the optimal trajectory (Fig. 7).

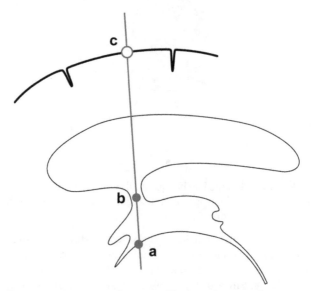

Fig. 7. Principle of stereotactic ventriculostomy. The coordinates of two points in the space were calculated, (a) at the level of the floor of the third ventricle and (b) at the level of the foramen of Monro. These two points defined a straight line in the space and thus implicitly also the trepanation point respectively the point (c) where the cortex was perforated.

Additionally these two target points determined implicitly the trepanation point. In most of the cases area thus defined trepanation point was within an area 1cm before till 1cm behind the coronar suture in the anterior posterior direction and 1.5 cm–3 cm laterally from the midline. For these stereotactic procedures originally a 6 mm diameter rigid Wolff cystoscope (Fig. 8) with four channels one 1.5 mm diameter working channel 2.3 mm optical channel, and two channels for rinsing were used. Because of their much better optical quality the rigid endoscopes were superior for neurosurgical purposes in the ventricles than the flexible fibrescopes.

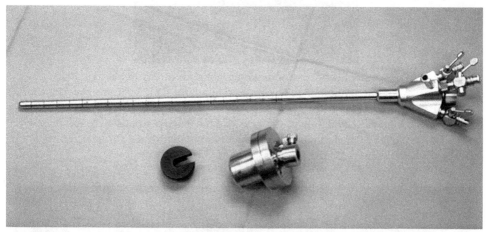

Fig. 8. First stereotactic endoscopic equipment in Mainz. Wolff 6mm cystoscope with 4 channels at the top. At the bottom: guiding block with the ball joint (right side) and a plastic disc for adjusting the endoscope in a coaxial direction of 0°.

After stereotactic calculation of the trajectory the head of the patient in the frame was fixed in the operating theatre by Mayfield adapter to the operating table in an inclination of 20°–30°. By this inclination the burr-hole was at the top and CSF leakage from the lateral ventricle during the endoscopy was minimal. This precaution guaranteed that the endoscope was advanced in the ventricles entirely within CSF and disturbing optical artefacts in form of mirror images could be avoided. After setting a burr-hole, opening of the dura mater a corticotomy was performed and slightly dilated on the surface to let easily introduce the endoscope into the brain substance. In the depth of 4.5 cm–5 cm the endoscope was fixed the trocar removed and the optic introduced. Usually at this level the endoscope tip was inside the lateral ventricle and a view of the lateral ventricle centred on the foramen of Monro was possible (Fig. 9).

Inside the lateral ventricle under visual control the endoscope was advanced to the foramen of Monro. To prevent injury during the passage through the foramen of Monro it was essential that the optical and mechanical axes coincided. For this reason during introduction of the endoscope the 0° optics was always used. At the level of the foramen the anatomical structures of the fornix and the deep intracerebral veins had to be respected. In the third ventricle the perforation was performed in front of the mamillary bodies and behind the dorsum sellae and the infundibular recessus (Fig. 10).

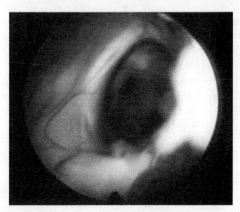

Fig. 9. Foramen of Monro during first endoscopic ventriculostomy in Mainz 1992. Endoscopic view of the right foramen of Monro confined medially by the fornix. The white spot in the image corresponds to a piece of ependyma wall sticking on the optics of the endoscope. It covers partialy the choroid plexus and the thalamostriatal vein. The floor of the third ventricle is visible through the foramen of Monro with a red vascularized spot corresponding to the infundibular recessus.

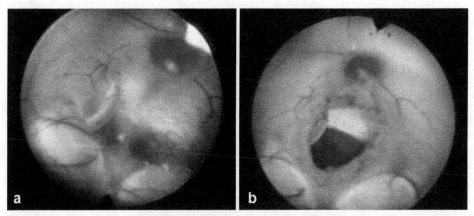

Fig. 10. Endoscopic view of the floor of the third ventricle during first ventriculostomy in Mainz 1992. Anatomy before perforation (a). Notice the mamillary bodies, and the posterior communicating artery. The red spot is the recessus infudibularis. Floor of the third ventricle after perforation (b). Notice the perforation between the dorsum sellae and in front of the mamillary bodies.

In patients with long lasting hydrocephalus the floor of the third ventricle was often thinned out to a translucent membrane. In these cases the whole anatomical structures laterally and under the floor of the third ventricle were visible including the basilar artery, the posterior communicating arteries and the occulomotor nerves. The perforation was performed bluntly with a Fogarty catheter or a forceps and dilated in steps with a balloon catheter till a diameter between 5 mm – 7 mm was reached.

The ventriculocysternostomies were very effective in the treatment of obstructive hydrocephalus. We performed the first 40 patients with the stereotactic framebased technique and the consecutive with free hand technique. From 150 evaluated patients operated between 1992–2000 best results with a long lasting success rate of 84% were obtained in adults with benign aqueduct stenosis followed by adults with a tumour obstructing the aqueduct with a success rate of 81.6%. Infants had less good outcome. A closure of the stoma was a rare event. In these patients we performed a reventriculostmy and were successful in 75% of the patients. Patients who had no profit of the ventriculostomy or worsened obtained a ventriculo-peritoneal shunt.

Comprehensive survey of the techniques and results of the third ventriculostomy in obstructive hydrocephalus can be found in the excellent review article of Hellwig published in the Neurosurgical Review (Hellwig et al 2005).

This above mentioned basic endoscopic technique with slight modifications was applied in the 90th for pellucidotomies in cases of unilateral dilatation of the lateral ventricle. Further the endoscopic technique was used for opening of cysts inside the ventricle or in the ventricle wall including the so called "captured fourth ventricle" in the posterior fossa. To prevent a secondary closure of the perforation for this last type of pathology a catheter was implanted through the aqueduct into the cyst in the fourth ventricle connecting the fourth ventricle with the third and lateral ventricles . Additionally in selected patients with thin good accessible membrane in the aqueduct an aqueductoplasty by opening and dilatation of the membrane inside the aqueduct was performed. However the complication rate of the aqueductoplasty was due to the nuclei and pathways in the midbrain immediately around the aqueduct higher than for the ventriculostomies. With higher experience and improved technology for hemostasis intraventricula lesions such as colloid cysts and intraventricular tumours were also removed or biopsied by minimally invasive endoscopic technique.

Hopf adapted the neuronavigation systems to endoscopes and the endoscopes could be used as apointers for planning the trajectory and for additional orientation during surgery (Hopf et al 1999). The second generation of endoscopes were already adapted to the neurosurgical requirements they were shorter and not so nose-heavy. This improved the handling of the endoscope by one person. With greater experience the frame based stereotactic technique was replaced by a free hand technique supported by holding arms. These were at the beginning two Leila retractor arms and later special arm holders which were attached to the operating table. The development of the endoscopes was pushed on ahead by the Storz, Wolff and Aesculap companies.

At the beginning of 90s Norbert Hüwel from Mainz used flexible endoscopes during syringostomies in the treatment of syringomyelia. He introduced the flexible endoscope into the syrinx cavity and fenestrated the membranes inside the syrinx in addition to the implantation of a syringo-subarachnoidal tube. However in patients with a syringomyelia due to Arnold Chiari II malformation the resection of the cerebellar tonsil with the aim to improve the CSF flow at the craniospinal level was superior to the endoscopic treatment.

In this time in Mainz Perneczky integrated the endoscope during microvascular procedures and resections of tumours to control the position of the aneurysma clip or with high degree optics "around the corner" to control the completeness of the tumour resection at the skull base. The idea was to use the endoscope during microsurgical interventions at a particular stage of the operation as a tool similar as any other surgical instrument such as the scalpel the suction or the drill. By means of the endoscope the illumination was transported into the depth of the operating area and complemented the view from the perspective of the microscope. By the endoscope more anatomical details could be distinguished. This proved to be valuable for instance during microvascular decompressions and all types of skull base surgery. Perneczky coined for this type of operations the term "endoscope assisted microsurgery"(Perneczky et al 1994, Pernecky & Fries 1998).

This idea of transportation of the illumination by means of an endoscope into the depth of the operating area was quickly picked up by neurosurgeons in the US and applied for transnasal pituitary surgery by Hae-Dong Jho (Jho 1996a, 1996b) 1996 in the endoscopic department of the centre for minimally invasive neurosurgery in Pittsburg. In Europe this type of endoscopic pituitary surgery was introduced 1998 by Cappabianca in Naples (Cappabianca et al 1998). By this minimally invasive endoscopic approach Amin Kassam (Kassam et al 2010) described removal also of lesions at the frontal skull base and clivus. In Mainz endoscopic pituitary and skull base surgery was introduced 2003 by the pupils of Perneczky, Robert Reisch and Patra Charalampaki. After both left Mainz, this work was continued by Ali Ayyad and Jens Conrad. Meanwhile the scope of endoscopic neurosurgical operations includes also spinal and periferal nerve surgery. Joachim Oertel coming from Hannover, where he was working with Gaab, introduced 2009 the spinal endoscopy also in Mainz.

3. Conclusion

From the historical point of view we can distinguish two periods in neuroendoscopy. An early period at the beginning of the modern neurosurgery in the 20s of the 20th century and an advanced period since the late 80s of the 20th century. In each period the clinical application was proceeded, accompanied and closely related to the technical development of the appropriate endoscopes. We can summarize this early neuroendoscopy period as a time of the first trials. They took place at different universities in the United States by pioneers of the modern neurosurgery. They recognized already in that time the potential use of the neuroendoscopy in the ventricles, but they gave up this technique after few trials due to technical and optical limitations of the available endoscopes. In contrary to the early period of neuroendoscopy the modern endoscopes fulfil all requirements and expectations regarding optical quality, safety and flexibility necessary also for neurosurgical applications. Therefore in this advanced period of neuroendoscopy the endoscopes became an accepted and permanent tool during neurosurgical interventions in a variety of neurosurgical fields.

4. Acknowledgment

The authors thank Stefan Kindel for his accurate, detailed and likewise artistically attractive illustrations.

5. References

Aschoff, A.; Kremer, P.; Hashemi, B. & Kunze S. (1999). The scientific history of hydrocephalus and its treatment. Neurosurg. Review 22: 67-93

Cappabianca, P.; Alfieri, A. & Devitiis, E. (1998). Endoscopic endonasal transspenoidal approach to the sella: towards functional endoscopic pituitari surgery (FEPS) Minim invas neurosurg. 41: 66-73

Caemaert, J.; Abdullah, J.; Calliaw, L.; Carton, D.; Dhooge, C. & Coster, R. (1992). Endoscopic treatment of suprasellar arachnoidal cysts. Acta neurochirurgica (Wien) 119: 68-73

Dandy, WE. & Blackfan, KD. (1913). An experimental and clinical study on internal hydrocephalus. JAMA. 61: 2216-2217

Dandy, WE. & Blackfan, KD. (1914). Internal hydrocephalus. An experimental clinical and pathological study. Am J. Dis Child 8: 406-482

Dandy, WE. (1918). Extirpation of the choroid plexus of the lateral ventricles in communicating hydrocephalus. Ann. Surg. 37: 569-579

Dandy, WE. (1921). The cause of so called idiopathic hydrocephalus Johns Hopkins Hosp. Bull. 32: 67-74

Dandy, WE. (1932). Practice of surgery, vol XII, chapter 1, (Dean Lewis ed.), WF Prior Company, Hagerstown

Dèsormeaux, AJ. (1865). De l'endoscope et de ses applications au diagnostique et au traitment de affections de l'urethre et de la vessie, JB Baillier, Paris

Doglietto, F.; Prevello, DM.; Jane, JA.; Han, J. & Laws ER. (2005). A brief history of endoscopic transsphenoidal surgery – from Philipp Bozzini to the first world congress of endoscopic skull base surgery. JNS Neurosurgical focus: vol 19(6) DOI: 10.3171/foc. 2005.19.6.4

Eppstein, M. & Marhic, ME. (1975) Fiber optic laser illumination.Proc IEEE 63: 727

Eppstein,M. (1980). Developments of optical instrumentation. Science 210:280-285

Fay, T. & Grant, FC. (1923). Ventriculoscopy and intraventricular photography in internal hydrocephalus. JAMA 80:461-463

Gaab, MR. & Schröder, HW. (1998). Neuroendoscopic approach to intraventricular lesions. J. Neurosurg. 88: 496-505

Hellwig, D.; Grotenhuis, JA.; Tirakotai, W.; Riegel, T.; Schulte, DM.; Bauer, BL. & Bertalanffy, H. (2005). Endoscopic third ventriculostomy for obstructive hydrocephalus. Neurosurg. Rev. 28: 1-34

Hellwig, D. & Bauer, BL. (1992). Minimally invasive neurosurgery by means of ultrathin endoscope. Acta neurochir Suppl. (Wien) 54: 63-68

Hellwig, D.; Benes, L.; Bertalanffy, H.&Bauer, BL. (1997). Endoscopic stereotaxy – an eight year experience. Stereotact. Funct. Neurosurg. 68: 90-97

Hirschowitz, BI.; Curtis, LE.; Peters, CW. & Pollard,HP. (1958). Demonstration of a new gastroscope the "fiberscope". Gastroenterology 35: 50-53

Hopf, N.; Grunert, P.; Darabi, K.; Busert, C. & Bettag, M. (1999). Frameless neuronavigation applied to endoscopic surgery. Minim. Invas Neurosurg. 42: 187-193

Hopkins, HH. (1950). Wave theory of aberrations. Oxford university press.

Hopkins, HH. & Kapany, NS. (1954). A flexible fiberscope using static scanning. Nature 1954; 173:39-41

Hopkins, HH. & Tiziani, HJ. (1966). A theoretical and experimental study of lens centring errors and their influence on image quality. Brit J. Appl. Phys. 17: 33-55

Huewel, N.; Perneczky, A.; Urban V.& Fries G. (1992). Neuroendoscopic technique for the operative treatment of septated syringomyelia. Acta Neurochir. Suppl. 54:59-62 Walter Dandy and neuroendoscopy. Historical vignette. JNS Neurosurgical Focus (3) DOI: 10.3171/2009.1. PEDS08342

Jho, HD. & Carau, RL. (1996). Endoscopy assisted transshenoidal surgery of pituitary adenoma. Technical note. Acta neurochirurgica. 138:1416-1425

Jones, RFC.; Stenting WA.& Brydon M.(1990). Endoscopic third ventriculostomy. Neurosurgery 26: 86-92

Kassam, AB.; Prevedello, DM.; Carau, RL.; Suyderman, CH.; Thomas, A. & Horowitz, MB. (2010). Endoscopic endonasal skullbase surgery. Analysis of complications in the author's initial 800 patients. J. Neurosurgery. PMID 21166570

Kelly, PJ.; Goerss, SJ.; Kall, BA. & Kispert, DB. (1986). Computed tomography based stereotactic third ventriculostomy: technical note. Neurosurgery. 18: 791-794

King, RB. (2003). Third ventriculostomy for internal hydrocephalus complicated by unrecognized subdural hygroma and hematoma: a case report of a patient treated by Walter Dandy. JNS. DOI: 10.3171/jns 2003.985.1136

Leiter, J. (1880). Elektro-Endoskopische Instrumente. Beschreibung und Instruction durch M. Nitze und J. Leiter. Wilhelm Braunmüller und Söhne Wien.

Mc Combie, CW. & Smith, J. (1998). Harold Horaz Hopkins. 6. December 1918–22. October 1994. Biographical memories fellows of the royal sociaty. 44: 239–252

WJ Mixter, WJ. (1923). Ventriculoscopy and puncture of the floor of the third ventricle. Boston med Surg J. 188: 277–278

Netzhat, C. (2005). Bozzini the beginning of early modern endoscopy, chapter 6 (a), the era Nitzechapter chapter 11(b) History of Endoscopy, http//laparoscopy.blogs.com /endoscopyhistory

Nitze, M. (1889). Lehrbuch der Kystoskopie. Technik und klinische Bedeutung. Von Bergmann Verlag, Wiesbaden

Northwestern university Feinberg school of medicine. Dept. of history. http//www. feinberg.northwestern.edu/neurosurgery/residency/history

Oertel, JM.; Baldauf, J.; Schröder, HW. & Gaab, MR. (2009). Endoscopic options in children: experience with 134 procedures J. Neurosurg. (Suppl. Pädiatr.) 3:81–89

Perneczky, A.; Cohen, A.; George, B. & Kanno, T. (1994). Editorial. Minimal. Invas. Neurosurgery. 37:1

Perneczky, A. & Fries, G. (1998). Endoscope-assisted brain surgery Part I. Evolution, basic concept and current technique. Neurosurgery. 42: 557-569

Sainte- Rose, C. (1992). Third ventriculostomy. Neuroendoscopy, Manwaring HK.& Crone KR.eds, Neuroendoscopy, Mary Ann Lieber, New York

Scarff, JE. (1936). Endoscopic treatment of hydrocephalus: description of the ventriculoscope and primary report of cases. Arch. Neurol.Psychiatry 35: 853-861

Scarff, JE.& B. Stookey, B. (1936). Treatment of obstructive hydrocephalus by third ventriculostomy. Report of two cases. Arch Neur. 36: 1400-1411

Scarff, JE. (1951). Treatment of obstructive hydrocephalus by puncture of lamina terminalis at the floor of the third ventricle. J. Neurosurg. 8: 204-213

Shah. J. (2002). Endoscopy through the ages. BJU International. 89: 645-652

Schultheiss, D.& Moll, F. (2009). Die Geschichte der Urologie in Dresden (The history of urology in Dresden), Springer Verlag, ISBN 9783642035937, Berlin

Verger-Kuhnke, AB.; Reuter, MA. & Beccaria,ML. (2007). Biography of Maximilian Nitze (1848–1906) and his contribution to urology. Acta Urol. Esp. 31: 697-704

10

Endoscopy in Intracranial Pathology

Marwan Najjar and Ali Turkmani
American University of Beirut
Lebanon

1. Introduction

The use of endoscopy in intracranial pathology may be divided into two main subsets of procedures. The first subset entails the use of the endoscope in the management and treatment of intracranial intra-ventricular pathologies such as hydrocephalus, arachnoid cysts, and intra-ventricular tumors. The second includes trans-nasal and sinus endoscopy to manage mostly pituitary tumors, and other skull base pathologies, in addition to endoscope assisted microsurgery. This chapter, thus, will be divided into two parts to shed light on these two main endoscopic techniques used in intracranial pathologies.

2. Intracranial intra-ventricular Endoscopy

The first part of this chapter on Endoscopy for Intracranial Pathology will focus mainly on intracranial intra-ventricular neuroendoscopy. As the brain is a solid organ, neuroendoscopy is mostly limited to intra-ventricular endoscopy in the cerebrospinal fluid filled ventricular cavities. This is particularly facilitated in the setting of dilated ventricles or hydrocephalus. Obstructive hydrocephalus is actually one of the most common indications for endoscopic management in modern neurosurgical practice. In addition to management of hydrocephalus, a variety of intra-ventricular and other deep seated intracranial lesions may be approached endoscopically.

2.1 History

Endoscopic management of hydrocephalus was attempted as early as 1910 when VL L'Espinasse, a urologist, used the cystoscope to cauterize the choroid plexus (Hellwig et al, 2005). Dandy later refined this method and coined the terms ventriculoscope and ventriculoscopy for the instrument and technique. Mixter then, in 1923, performed the first successful endoscopic third ventriculostomy (ETV), and proposed ETV as a treatment option in occlusive hydrocephalus. Putnam later, in 1934 and then Scarff in 1936 reported on their series of patients treated with endoscopic coagulation of the choroid plexus using the special coagulation-endoscope. The mortality and morbidity of the choroid plexus coagulation procedures was high, and with the introduction of valved shunts in 1949, endoscopic management of hydrocephalus fell out of favor. With improved optics over the past two decades, and since the use of valved shunts is fraught with several known complications, endoscopic management of hydrocephalus regained intense interest.

2.2 Endoscopic third ventriculostomy for hydrocephalus

Endoscopic third ventriculostomy (ETV) is emerging now as one of the preferred treatment modalities for obstructive hydrocephalus (Schroeder & Niendorf, 2002) .The conventional ventriculostomy is simply a ventriculo-subarachnoidal shunt through a minimally invasive endoscopic approach with excellent endoscopic exposure and handling. The progress in magnetic resonance imaging (MRI) and Cine–Phase Contrast MRI in particular offers a reliable method for pre- and post-operative assessment of the patients (Fukuhara et al, 1999; Schroeder et al, 2000).

The surgical technique entails entering the foramen of Monroe after cannulating the lateral ventricle via a coronal burr hole and then after inspecting the floor of the third ventricle, perforating the floor with a blunt stylet or instrument and enlarging the perforation using a fogarthy balloon catheter or the endoscopic forceps. Inspection of the pre-pontine cistern is then performed and obstructing membranes may be similarly opened. A rigid neuroendoscope is usually placed through the burr hole performed approximately 2-3 cm lateral to the midline and just anterior to the coronal suture. Although flexible fiberscopes have been used for ETV, they offer a considerably inferior image quality and there is usually difficulty with their orientation, guidance, and fixation (Kamikawa et al, 2001). Before surgery, the relationship between the floor of the third ventricle and the tip of basilar artery is carefully evaluated on the sagittal MRI to reduce the risk of injury to the basilar artery (Wilcock et al, 1997).

ETV is considered a simple, fast, and safe procedure (Schroeder et al, 2002). Obstructive hydrocephalus represents the most important indication for ETV (Jones et al, 1994). Shunt independence, is the ultimate measure of the successful outcome of ETV. ETV for obstructive hydrocephalus has a failure rate of 20–40% in various series (Siomin et al, 2002). The failure rate, however, is markedly reduced, if certain selection criteria are taken into consideration, and these include obstructive hydrocephalus, age more than one year, history free of meningitis and subarachnoid hemorrhage, normal ventricular anatomy, tectal gliomas, posterior fossa tumors, and pineal region tumors (Bargallò et al, 2005; Li et al, 2005; O Brien et al, 2006; Oi et al, 2001; Pople et al, 2001; Sainte-Rose et al, 2001; Wellons et al, 2002).

Patients with obstructive hydrocephalus secondary to idiopathic aqueductal stenosis, tectal gliomas, and third or fourth ventricular tumors seem to have the best outcome after ETV (figure 1a&b) Communicating hydrocephalus secondary to meningitis or intra-ventricular or subarachnoid hemorrhage is associated with a higher failure rate (Siomin et al, 2002). Age seems also to be a very important factor, where infants less than 1 year of age have a higher failure rate, and in some series, under 6 months in particular. Studies have demonstrated a gradual decrease in ventricle size over months to years postoperatively, coinciding with clinical improvement (Buxton et al, 2002). The size of the ventricles is not a good predictor to use in the evaluation of the outcome within three months of surgery (Feng et al, 2004). In the early postoperative period, a decrease in the size of the ventricles is often minimal and not visible before three to four weeks. Cine-phase contrast MRI may be used to determine the patency of the stoma and may be used in follow up and has been demonstrated to correlate with patency of the stoma intraoperatively, where minor flow appears to be an early sign of closure (Fukuhara et al, 1999).

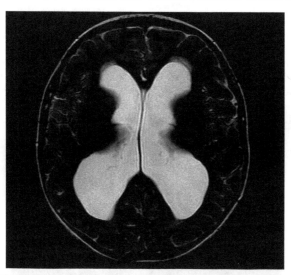

Fig. 1. a. Axial T2W MRI sequence demonstrating hydrocephalus secondary to tectal glioma. The child underwent endoscopic 3rd ventriculostomy with good outcome.

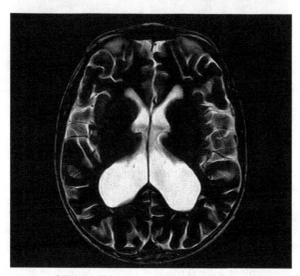

Fig. 1. b. Post operative axial T2W MRI sequence one year after surgery showing reduced ventricular size compared to the pre-operative examination.

A complication rate range of 0-20% is reported (Schroeder et al, 2002). The most serious complication of ETV is the injury to the basilar artery. The correct fenestration site is crucial for ETV success, which is recommended to be halfway between the infundibular recess and the mammillary bodies in the midline, just behind the dorsum sellae. Other complications reported are subdural hygroma (figure 2), CSF leakage, ventriculitis, diabetes incipidus, and third cranial nerve injury (Buxton et al, 2002; Fukuhara et al, 1999; Sainte-Rose et al, 2001). In one series of 193 ETVs done in 188 patients, permanent morbidities occurred in 1.6%, and 7.8% had transient morbidities (Schroeder et al, 2002). There were two deaths (1%). It was noted that during the course of the study, the complication rate dropped significantly, and no deaths or permanent morbidities occurred in the last 100 patients. In our unpublished series of 42 ETV procedures done for various causes of hydrocephalus, we had no procedure related complications, other than stoma occlusion in 4 of the patients necessitating ventriculo-peritoneal shunting. When done by an experienced endoscopist, and for the proper indications, we feel that ETV has a high success rate with a minimal chance of complications.

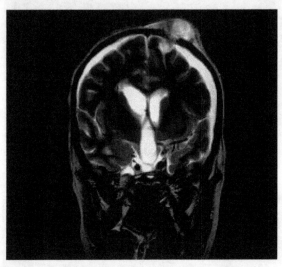

Fig. 2. Coronal T2W MRI sequence showing bilateral subdural hygromas and subcutaneous collection post endoscopic 3rd ventriculostomy for hydrocephalus. The stoma later blocked and a shunt was placed.

Whereas endoscopic 3rd ventriculostomy has a definite role in the management of 3rd ventricular, pineal region, thalamic, and tectal lesions, allowing simultaneous treatment of hydrocephalus and biopsy of the lesion, the role of ETV as a routine preoperative measure to treat hydrocephalus in posterior fossa tumors is less defined. In one study where patients with hydrocephalus and posterior fossa tumors either received ETV before resective surgery or conventional management, ETV dropped the need for a shunt from 20% to 6% (Sainte-Rose et al, 2001). Other authors confirm that ETV is an efficient procedure for controlling hydrocephalus associated with posterior fossa tumors, but find that the low rate of persistent hydrocephalus after tumor removal (9-12%) does not justify adopting routine preoperative third ventriculostomies (Fritsch et al, 2005; Morelli et al, 2005). Despite being successful, the two ETV procedures done before microsurgical resection in our previously reported series do not provide sufficient evidence to support performing ETV as a routine preoperative procedure (Najjar et al, 2010).

2.3 Endoscopic management of intra-ventricular lesions
Intra-ventricular lesions are often deep seated intra-cranial pathologies that pose a diagnostic and therapeutic challenge. They are often associated with hydrocephalus, and dealt with via stereotactic or open biopsies along with a CSF diversion procedure such as

ventriculo-peritoneal shunting. Endoscopy is quickly rising as a minimally invasive technique that is extremely helpful in the management of certain intraventricular lesions thru the ability to get pathological tissue diagnosis, CSF markers, and treat the accompanying hydrocephalus, all in the same procedure. As just mentioned, these patients often undergo at least 2 different procedures such as stereotactic biopsies, shunts, and even bilateral shunts. The endoscopic procedure may be the only procedure needed in many of these patients who harbor chemosensitive or radiosensitive tumors that do not need further removal surgery. In others, endoscopic resection of cystic or small intraventricular lesions may be the definitive surgical management.

Endoscopic tumor management was successful in up to 96% of the cases in one series where 23 out of 24 biopsies and 2 out of 2 resections were successful (Souweidane 2005). In another series of 34 patients with pineal region tumors, histological diagnosis was obtained in 94% of the cases (Pople et al, 2001). Definitive treatment was then designed for each tumor according to the diagnosis. In our reported series, 8 out of 9 endoscopic biopsies were successful (89%), and the procedure was definitive in all the patients, where none required additional surgery (Najjar et al, 2010). Neuroendoscopic procedures, thus, have a great advantage in chemo- or radiosensitive tumors, such as germinomas, pineoblastomas, and primitive neuroectodermal tumors and are the preferential management option in most pineal region and posterior third ventricular tumors, since they guide further management whether microsurgical resection or other non-surgical therapies (Gangemi et al, 2001).

Some tumors may, on the other hand, be treated observantly. Certain thalamic gliomas that are beyond surgical resection may be observed, and others may be irradiated, depending on the grade of the tumor (Selvapandian 2006). An endoscopic biopsy, along with 3rd ventriculostomy to treat associated hydrocephalus, may easily attain the diagnosis (figure 3). A biopsy is not even necessary in tectal gliomas, since these lesions are usually indolent and the mere treatment of hydrocephalus and endoscopic inspection of the benign mass are enough according to several authors (Li et al, 2005; Ternier et al, 2006; Wellons et al, 2002). We had 4 patients with small tectal lesions who were successfully treated with endoscopic 3rd ventriculostomy, and had stable tumors and patent ventriculostomies through out the follow up period (Najjar et al, 2010).

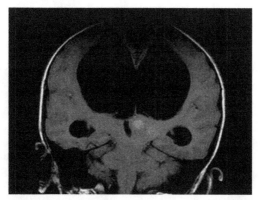

Fig. 3. Coronal T1W MRI sequence showing a small left thalamic lesion with hydrocephalus. The child underwent endoscopic 3rd ventriculostomy and biopsy. Symptomatic hydrocephalus was thus treated and the low grade tumor proven at biopsy was stable and followed with imaging.

Colloid cysts, simple pineal cysts, and small intraventricular tumors may be removed or debulked endoscopically. Colloid cyst endoscopic surgery is described widely in the literature and is becoming a popular surgical technique in the management of these lesions (Grondin et al, 2007; Horn et al, 2007; Schroeder & Gaab 2002). Navigation assisted endoscopy may be needed in some of these patients, especially when there is no accompanying hydrocephalus (Souweidane 2005). Navigation could be also of great value in colloid cyst surgery, especially in selecting the entry point necessary for the optimal working angle (Schroeder & Gaab 2002).

Intra-ventricular arachnoid cysts such as suprasellar cysts and quadrigeminal plate cysts are optimal targets for endoscopic surgical management (Greenfield 2005). The cyst is usually fenestrated at two points to communicate it with the ventricular system and the adjacent arachnoid cisterns (ventriculo-cysternal and cysto-arachnoid communication). The success rate is quite high, and the simple procedure helps avoid implanatation of a permanent cysto-peritoneal shunting device in most patients. The more common temporal extraparenchymal arachnoid cysts, however, pose a more difficult endoscopic task. The anatomy is often more difficult and the fenestration site is close to critical structures. These temporal cysts may also be managed by microsurgical removal and/ or cysto-peritoneal shuting with similar results, and there is no consensus on their management (Tamburrini 2007).

Most patients with intraventricular lesions have associated symptomatic hydrocephalus. As mentioned earlier, endoscopic 3rd ventriculostomy (ETV) has a high success rate in tumor related obstructive hydrocephalus with long term patency ranging from 70-90%, and minimal complications. The ventriculostomy is usually done through the standard frontal burr hole, which may be adjusted to a more anterior position so the biopsy procedure can be done concomitantly (O'Brien 2006). Other authors advocate a 2 burr hole technique for optimal results, but we have found a single burr hole sufficient to perform the 3rd ventriculostomy and access most lesions in the 3rd and lateral ventricles to get a biopsy or perform a resection or debulking procedure. We also prefer to perform the ETV first, as preferred by most authorities, to avoid obscuring the operative field with blood-stained CSF after the biopsy. Smaller ventricles, presence of void signal on sagittal T2W MRI images, and presence of flow on cine-phase-contrast MR flow imaging, are helpful indicators of ventriculostomy patency, and when absent, close follow up is advised depending on the clinical condition (figure 4).

2.4 Conclusion

In summary, intra-ventricular neuroendoscopic techniques have rapidly become invaluable in the management of intra-ventricular brain lesions and hydrocephalus. In experienced hands, and after careful planning, biopsies can be taken safely, and adequately, outlining further management, especially in chemo and/or radio sensitive tumors. Other lesions may be resected, or debulked, and some may be observed. Cystic lesions, such as arachnoid cysts, may be resected or fenestrated, and the accompanying hydrocephalus is often treated in the same procedure, either with 3rd ventriculostomy, or with shunting after fenestration of the septum pellucidum in patients with large 3rd ventricular lesions. Thus, endoscopic procedures provide a minimally invasive approach to these pathologies, and might overcome complications that are usually associated with the conventional therapeutic strategies. These endoscopic procedures have simply become an indispensable part of our neurosurgical armamentarium available for the management of intra-ventricular pathologies.

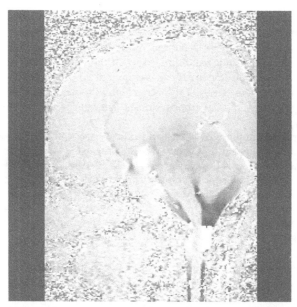

Fig. 4. Post-operative cine-phase contrast MR flow study for the child shown in figure 2 demonstrating good flow of CSF at the level of the ventriculostomy (central white signal).

3. Endoscopic endonasal transsphenoidal & extended skull base approaches

The second part of this chapter deals with endoscopic skull base approaches, with special emphasis on their most common application: the endoscopic transphenoidal approach to sellar and pituitary tumors. This surgery has continuously evolved in the past century, and its history is a complex tale of development of innovative ideas coupled with periods of extensive surgical experimentation, striving to attain the best surgical results with minimal morbidity.

3.1 Historical perspective

The pituitary tumor resection performed by Canton and Paul, and via a temporal approach as advised by Homsley in 1893, is often sited as the first transcranial approach to pituitary tumors. Soon after, and in 1907, Schloffer attempted the first transsphenoidal surgery (Schloffer 1907). During that period, multiple variations of the inferior transnasal exposure were developed, and among the most popular were Cushing's sublabial route, and Hirsch's transnasal approach (Hirsch 1910). These approaches, however, and especially the latter, were sometimes extensive, and suffered significant technical difficulties, especially in the field of illumination. In 1956, Dott, and later Guiot, revived the interest in transsphenoidal pituitary surgery, and established its basic techniques. It was only till Hardy introduced the operating microscope in 1965, however, that the procedure gained wide acceptance, and became the work horse of pituitary surgery (Gandhi et al, 2009).

Variations of the sublabial transsphenoidal technique were then developed, with transnasal transseptal route, and other approaches aiming at a deeper mucosal incision to avoid nasal and dental complications. Despite the marked improvement in stereoscopic visualization afforded by microscopic surgery, deeper incisions were difficult to perform because of the narrow surgical field. In 1977, Apuzzo described the use of the endoscope as an adjunct to the microscope in tumors with extrasellar extension, to afford better visual control around the corners, and to help obtain a panoramic view in the depth of the field (Appuzo et al, 1997). This was an essential step in the development of the extended transsphenoidal approach, expanding the boundaries of the surgical field to include lesions extending to the cribriform plate anteriorly, the cavernous sinuses laterally, and the clivus and foramen magnum inferiorly.

The pure endoscopic technique was described in the 1990s, first by Jankowski in 1992, and then three years later by Jho and Carrau who are regarded as the pioneers of the pure endoscopic endonasal approach (Jho & Carrau, 1997). In 1998, Cappabianca introduced the term functional endoscopic pituitary surgery (Cappabianca et al, 1999). The advantages of the pure endoscopic technique include the reduction of nasal complications, better visualization of the blind corners with angled telescopes, and the ability to change perspectives between close-up and panoramic views. The endoscopic technique has since spread and is being practiced in many centers around the world.

3.2 Endoscopic endonasal approaches: Technical considerations

The endoscopic endonasal transphenoidal approach can be divided into 3 phases: the nasal phase, the sphenoidal phase, and the sellar phase. In the nasal stage, the rigid endoscope is introduced along the floor of the nasal cavity reaching the choana which is a fundamental finding in this phase. Its medial aspect represents the vomer which confirms the midline of the approach, while its roof takes the shape of the sphenoid sinus's floor. Proceeding with the endoscope in a superior direction, the middle turbinate is encountered and dislocated laterally to ensure an adequate surgical pathway. Then, the endoscope can be angled along the spheno-ethmoid recess reaching the sphenoid ostium . This heralds the beginning of the next phase; the sphenoidal phase. After identifying the sphenoid ostium , the mucosa covering the ethmoid recess has to be cauterized to reduce possible annoying bleeding from the septal branches, exposing the whole anterior wall of the sphenoid sinus . The ostium is enlarged completing the anterior sphenoidectomy step (figure 5). Reviewing the anatomy of the sphenoid sinus septae on the pre-op CT scan helps understanding the sellar floor and the medial extent of the cavernous sinus. Preservation of the sphenoidal mucosa is important to ensure an adequate muco-ciliar transport which plays a major role in the physiology of the naso-sinusal ventilation (Kalushar 1997). Moreover, the proximity of the internal carotid artery (ICA) and the sphenoid sinus must be considered while removing the sphenoid sinus mucosa as the bone covering its anterior loop might be missing in 4-8% (Fujii et al 1979). Now, the posterior wall of the sphenoid sinus with the sellar floor at its center is recognizable and we can fix the endoscope to its holder freeing the surgeon hands for the next step (figure 6). The sellar phase starts with opening of the sellar floor by means of microdrill or a kerrison's rongeur depending on its consistency and it may be extended as required by the specific pathology reaching the sphenoid planum above, the anterior limit of the cavernous sinus on the side or the clivus inferiorly. Then, the dura is incised and care should be applied not to reach the perisellar sinus or the ICA itself. Before removing the adenoma, the pituitary gland should be identified and preserved. Removal of macroadenomas should be performed sequentially starting laterally to avoid premature delivery of the redundant diaphragm into the operating field. After emptying the intrasellar adenoma, an angled endoscope may be advanced for a better inspection of the supra and retrosellar compartments.

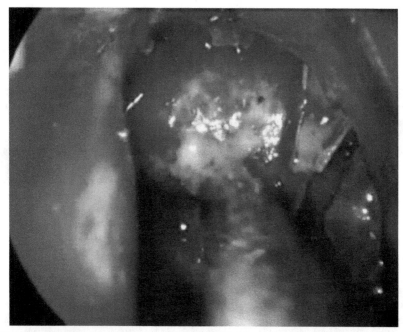

Fig. 5. Endoscopic view of the sellar floor during the sphenoidal phase

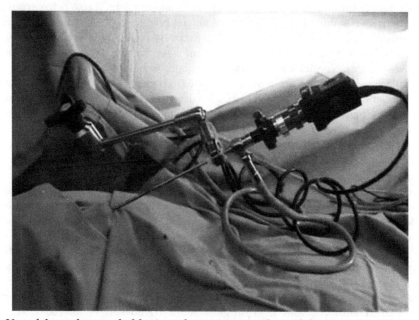

Fig. 6. Use of the endoscope holder in endoscopic transsphenoidal surgery for pituitary adenomas

A variation of the technique described above entails using both nostrils and the dynamic process of the two surgeons working together without the endoscope holder (2 nostril, 4 hand technique). Although many centers have moved towards adopting this more dynamic technique, we feel that it entails more aggressive work in the nose, often not needed in the soft, easy to remove pituitary adenomas. This technique becomes necessary, however, for more extensive skull base pathology. With the recent revolution of skull base surgery, the endoscope is increasingly used for attacking skull base lesions from below. The same rules of endoscopic endonasal transphenoidal approach may be applied but in an extended fashion to treat a wide variety of pathologies involving the cribriform plate, the planum sphenoidale , the cavernous sinus, the sellar and parasellar compartments, the clivus, down to the foramen magnum and C2 level. The ethmoido-pterygo-sphenoidal approach allows a rapid, wide, extracerbral, and direct exposition of the skull base floor. Yet, CSF leak and the inability to cross nerves, represent major challenges that limit its widespread use. In a series of 16 craniopharyngiomas, Gardner reported high rates of preservation of endocrine function without sacrificing the extent of resection using the extended endoscopic approach (Gardner et al, 2008). A high rate of post-op CSF leak was noted (58%) though, highlighting the importance and complexity of skull base reconstruction in these patients.

3.3 Endoscopic endonasal surgery: Advantages

The main advantages of the endoscopic technique may be divided into nasal and neurological (Har-El 2005). In addition to an excellent view of the bony and soft tissues in the nose, the endoscopic approach helps avoid several complications commonly seen in the transseptal microscopic approach, such as perforation, septal deformity, saddle nose deformity, nasal obstruction, and long term epistaxis and crusting. It also helps avoid dental complications seen at times after the sublabial microscopic approach including hypoesthesia or anesthesia of the incisor teeth (Har-El 2005). Recovery from an otolaryngologic aspect of the surgery is often rapid, with no swelling or oral wounds that contribute to postoperative pain and discomfort. Normal food intake is immediate, and hospital stay is shorter.

The neurological advantages are mostly related to superior visualization in the intrasellar cavity, especially when the angled telescopes are used to look for residual tumor in the blind corners and suprasellar area. When judging any new surgical technique, it must be compared with the current gold standard on the most important key indicators: oncological and endocrine outcomes, re-operation rates, and complications. In a meta-analysis on over 800 pts from studies published prior to 2006, both safety and efficacy of the endoscopic approach was demonstrated with high rates of gross total removal of tumors and normalization of endocrine function with improved vision (Tabaee et al, 2009a). In another study, an angled endoscope was used to evaluate 40 patients who underwent a microscopic resection of a pituitary tumor (Helal 1995). A large percentage (40%) had residual tumor. The same result was reproduced by Jarrahy's assessment of the efficacy of endoscopy in pituitary adenoma resection (Jarrahy et al, 2000). Others authors, using a hybrid technique, have agreed that the endoscopic view is superior when compared to the microscopic view (Baussart et al, 2005). Dehdashti et al reported on the early surgical results in 200 patients who had the pure endoscopic endonasal approach for their pituitary adenomas and compared them with previous microsurgical series (Dehdashti et al, 2008). He found comparable rates of gross total resection at 98% for intrasellar tumors and 96% for tumors with suprasellar extention (figure 7a&b).

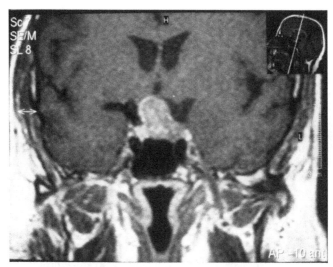

Fig. 7. a. Coronal T1W MRI sequence of the brain with gadolinium showing a large pituitary macroadenoma displacing the optic chiasm superiorly and the pituitary gland to the right side. The patient suffered visual field disturbances.

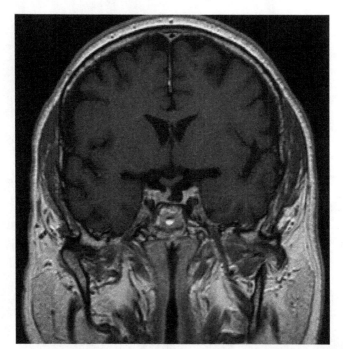

Fig. 7. b. Post-operative coronal T1W sequence of the brain with gadolinium for the same patient showing complete removal of the tumor. The patient's visual field defect resolved after surgery.

A multitude of studies support excellent endocrinologic outcomes following endoscopic surgery for secreting pituitary adenomas. D'Haens et al assessed 120 patients with functioning adenomas in a retrospective study (D'Haens et al, 2009). The remission rate of hypersecretion was significantly better in the endoscopic group (63 vs 50%). Kabil et al reported on 300 pts undergoing endoscopic resection with a similar cure rate of 87% in GH secreting adenomas, 86% in Cushing's disease and 80% in prolactinomas (Kabil et al, 2005). We have also noted a high cure rate in our endoscopic series of patients treated for Cushing's disease (figure 8a&b). A 90% biochemical cure in a purely endoscopic series of 21 patients was also reported in another series (Tabaee et al, 2009b). In patients with macroadenomas with visual field cuts, complete normalization of preoperative visual defect was noted in 50% of endoscopically approached tumors in one study, with an additional 39% having improvement (Dehdashti et al, 2008). Zhang et al achieved 70% recovery of preoperative visual defects in over 300 cases (Zhang et al, 2008). These reported rates of visual recovery in the endoscopic literature are slightly higher than those traditionally reported for microscopic approaches (Schaberg et al, 2010).

Length of stay has been shown to be decreased in multiple series (O'Malley et al, 2008). Patients were able to return home 2 days earlier on average (Higgins et al, 2008). We have had a similar experience in our patient series, where the average hospital stay was 2 or 3 days. In one review, the endoscopic group had a statistically significant reduction in their hospital stay: 3.4 vs 8.3 days (Neal et al, 2007). Similarly, a number of studies demonstrated an operative time that is significantly less on average by about 1hour (O'Malley et al, 2008).

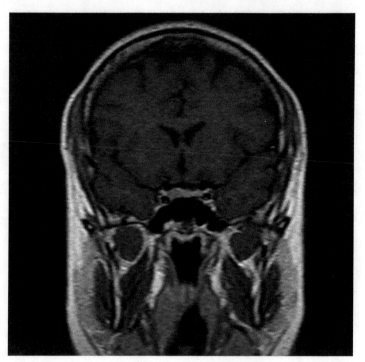

Fig. 8. a. Coronal T1W MRI sequence of the brain showing a hypointense lesion in the right sellar area indicating a pituitary microadenoma. The patient had Cushing's disease.

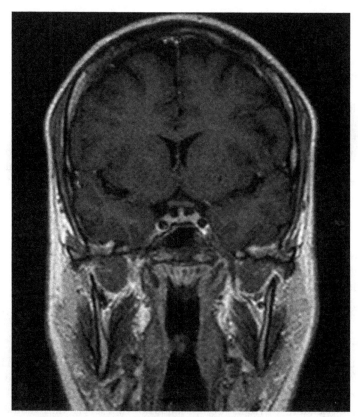

Fig. 8. b. Post-operative coronal T1W MRI sequence of the brain with gadolinium at 1 year after endoscopic removal of the adenoma indicating complete removal with no recurrence. The patient had endocrinological cure by blood testing as well.

3.4 Complications and disadvantages

The major complications, which are quite rare, are similar to those seen in the routine microscopic surgery and include CSF leak, vascular injuries, intracranial injury, endocrine abnormalities, meningitis, and death. The complications rates have been comparable between the two techniques. O'Malley et al reported on 50 pts, half of them undergoing microscopic approaches and half undergoing endoscopic approaches, and showed comparable complication rates between the two groups for both CSF leak and incidence of diabetes insipidis with a trend toward less diabetes incipidus (DI) in the endoscopic group (O'Malley et al, 2008) . Kabil et al demonstrated a 2% CSF leak in a series of over 650 patients undergoing endoscopic resection (Kabil et al, 2005). Minor complications include septal perforation, trauma to external nose and sinusitis. The nasal complications are much less in the endoscopic approach when compared to microsurgical sublabial approaches as mentioned earlier.

The development of a new surgical technique often begets criticism due to the possibility of a learning curve. In modern medicine, there is a distinct advantage to a multidisciplinary team approach with otolaryngologists and neurosurgeons working together in the surgical management of these cases. Another controversy is the lack of stereoscopic vision .Yet, novel 3D endoscopy provides stereoscopic view and may help overcome this obstacle. The next step in the evolution of endoscopic transphenoidal surgery is linked to ongoing work utilizing intra-operative magnetic resonance imaging and robotics, and to the miniaturization of the optical systems in terms of chip-stick technology, and the cooperation between different technologies and industries (Cappabianca et al, 2008).

3.5 Conclusion

In summary, the endoscopic techniques used in anterior skull base surgery have caused a revolution in the management of pituitary tumors and several other lesions in the anterior skull base and clival regions. The approach is minimally invasive, and affords excellent visualization of deep structures. The endoscopic technique is moving to be the standard technique for pituitary tumors and other sellar lesions. Patients have much less nasal complaints, and stay less in the hospital. Most authorities report superior visualization of small tumor remnants in the corners, usually blind in microscopic surgery. For more extensive lesions of the anterior skull base and clivus on the other hand, the significant CSF leak rate, though reduced with recent nasal flap techniques, and significant nasal side effects seen in the more extensive extended endoscopic approaches, have stalled their widespread acceptance. The technology is continuously evolving, however, and much is to be expected in a very exciting and rapidly evolving field.

Note: All the figures listed are original figures.

4. References

Hellwig, D.; Grotenhuis, J.A.; Tirakotai W.; Riegel, T.; Schulte, D.M.; Bauer, B.L.; Bertalanffy, H. (2005). Endoscopic third ventriculostomy for obstructive hydrocephalus. *Neurosurg Rev*, Vol. 28, pp. 1-34

Schroeder, H & Niendorf, W. (2002). Complications of endoscopic third ventriculostomy, *J Neurosurg*, Vol 96, No. 6, pp. 1032-1040

Fukuhara, T; Vorster, S; Ruggieri, P; Luciano, M. (1999). Third ventriculostomy patency: comparisons of findings at cine phase-contrast MR imaging and at direct exploration, *American Journal of Neuroradiology*, Vol. 20, No. 8, pp. 1560-1566

Schroeder, H; Schweim, C; schweim,K; Gaab, M. (2000). Analysis of aqueductal cerebrospinal fluid flow after endoscopic aqueductoplasty by using cine phase-contrast magnetic resonance imaging, *J Neurosurg*, Vol. 93, No. 2, pp. 237-244

Kamikawa, S; Inui, A; Tamaki, N; Kobayashi, N; Yamadori, T. (2001). Application of flexible neuroendoscopes to intracerebroventricular arachnoid cysts in children: use of videoscopes, *Minim Invasive Neurosurg*, Vol. 44, No. 4, pp. 186-189

Wilcock, D.J.; Jaspan, T; Worthington, B.S.; Punt, J. (1997). Neuro-endoscopic third ventriculostomy: evaluation with magnetic resonance imaging, *Clinical Radiology*, Vol. 52, No. 2, pp. 50-54

Schroeder, H.W.; Niendorf, W.R.; Gaab, M.R. (2002). Complications of endoscopic third ventriculostomy. *J Neurosurg*, Vol. 96, No.4 , pp.1032-1040

Jones, R.F.; Kwok, B.C.; Stening, W.A.; Vonau, M. (1994). The current status of endoscopic third ventriculostomy in the management of non-communicating hydrocephalus, *Minim Invasive Neurosurg*, Vol. 37, No. 1, pp. 28-36

Siomin, V.; Cinalli, G.; Grotenhuis, A.; Golash, A.; Oi, S.; Kothbauer, K.; Weiner, H.; Roth, J.; Beni-Adani, L.; Pierre-Kahn, A.; Takahashi, Y.; Mallucci, C.; Abbott, R.; Wisoff, J.; Constantini, S. (2002). *J Neurosurg*, Vol. 97, No. 3, pp. 519-524

Bargalló, N.; Olondo, L.; Garcia, A.; Capurro, S.; Caral, L; Rumia, J. (2005). Functional analysis of third ventriculostomy patency by quantification of CSF stroke volume by using cine phase-contrast MR imaging, *AJNR Am J Neuroradiol*, Vol. 26, No. 10, pp. 2514-2521

Li, K.W.; Roonprapunt, C.; Lawson, H.C.; Abbot, I.R.; Wisoff, J.; Epstein, F.; Jallo, G.I. (2005). Endoscopic third ventriculostomy for hydrocephalus associated with tectal gliomas, *Neurosurg Focus*, Vol. 18,   No. 6A, pp. E2

O Brien, D.F.; Hayhurst, C.; Pizer, B.; Malluci, C.L. (2006). Outcomes in patients undergoing single-trajectory endoscopic third ventriculostomy and endoscopic biopsy for midline tumors presentingwith obstructive hydrocephalus, *J Neurosurg*, Vol. 105, No. 3 Suppl, pp. 219-226

Oi, S.; Kamio, M.; Joki, T.; Abe, T. (2001). Neuroendoscopic anatomy and surgery in pineal region tumors: role of neuroendoscopic procedure in the "minimally-invasive preferential" management, *J Neurooncol*, vol. 54, No. 3, pp. 277-286

Pople, I.K.; Athanasiou, T.C.; Sandeman, D.R.; Coakham, H.B. (2001). The role of endoscopic biopsy and third venrticulostomy in the management of pineal region tumors, *Br J Neurosurg*, Vol. 15, No. 4, pp. 305-311

Sainte-Rose, C.; Cinalli, G.; Roux, F.E.; Maixner, R.; Chumas, P.D.; Mansour, M.; Carpentier, A.; Bourgeois, M.; Zerah, M.; Pierre-Kahn, A.; Renier, D. (2001). Management of hydrocephalus in pediatric patients with posterior fossa tumors: the role of endoscopic third ventriculostomy, *J Neurosurg*, Vol, 95, No. 5, pp. 791-797

Wellons, J.C. 3rd; Tubbs, R.S.; Banks, J.T.; Grabb, B.; Blount, J.P.; Oakes, W.J.; Grabb, P.A. (2002). Long-term control of hydrocephalus via endoscopic third ventriculostomy in children with tectal plate gliomas, *Neurosurgery*, Vol. 51, No. 1, pp. 63-67

Buxton, N.; Turner, B.; Ramli, N.; Vloeberghs, M. (2002). Changes in third ventricular size with neuroendoscopic third ventriculostomy: a blinded study, *J Neurol Neurosurg Psychiatry*, Vol. 72, No. 3, pp. 385-387

Feng, H.; Huang, G.; Liao, X.; Fu, K.; Tan, H.; Pu, H. (2004). Endoscopic third ventriculostomy in the management of obstructive hydrocephalus: an outcome analysis, *J Neurosurg*, Vol. 100, No. 4, pp. 626-633

Fritsch, M.J.; Doerner, L.; Kienke, S.; Mehdorn, H.M. (2005). Hydrocephalus in children with posterior fossa tumors: role of endoscopic third ventriculostomy, *J Neurosurg*, Vol. 103, No. 1 (Suppl), pp. 40-42

Morelli, D.; Pirotte, B.; Lubansu, A.; Detemmerman, D.; Aeby, A.; Fricx, C.; Berré, J.; David, P.; Brotchi, J. (2005). Persistent hydrocephalus after early surgical management of posterior fossa tumors in children: is routine preoperative endoscopic third ventriculostomy justified? *J Neurosurg*, Vol. 103, No. 3 (Suppl), pp. 247-252

Najjar, M.W.; Azzm, N.I.; Baghdadi, T.S.; Turkmani, A.H.; Skaf, G. (2010). Endoscopy in the management of intra-ventricular lesions: preliminary experience in the Middle East, *Clin Neurol Neurosurg*, Vol. 112, No. 1, pp. 17-22

Souweidane, M.M. (2005). Endoscopic management of pediatric brain tumors, *Neurosurg Focus*, Vol. 18, No. 6A, pp. E1

Gangemi, M.; Maiuri, F.; Colella, G.; Buonamassa, S. (2001). Endoscopic surgery for pineal region tumors, *Minim Invasive Neurosurg*, Vol. 44, pp. 70-73

Selvapandian, S. (2006). Endoscopic management of thalamic gliomas, *Minim Invasive Neurosurg*, Vol. 49, pp. 194-196

Ternier, J.; Wray, A.; Puget, S.; Bodaert, N.; Zerah, M.; Sainte-Rose, C. (2006). Tectal plate lesions in children. *J Neurosurg*, Vol. 104, No. 6 (Suppl), pp. 369-376

Grondin, R.T.; Hader, W.; MacRae, M.E.; Hamilton, M.G. (2007). Endoscopic versus microsurgical resection of third ventricle colloid cysts, *Can J Neurol Sci*, Vol. 34, pp. 197-207

Horn, E.M.; Feiz-Erfan, I.; Bristol, R.E.; Lekovic, G.P.; Goslar, P.W.; Smith, K.A.; Nakaji, P; Spetzler, R.F. (2007). Treatment options for third ventricular colloid cysts: comparison of open versus endoscopic resection, *Neurosurgery*, Vol. 60, No. 4, pp. 613-618

Schroeder, H.W. & Gaab, M.R. (2002). Endoscopic resection of colloid cysts, *Neurosurgery*, Vol. 51, No. 6, pp.1441-1445

Greenfield, J.P.; Souweidane, M.M. (2005). Endoscopic management of intracranial cysts, *Neurosurg Focus*, Vol. 19, No. 6, pp. E7

Tamburrini, G.; Dal Fabbro, M.; Di Rocco, C. (2008). Sylvian fissure arachnoid cysts: a survey on their   diagnostic workout and practical management, *Childs Nerv Syst*, Vol. 24, No. 5, pp. 593-604

Schloffer, H. (1907). Erfolgreiche operation eines hypophysentumors auf nasalem wege, *Wein Klin Wochenschr*, Vol. 20, pp. 621-624

Hirsch, O. (1910). Demonstration eines nach einer neuen method operiten hypophysentumors, *Verh Dtsch Ges Chir*, Vol. 39, pp. 51-56

Gandhi, C.D..; Christiano, L.D..; Eloy, J.A..; Prestigiacomo, C.J..; Post, K.D. (2009). The historical evolution of transsphenoidal surgery : facilitation by technological advances, *Neurosurg Focus*, Vol. 27, No. 3,   pp. E8

Apuzzo, M.L.J.; Heifetz, M.; Weiss, M.H.; Kurze, T. (1977). Neurosurgical endoscopy using the side-viewing telescope.technical note, *J Neurosurg*, Vol. 16, No. 3, pp. 398-400

Jho, H.D.; Carrau, R.L. (1997). Endoscopic endonasal transsphenoidal surgery: experience with 50 patients, *J Neurosurg*, Vol. 87, pp. 44-51

Cappabianca, P.; Alfieri, A.; Colao, A.; Ferone D.; Lombardi, G.; de Divitiis, E. (1999). Endoscopic endonasal transsphenoidal approach: an additional reason in support of surgery in the management of pituitary lesions, *Skull Base Surgery*, Vol. 9, No. 2, pp. 109-117

Kaluskar, S.K. (1997). Pre- and postoperative mucociliary clearance in functional endoscopic sinus surgery, *Ear Nose Throat J*, Vol. 76, No. 12, pp. 884-886

Fujii, K.; Chambers, S.M.; Rhoton, A.L.Jr. (1979). Neurovascular relationships of the sphenoid sinus. A microsurgical study, *J Neurosurg*, Vol. 50, No. 1, pp. 31-39

Gardner, P.A.; Kassam, A.B.; Snyderman, C.H.; Carrau, R.L.; Mintz, A.H.; Grahovac, S.; Stefko, S. (2008). Outcomes following endoscopic, expanded endonasal resection of suprasellar craniopharyngiomas: a case series, *J Neurosurg*, Vol. 109, No.1, pp. 6-16

Har-El, G. (2005). Endoscopic transnasal transsphenoidal pituitary surgery-Comparison with the traditional sublabial transseptal approach, *Otolaryngol Clin N Am*, Vol. 38, pp. 723-735

Tabaee, A.; Anand, V.K.; Barrón, Y.; Hitzik, D.H.; Brown, S.M.; Kacker, A.; Mazumdar, M; Schwartz, T.H. (2009a).Endoscopic pituitary surgery: a systematic review and meta-analysis, *J Neurosurg*, Vol. 111, No. 3, pp. 545-554

Helal, M.Z. (1995). Combined micro-endoscopic trans-sphenoidal excisions of pituitary macroadenomas. *Eur Arch Otorhinolaryngol*, Vol. 252, No. 3, pp.186-189

Jarrahy, R.;Berci, G.;Shahinian, H.K. (2000). Assessment of the efficacy of endoscopy in pituitary adenoma resection, *Arch Otolaryngol Head Neck Surg*, Vol. 126, No. 12, pp. 1487-1490

Baussart ,B.; Aghakhani, N.; Portier, F.; Chanson, P.; Tadié, M.; Parker, F. (2005). Endoscope-assisted microsurgery for invasive endo-and suprasellar pituitary macroadenomas: a consecutive retrospective study with 13 patients, *Neurochirurgie*, Vol. 51, No.5, pp.455-463

Dehdashti, A.R.; Ganna, A.; Karabatsou, K.; Gentili, F. (2008). Pure endoscopic endonasal approach for pituitary adenomas: early surgical results in 200 patients and comparison with previous microsurgical series, *Neurosurgery*, Vol. 62, No. 5, pp. 1006-1015.

D'Haens, J.; Rompaey, K.V.; Stadnik, T.; Haentjens, P.; Poppe, K.; Velkeniers, B. (2009). Fully endoscopic transsphenoidal surgery for functioning pituitary adenomas: a retrospective comparison with traditional transsphenoidal microsurgery in the same institution, *Surg Neurol*, Vol. 72, No. 4, pp. 336-340.

Kabil, M.S.; Eby, J.B.; Shahinian, H.K. (2005). Fully endoscopic endonasal vs transseptal transphenoidal pituitary surgery, *Minim Invasive Neurosurg*, Vol. 48, No. 6, pp. 348-354

Tabaee, A.; Anand, V.K.; Barrón, Y.; Hitzik, D.H.; Brown, S.M.; Kacker, A.; Mazumdar, M; Schwartz, T.H. (2009b). Predictors of short-term outcomes following endoscopic pituitary surgery, *Clin Neurol Neurosurg*, Vol. 111, No. 2, pp. 119-122

Zhang, Y.; Wang, Z.; Liu, Y.; Zong, X.; Song, M.; Pei, A.; Zhao, P.; Zhang, P.; Piao, M. (2008). Endoscopic transsphenoidal treatment of pituitary adenomas, *Neurol Res*, Vol. 30, No. 6, pp. 581-586

Schaberg, M.R.; Anand, V.K.; Schwartz,T.H.; Cobb,W. (2010). Microscopic versus endoscopic transnasal pituitary surgery, *Curr opin otolaryngol head neck surg*, Vol. 18, No. 1, pp. 8-14

O'Malley, B.W. Jr.; Grady , M.S.; Gabel, B.C.; Cohen, M.A.; Heuer, G.G.; Pisapia, J.; Bohman, L.E.; Leibowitz, J.M. (2008). Comparison of endoscopic and microscopic removal of pituitary adenomas: single-surgeon experience and the learning curve, *Neurosurg Focus*, Vol. 25, No. 6, pp. E10

Higgins, T.S.; Courtemanche, C.; Karakla, D.; Starsnick, B.; Singh, R.V.; Koen, J.L.; Han, J.K. (2008).Analysis of transnasal endoscopic versus transseptal microscopic approach for excision of pituitary tumors, *Am J Rhinol*, Vol. 22, No. 6, pp. 649-652

Neal, J.G.; Patel, S.J.; Kulbersh, J.S; Osguthorpe, J.D.; Schlosser, R.J. (2007). Comparison of
    techniques for transsphenoidal pituitary surgery, *Am J Rhinol*, Vol. 21, No. 2, pp.
    203-206
Cappabianca, P.; Cavallo, L.M.; de Divitiis, O.; Solari, D.; Esposito, F.; Colao, A.(2008).
    Endoscopic pituitary surgery, *Pituitary*, Vol. 11, No. 4, pp. 385-390

11

Minimally Invasive Endoscopic and Endoscopy-Assisted Microsurgery of Vestibular Schwannoma

Betka Jan et al.[*]
Charles University in Prague, 1st Faculty of Medicine,
Department of Otorhinolaryngology and Head and
Neck Surgery, Faculty Hospital Motol, Prague,
Czech Republic

1. Introduction

Endoscopic techniques have revolutionized the practice of surgery in a number of specialities. Endoscopes have the ability to provide high magnification and illumination of the operative field, as well as the possibility to look around the corner past obstructing tissues and structures, thus allowing for more radical and safer surgeries. With several clinical applications, smaller incisions and surgical approaches are now possible, resulting in decreased postoperative pain, faster rehabilitation, better cosmetic results, and shorter hospitalization.

Similar to other specialities the endoscope represents an established component of the contemporary skull base surgery armamentarium. Its application in various skull base, otologic and neurosurgical procedures, either as a sole visualizing tool or as an adjunct to the microscope, is constantly expanding. The aim of this chapter is to review the application of endoscopic techniques in the treatment of vestibular schwannoma.

2. Vestibular schwannoma

Vestibular schwannomas are benign, slow-growing tumors which arise from the sheath of the eighth cranial nerve. The transition zone (Obersteiner–Redlich zone) of the superior or inferior vestibular nerves where the covering myelin changes from a central to a peripheral type or vestibular ganglion are estimated to be the site of pathologic proliferation of Schwann cells leading to tumor (Tallan et al. 1993, Zverina, 2010). Thus acoustic neuroma or

[*] Chovanec Martin[1,2], Zverina Eduard[1,3], Profant Oliver[1,4], Lukes Petr[1], Skrivan Jiri[1],
Kluh Jan[1] and Fik Zdenek[1,2]
[1]*Charles University in Prague, 1st Faculty of Medicine, Department of Otorhinolaryngology and Head and Neck Surgery, Faculty Hospital Motol, Prague, Czech Republic*
[2]*Charles University in Prague, 1st Faculty of Medicine, Institute of Anatomy, Prague, Czech Republic*
[3]*Charles University in Prague, 3rd Faculty of Medicine, Department of Neurosurgery, Faculty Hospital Kralovske Vinohrady, Prague, Czech Republic*
[4]*Department of Auditory Neurosciene, Institute of Experimental Medicine AS CR, Prague, Czech Republic*

neurinoma represent misnomers. The proportion of tumors arising from each of the two vestibular nerves superior or inferior has been reported to be equal (Clemis et al. 1986). There are two distinct clinical presentations for vestibular schwannomas: Sporadic unilateral tumor is the most common form occurring in 95% of cases, and the rare hereditary bilateral tumors which are typically a sign of neurofibromatosis type 2.

Vestibular schwannomas have an incidence of 10 to 15 per million per year and represent the most common tumor in neurotology (Myrseth et al. 2007, Zverina, 2010). These tumors account for approximately 10% of all intracranial and 80 to 95% of cerebellopontine angle tumors (Springborg et al. 2008). Most commonly vestibular schwannomas occur during the fourth and fifth decades of life and with slightly higher incidence among females than males. The reported increasing incidence along with the higher prevalence of smaller tumors being diagnosed during the last decades probably reflect improvements in diagnostic methods and growing awareness of both patients and specialists rather than a true increase in tumor incidence (Stangerup et al. 2010).

The diagnosis is either made or suspected based on clinical symptoms at presentation, audiometric testing, or imaging methods. Symptoms and signs associated with vestibular schwannomas have been known for over 150 years and are due to direct tumor compression, invasion or vascular compromise of the surrounding structures (Betka et al. 2008).

Hearing loss is the most common and also most frequent initial symptom and reason for patients to seek medical care. Typically, patients will develop a slowly (over months or years) progressive hearing loss. Despite not being specific, progressive sensorineural hearing loss at the high frequencies is the most common finding. Sudden onset of hearing loss is found in 12–22% of patients (Myrseth et al. 2007). Normal hearing is reported in about 5% of patients. Tinnitus is the second most frequent symptom of vestibular schwannoma. Its incidence usually coincides with hearing loss. Tinnitus may be constant or fluctuating in quality and quantity. Rarely is tinnitus the only symptom. Hearing loss indicates either damage of the cochlear nerve or occlusion of the labyrinthine artery. The origin of tinnitus is uncertain as it can be present even in the deaf ear. In conclusion, any unilateral or asymmetric sensorineural hearing loss and unilateral tinnitus deserve attention (Betka et al. 2008).

Vestibular symptoms are found in 40–60% of patients who may report a combination of vertigo, dizziness and unsteadiness. Balance problems are minor in the majority of patients probably reflecting very slow destruction of the vestibular nerve during the tumor growth however, once the tumor becomes expansive symptoms tend to worsen. Dysequilibrium is the most common vestibular symptom. Initially it is due to reduced or abolished unilateral peripheral vestibular function and incomplete compensation due to the tumor. It tends to be constant in nature, progressive in severity and aggravated by head movements. True vertigo, occurring in about 5-10% of cases, typically occurs early in the history of the tumor growth and may last for several days and weeks before resolving due to compensation of the acute peripheral vestibular function loss (Betka et al. 2008). Persistent vertigo is associated with a significant reduction in quality of life among vestibular schwannoma patients (Myrseth et al. 2007, Saman et al. 2009). In patients with large tumors, dysmetria and ataxia due to cerebellar and brainstem compression are common signs.

Headache is recalled by 10-30% of patients. It is typically described as a fullness or pressure in the ear or retroauricular region ipsilateral to the tumor. Trigeminal nerve compression and stretching may manifest as a paresthesia, hypesthesia or neuralgia occurring in about 5-10% of cases. Clinically apparent facial nerve dysfunction is a relatively rare finding as facial nerve tolerates a large degree of compression, stretching and distortion (Betka et al. 2008).

The growth rate of vestibular schwannoma varies and can be categorized into one of three patterns: slow (1-2 mm/year), medium (2-4 mm/year), and fast (1-2 cm/year). The majority of tumors grow slowly and in some cases spontaneous regression was reported (Zverina et al. 2010).

If not treated, vestibular schwannomas can reach a remarkable size causing severe compression of the brainstem and cerebellum eventually leading to hydrocephalus and intracranial hypertension (Zverina, 2010). However, many of these tumors fail to become symptomatic during a patient's life (Betka et al. 2008).

There are three treatment options for patients with a vestibular schwannoma: observation, radiosurgery/radiotherapy, and microsurgery.

The concept of observation (wait and scan) is based on two main principles. First, a high proportion of vestibular schwannomas do not grow or grow very slowly following the diagnosis. Second, there is little evidence that active treatment of a non-growing lesion is beneficial to the patient, but it is well documented that active treatment may cause additional complaints and decrease quality of life (Martin et al. 2001, Myrseth et al. 2006, Cheng et al. 2009, Myrseth et al. 2009). Therefore, in spite of increasing hearing loss in many patients, the conservative approach may be a reasonable option for patients with small and medium sized tumours (Yamakami et al. 2003, Sandooram et al. 2004, Zverina, 2010, Sughrue et al. 2011). For the success of observation close follow up and patient´s compliance are crucial. The failure rate (e.g. continuous growth or new and progressive symptoms) that need conversion to active treatment is reported to be 15-50% (Wackym, 2005, Myrseth et al. 2007, Betka et al. 2008).

Although there are enthusiastic supporters for both arms of active treatment (e.g. radiosurgery/radiotherapy and microsurgery), the data on which to base an objective opinion are incomplete (Yamakami et al. 2003, Myrseth et al., 2007, Myrseth et al. 2009, Zverina, 2010). Radiosurgery refers to the delivery of a therapeutic radiation dose in a single fraction while radiotherapy represents the delivery of a therapeutic radiation in multiple fractions. Radiosurgery represented by the Leksell´s gamma knife surgery (GKS) represents the treatment strategy with the biological chance of achieving permanent tumor control for late-responding and slowly proliferating tumors as vestibular schwannoma (Linskey, 2000). Other methods of stereotactic radiosurgery such as linear accelerator (LINAC) and cyber knife, and fractionated radiotherapy are employed for treatment of vestibular schwannomas with similar results (Wackym, 2005, Sakamoto et al. 2009). Radiosurgery does not attempt to eliminate the tumor or cure patients thus it is difficult to compare with microsurgery. Ideal results of radiosurgery are control/no further growth of tumor, preservation of facial nerve function and hearing without any complications. This form of treatment is not appropriate for patients with tumors larger than 3 cm in diameter, as radiosurgery is problematic in larger tumors. Indications in patients with intrameatal tumors, tumors indenting the brainstem and patients with balance problems is also speculative (Wackym, 2005, Zverina, 2010, Cakrt et al. 2010).

The majority of centers report tumor control rates between 90 and 100%, but few report observation periods longer than five years (Myrseth et al. 2007). Useful hearing preservation is reported in about half of cases approaching 3–4 years after radiosurgical treatment (Yang et al., 2010). The effect on tinnitus and vertigo is largely unknown (Wackym et al. 2008, Gerosa et al. 2010). Post-irradiation facial and trigeminal nerve dysfunction decreased to less than 5% as the treatment dose to the tumor margin has been gradually lowered during the last decades thus making the treatment very attractive for the patients and physicians (Myrseth et al. 2007, Myrseth et al. 2009). Hydrocephalus after stereoradiosurgical treatment is reported in 2–4% of patients. The mechanism of its development remains controversial. Frequent monitoring and early intervention is highly recommended to prevent irreversible cerebral damage (Myrseth et al. 2007). Induction of secondary neoplasia and malignant transformation of vestibular schwannoma has been reported rarely (Zverina, 2010).

Despite the fact that published data are difficult to interpret, mainly due to lack of long-term follow up, changing treatment protocols, lack of control groups, limited understanding of the natural history of treated tumors, insufficient stratification of patients and incomplete reporting results, there is little debate that radiosurgery has the ability to achieve tumor control with short-term low complication rates and a shorter hospital stay, and its role in the treatment of vestibular schwannoma is expanding (Wackym, 2005, Myrseth et al. 2007).

The objectives of surgical management are radical resection of the tumor, preservation of facial nerve function, conservation of hearing, and preservation of neighbouring neurovascular structures. Surgical treatment is technically challenging with gradual learning curve (Roser & Tatagiba, 2010). In many contemporary centres, vestibular schwannoma patients are operated on by a multidisciplinary team consisting of neurootologist and neurosurgeon. Ideally, it is a true team with each participant capable of performing the entire operation (Skrivan et al. 2004, Myrseth et al. 2007). This unique cooperation among the two disciplines has allowed each to bring the best of their speciality to the management of vestibular schwannoma (Zverina et al. 2010).

Three different approaches (e.g. translabyrinthine, middle fossa and retrosigmoid) were developed for the microsurgical treatment of vestibular schwannoma. Debate continues as to which of the three approaches is best suited for large and for small tumors, and which technique allows for best results. Several articles have eloquently outlined the advantages and disadvantages of each approach (Colleti & Fiorino, 2005, Wackym, 2005, Myrseth et al. 2007, Betka et al. 2008, Sughrue et al. 2010a, Sughrue et al. 2010b). The translabyrinthine and the retrosigmoid approaches can be used for all tumor sizes, whereas the middle fossa approach is useful only for removal of intrameatal tumors. Hearing preservation can be achieved only through the retrosigmoid and middle fossa approaches. The approach is chosen based on criteria such as tumor size, internal auditory canal extension, preoperative hearing level, and the surgeon's experience. Many teams employ all three approaches in an effort to take advantage of each of them and to achieve the best outcome for each patient. Radical tumor removal can be achieved in the majority of cases, and there is a seldom role for partial resection (e.g. preservation of functional neural structures, advanced patient age, hearing status in the contralateral ear).

The morbidity associated with vestibular schwannoma surgery has declined steadily since the first successful operation was performed more than 100 years ago. The development of the surgical microscope in the 1960s revolutionized the field of its treatment.

Recent results following microsurgical removal of vestibular schwannomas are in general excellent although mortality and morbidity are not completely eliminated. Today most large series report mortality rates of 1% or less (Yamakami et al. 2003, Myrseth et al. 2007, Zverina et al. 2010). Facial nerve injury, hearing loss, postoperative balance problems, cerebrospinal fluid leak and headache are among the main risks of surgical treatment of vestibular schwannoma.

With the routine use of intraoperative neuromonitoring anatomic preservation of facial nerve in the large series from the centers ranges from 90% to 100% (Wackym, 2005, Myrseth et al. 2007). Even if facial nerve is anatomically and physiologically intact after tumor resection, paresis may develop during the early postoperative period with improvement of function gradually over the next months. The single most important predictive factor of facial nerve preservation is the size of the treated tumor. In the group of surgically treated small and medium size tumors normal function of the facial nerve can be achieved in the vast majority of cases. Immediate postoperative normal function was shown to be better in cases of retrosigmoid and translabyrinthine approaches (Colleti & Fiorino, 2005). In the group of large tumors immediate postoperative normal facial nerve function can be achieved in about 50% of cases treated by the experienced team with subsequent improvement to normal or near normal (House Brackmann grade I and II) in about 60 to 80% of cases (Magnan et al. 2002, Zverina, 2010). Tumor adherence to the facial nerve, intraoperative monitoring and age represent also important prognostic markers of facial nerve preservation (Sughrue et al. 2010b).

Type of surgical approach, tumor size, younger age of the patient, and the use of intraoperative monitoring have all been implicated as predictive factors of hearing preservation. Beside surgical experience and skill, the chance for hearing preservation is influenced by the proper identification of the cochlear nerve and tumor adhesion to the cochlear nerve. Hearing preservation in patients with large tumors is difficult and less likely to succeed compared with small or medium-sized tumors. Reported hearing preservation in the case of tumors > 2 cm ranges from 5 to 53% (Wanibuchi et al. 2009). The success rate in the group of small tumors is significantly better ranging from 17 to 100% in some series. In a recent review of results of hearing preservation after microsurgical resection the hearing preservation rate was 64% in tumors < 1 cm and 61% in tumors 1-1.5 cm. The results of this multivariate analysis have shown the middle fossa approach to be more effective for preservation of hearing. The increased risk of surgically related hearing loss with retrosigmoid approach possibly reflect the fact that in this approach the cochlear nerve usually presents on the microscopically blind anterior side of tumor, and is encountered late, while the middle fossa approach permits earlier identification of the nerve, which can subsequently be safely avoided during tumor resection (Sughrue et al. 2011).

Following surgery, patients may develop balance problems, but eventually most recover well. Vestibular compensation after tumor removal and vestibular nerve sectioning can take weeks to months. Large tumor size, postoperative rehabilitation, central vestibular pathology and cerebellar dysfunction, surgical approach, impairment of vision a depression are among the main factors that influence the eventual level of compensation and the time taken to achieve this (Saman et al. 2009, Cakrt et al. 2010).

Some pain is expected in most patients immediately after surgery. Headache that persists weeks to months after surgery is not a major problem in the majority of patients but in some cases it can be incapacitating and decreasing quality of life. The reported incidence of postoperative headache has ranged from 0% to 73% depending on the type of surgical approach, technique used, and interval since surgery. The retrosigmoid approach was associated with higher incidence of debilitating persistent postoperative headache when compared with the translabyrinthine or middle fossa approaches. There is evidence indicating that a standard craniectomy may be associated with significant postoperative headache, which may be reduced with minimal bone removal during craniectomy (Magnan et al. 2002, Ryzenman et al. 2005, Wackym et al. 2005, Myrseth et al. 2007).

Recurrence rates after radical tumor removal, regardless of the type of approach used is less than 2%. There are compelling reasons to conclude that the recurrence rate is higher if hearing preservation approaches are employed reflecting possibly incomplete tumor removal, especially at the fundus of the internal auditory canal (Yamakami et al., 2003, Zverina, 2010).

Cerebrospinal fluid leak is the most common postoperative complication with the rate of around 10 to 20% of patients. It is associated with a higher risk of meningitis and must therefore be recognized and treated promptly. According to some works leakage after retrosigmoid or middle fossa approaches are more likely to require surgical intervention than a leak after a translabyrinthine approach. The majority of leaks are a result of poor intraoperative identification of exposed air cells within the temporal bone (Wackym et al. 1999, Zverina, 2010)

3. Historical perspective of endoscopic surgery of the cerebellopontine angle

Development of endoscopic surgery of vestibular schwannoma parallels application of endoscopes for other procedures in the cerebellopontine angle (e.g. diagnostic cisternoscopy, vestibular neurectomy, microvascular decompression) thus it must be understood in its broader context.

Urologist L'Espinase through use of a cystoscope attempted fulguration of the choroid plexus bilaterally in two infants with hydrocephalus in 1910 (Ozluoglu & Akbasak, 1996, as cited in Davis 1936). Doyen, who reported an endoscopic approach to the fifth cranial nerve by means of a retrosigmoid craniectomy in 1917, is credited with being the first to use an endoscope for the cerebellopontine angle surgery. He also developed instruments for the endoscopic division of the sensory roots of the nerve (Doyen, 1917).

In the late 1940s and early 1950s, the development of a coherent fiber optic bundles for image transmission, and an incoherent bundle for light transmission by Hopkins greatly aided the improvement of endoscopes that are used in modern surgical practice (Prott, 1974, Griffith, 1975, Mer et al. 1967). Later on the endoscopic anatomy of the cerebellopontine angle via translabyrinthine end retrosigmoid approach was described in detail by Prott and Opel (Prott, 1974, Opel, 1974, 1981, O'Donough et al. 1993).

Bremond and co-workers were the first reported minimally invasive retrosigmoid approach to treat the cerebellopontine angle pathologies. The authors had established that the procedure requires only a small retroauricular incison and craniectomy and the risk of the this appears to be minimal (Bremond et al. 1974, Bremond et al. 1975). Similary Fukushima used the endoscope to explore the cerebellopontine angle, cisterna magna, C1-C2 space and Meckel's cave from small burr hole and stated that cisternoscopy could be useful for the differential diagnosis of small tumors, vascular abnormalities or neurovascular compression syndromes (Fukushima, 1978).

In the 1990s few teams supported the employment of endoscopy during the retrosigmoid or retrosigmoid-retrolabyrinthine microsurgery of vestibular schwannoma. Endoscope was shown to be an ideal adjunct to hearing-preserving microsurgery of vestibular schwannomas, enabling direct control of the lateral aspects of the internal auditory canal, intrameatal portion of tumor and nerves while decreasing the rate of potential complications (Magnan et al. 1993, McKennan 1993, Magnan et al. 1994, Rosenberg et al. 1994, Tatagiba et al. 1996, Goksu et al. 1999, King & Wackym, 1999, Wackym et al. 1999). Benefits of the endoscope during microsurgical vestibular neurectomy to treat intractable vertigo (e.g.

Meniere´s disease) were described at the same time. It was shown that endoscopy allows improved identification of the nervus intermedius, facial, cochlear, and vestibular nerves and adjacent neurovascular relationships without the need for significant brain retraction. In addition, endoscope was shown to be beneficiary for identification of the cleavage plane between the cochlear and vestibular nerves.

Endoscopy was also evaluated for the placement of an auditory brainstem implant via the translabyrinthine, retrosigmoid, and middle cranial fossa approaches. Authors stated that endoscopy provided superior visualization of the lateral recess of the fourth ventricle than the operating microscope with all approaches and recommended the retrosigmoid approach as it provides the best view of the implantation site and the easiest angle for placement of the neuroprosthesis (Friedland & Wackym, 1999).

Endoscopic technique and assistance during microvascular decompression of the facial nerve for hemifacial spasm, trigeminal nerve for trigeminal neuralgia, glossopharyngeal nerve for glossopharyngeal neuralgia, and cochlear nerve for incapacitating tinnitus were shown to add additional accuracy rate in identifying nerve-vessel conflicts and even revealed a significant number of persistent nerve compression in despite negative binocular microscopic evidence (Magnan et al. 1993, Magnan et al. 1997, Jarrahy et al. 2000, Badr-El-Dine et al. 2002, El-Garem et al. 2002, Miyazaki et al. 2005, Chen et al. 2008, Guevarra et al. 2008).

Growing experience with endoscopic control and assistance for microsurgical management of other cerebellopontine angle pathologies led to a broader application of these techniques for tumor treatment including vestibular schwannomas, meningiomas and epidermoids (Magnan et al. 1993, King & Wackym, 1999, Wackym et al. 1999, Magnan et al. 2002, Schroeder et al. 2004, Hori et al. 2006, de Vitiis et al. 2007). Progressive implementation of rigid endoscopy in cerebellopontine angle surgery, has revealed it to be an equal if not superior imaging tool in this anatomic region. Cerebellopontine angle endoscopy was no longer seen as a risky procedure (Ozluoglu & Akbasak, 1996, Fries & Pernecki, 1998, Pernecki & Fries, 1998, Wackym et al. 1998, Miyazaki et al. 2005, Koval, 2009). Although its use has been described as an adjunctive imaging modality in many surgical procedures the use of endoscopy as the sole means of intra-operative imaging in this setting has not been reported at that time.

Microvascular decompressions were the first fully endoscopic procedures reported (Eby et al. 2001, Jarrahy et al. 2002a, Jarrahy et al. 2002b, Kabil et al. 2005, Cheng et al. 2008). The first report of fully endoscopic resection of vestibular schwannoma was by Shainian and coworkers in 2004 (Shahinian et al. 2004). Kabil and Shahinian in 2006 have presented 112 fully endoscopic procedures performed via 1.5 cm retrosigmoid craniotomy with excellent results. 95% tumors were completely removed. Subtotal removal was performed in 5% of patients in an attempt to preserve their hearing. Anatomical preservation of the facial nerve was achieved in all patients and of the cochlear nerve in 82% of hearing ears. Some or serviceable hearing was preserved in 58% of preoperative cases. There were no major neurological complications (Kabil & Shahinian, 2006).

Recently, the first high-definition (HD) cameras designed for endoscopic surgery have been developed. They provide the HD Television (HDTV) image format that provides an image with improved color fidelity and enhanced image resolution that is comparable to the image obtained when looking through the microscope. Their application in the cerebellopontine angle surgery is promising. Comparing the standard three-chip camera with a HD three-chip camera for video-assisted vestibular schwannoma surgery and microvascular decompression has provided a more detailed image with improved resolution of tissue and vasculature of the tumor, nerves and brainstem (Schroeder and Nehlsen, 2010).

4. Rationale for endoscopic surgery of the vestibular schwannoma

The main goals in vestibular schwannoma surgery are complete tumor removal with preservation of neurovascular structures and their function (e.g. facial nerve, hearing), and minimization of the sequelae of surgery and its complications (e.g. persistent balance problems, headache, cerebrospinal fluid leaks). The development of the surgical microscope in the 1960s revolutionized the field of both otology and neurosurgery as it provided accurate and detailed imaging of very restricted spaces, with simultaneous possibility of bimanual dissection. Despite the fact that endoscopic technique is applicable for each type of vestibular schwannoma surgical approach its benefits were predominantly shown to overcome some of the main disadvantages of the microsurgical retrosigmoid approach (Low 1999a).

Compared with the surgical microscope, endoscopes provide a wide angle of view with superb illumination in the depth and an increased depth of focus even with high magnification. Employment of endoscopic technique allows unobstructed visualization of all critical neurovascular structures of the cerebellopontine angle with simultaneous reduction in the craniotomy size, thus eliminating or at least reducing the need for retraction of the cerebellum. Both factors might reduce the number of complications resulting from dissection in this region (Magnan et al. 2002, Goksu et al. 2006).

Furthermore, angled optics expand the lateral boundaries of the microsurgical view. Endoscopes with angles of 30°, 45° and 70° can be used for early identification of the relationship between the tumor and neighboring structures in the cisternal part of dissection. The early identification of the brainstem and neurovascular structures (e.g. early identification of the position of the facial nerve to tumor or inspection of relationship between the tumor and brain or vessels) in the case of large tumors may be important in order to plan subsequent surgical steps (Fries & Pernecki 1998, Gerganov et al. 2009).

Using the surgical microscope with its direct forward view, it is virtually impossible to look around the corner due to the oblique angle of the internal auditory canal in relation to the trajectory of the dissection. Inability to completely visualize the lateral extent of the tumor as well as incomplete visualization of the exposed air cells are among the main disadvantages of the retrosigmoid approach. Excessive drilling of the petrous bone that is necessary in tumors extending to the lateral parts and fundus of internal auditory canal needed to achieve safe and radical tumor removal, might hamper the chance for hearing preservation as a consequence of injury of the posterior semicircular canal or labyrinth (Koval et al. 1993, Low 1999b, Goksu et al. 2005). Simultaneously, extensive drilling of the posterior meatal wall with improper sealing of the opened pneumatic system is associated with increased risk of cerebrospinal fluid leak (Valtonen et al. 1997). All these disadvantages can be alleviated by angled endoscopes that can be used for both inspection and visualization of the tumor and neurovascular structures during dissection within the internal auditory canal. Moreover, after completion of tumor removal the endoscope can be used to inspect the fundus for residual tumor and integrity of labyrinthine artery, facial and cochlear nerve. Similarly endoscopes are used for visualization of the drilled-out portion of the petrous bone for opened air cells that might need sealing. Some authors report that the risk of cerebrospinal fluid leaks have been lowered or even completely avoided (Valtonen et al. 1997, Wackym et al. 1999, Wackym et al. 2002, Gerganov et al. 2010). Under specific anatomical conditions angled endoscopes can be beneficial to identify and manage high jugular bulb (Betka et al. 2010). Minimally-invasive approach with limited bony removal is advantageous for the case of eventual Bone Anchored Hearing Aid implantation in case of single sided deafness rehabilitation.

Endoscopic approach for vestibular schwannoma surgery has some potential disadvantages as well. The two-dimensional view obtained by the endoscope instead of the three-dimensional view of the microscope represents an often cited disadvantage. Compared to the static imaging obtained by the surgical microscope, endoscopes of varying diameter, length and angulation allow surgeons to dynamically rotate and alter their perspective of the surgical field to compensate for the two-dimensional view. This amounts to a greater appreciation of the three-dimensional relationships between the tumor and the surrounding structures (Kabil & Shahinian, 2006). Furthermore novel binocular three-dimensional endoscopical technique during skull base surgery facilitating depth perception has been described recently.

Because angled endoscopes have a sharp front edge compared with a 0° endoscope, the surgeon cannot see the insertion trajectory directly. It is necessary to keep in mind that there could be a risk of damaging the neurovascular structures (Hori et al., 2006). Cerebellum can be protected during the procedure by covering it with a neurosurgical cotton, piece of Penrose drain or artificial dura. However working with 30° endoscopes has been repeatedly shown to be safe (Magnan et al. 2002, Goksu et al. 2005, Miyazaki et al. 2005). Risk of injury with insertion of 45° and 70° endoscopes is probably higher, but this can best alleviated by microscopic control. Complications due to inadvertent injury of healthy tissues have not been reported reflecting judicious use of the instruments.

As the delicate bimanual dissection is crucial for safe management of neurovascular structures of the cerebellopontine angle, a significant number of experts always struggled against the possibility of compromising one of their hands in endoscopic handling. However this potential problem was solved with introduction of either rigid pneumatic holding arms for the endoscope or freehand endoscopic technique with the endoscope being moved and held by a second surgeon. Both techniques were shown to be safe at allowing bimanual surgical dissection (Eby et al. 2001, Jarrahy et al. 2002a, Jarrahy et al. 2002b, Schroeder et al. 2004, Kabil & Shahinian, 2006, de Vitiis et al. 2007). Another important step forward was the introduction of an irrigation system, eliminating the time consuming and unsafe practice of removing and reinserting the endoscope.

Among the main drawbacks of endoscopic surgery of vestibular schwannoma is the risk of injury of very sensitive and critical structures of the cerebellopontine angle as the endoscope does not see the instrument used before it passes in front of the lens. Thus it is mandatory to achieve synchronized, in-and-out movements of the endoscope together with the instruments (Jarrahy et al. 2002a, Jarrahy et al. 2002b, Kabil & Shahinian, 2006, de Vitiis et al. 2007). Using the video-endoscopy assisted microsurgical technique the handling of instruments is controlled by the microscope before coming in front of the lens of the endoscope (Magnan et al. 2002, Miyazaki et al. 2005, Betka et al. 2010, Gerganov et al. 2010).

Another potential risk of the endoscopic technique is possibility of heat injury from prolonged use of the endoscope too close to the cranial nerves and other brain structures (Betka et al. 2010, Gerganov et al. 2010). Thus it is of the utmost importance to irrigate the operating field regularly, because the tip of the endoscope may become very hot (Wackym et al. 2002, Magnan et al. 2002, Goksu e al. 2005, Hori et al. 2006, Betka et al. 2010, Gerganov et al. 2010).

5. Endoscopic anatomy of the cerebellopontine angle

O'Donoghue and O'Flynn divided the CPA area into four levels on the basis of neuroendoscopic inspection of 10 fresh cadaver heads (O'Donoghue & O'Flynn, 1993). Level 1 contains the trigeminal and abducens nerves, Meckel's cave, superior cerebellar artery and superior petrosal vein. Level 2 contains the acousticofacial bundle and anterior inferior cerebellar artery. Level 3 contains the lower cranial and posterior inferior cerebellar artery. Level 4 contains the lower medulla, spinal cord, spinal root of the accessory nerve and hypoglossal nerve.

The majority of authors rather divide the region of cerebellopontine angle into three neurovascular complexes with no distinct borders (Rhoton, 2000a, Yuguang et al. 2005). The upper complex is related to the superior cerebellar artery, a middle complex related to the anterior inferior cerebellar artery and a lower complex related to the posterior inferior cerebellar artery (Fig.1). Each neurovascular complex includes one of the three parts of the brainstem (midbrain, pons, medulla), one of the three surfaces of the cerebellum (e.g. tentorial, petrosal and occipital), one of the three cerebellar peduncles, and one of the three major fissures between the cerebellum and the brainstem. In addition, each neurovascular complex contains a group of cranial nerves.

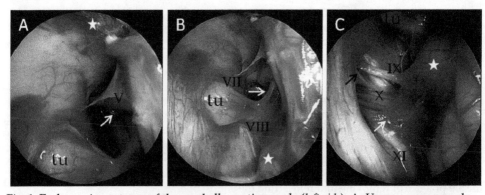

Fig. 1. Endoscopic anatomy of the cerebellopontine angle (*left side*). A: Upper neurovascular complex with the superior cerebellar atery (arrow) over the trigeminal nerve (V) and superior petrosal vein (asterisk); B: Middle neurovascular complex with the anterior inferior cerebellar atery (arrow), bundle of the facial (VII) and vestibulocochlear (VIII) nerves is distorted by the tumor (tu), floculus (asterisk); C: Lower neurovascular complex with the posterior inferior cerebellar atery (white arrow) over the lower cranial nerves. The spinal accessory fibers (IX) enter the jugular foramen bellow the cranial fibers of the eleventh cranial nerve that is in contact with the vagus nerve (X). Glossopharyngeal nerve at the level of the jugular foramen enters the glossopharyngeal meatus, that is separated by a dural septum (black arrow) from the vagal meatus.

The upper neurovascular complex includes the superior cerebellar artery, midbrain, cerebellomesencephalic fissure, superior cerebellar peduncle, tentorial surface of the cerebellum, and the oculomotor, trochlear, and trigeminal nerves (Fig.1) (Rhoton, 2000a, Cappabianca et al. 2002, Yuguang et al. 2005).

The superior cerebellar artery (SCA) arises in front of the midbrain, usually from the basilar artery near its apex. The artery passes below the oculomotor nerve, but may infrequently arise from the proximal posterior cerebral artery and pass above the oculomotor nerve. Close to its origin superior cerebellar artery encircles the brainstem near the pontomesencephalic junction, passing below the trochlear nerve and above the trigeminal nerve. Its proximal portion courses medial to the free edge of the tentorium cerebelli, and its distal part passes below the tentorium. After passing above the trigeminal nerve, it reaches the cerebellomesencephalic fissure, where it runs on the superior cerebellar peduncle and terminates by supplying the tentorial surface of the cerebellum (Rhoton, 2000a, Rhoton 2000b, Rhoton, 2000c).

The trigeminal nerve joins the brainstem about halfway between the lower and upper borders of the pons. Junction of the sensory rootlets of the nerve (e.g. main cone) with the brainstem is frequently obscured by little projection of cerebellum. There may be aberrant sensory rootlets that penetrate the pons outside the main sensory cone. These are typically rostral to the main cone and related to the first division of the nerve. Motor rootlets arise even more rostral to the main sensory cone. The trigeminal nerve runs obliquely upward from the lateral part of the pons toward the petrous apex. Fibres of the third-division remain caudolateral while the fibres of the first-division remain rostromedial during the course from the pons to the trigeminal ganglion. The fifth nerve exits the posterior fossa to enter the middle cranial fossa by passing forward and beneath the tentorial attachment to enter Meckel's cave, which sits in the trigeminal impression on the upper surface of the petrous part of the temporal bone (Rhoton, 2000a).

The superior petrosal vein (SPV) is one of the most frequently encountered veins during vestibular schwannoma surgery. SPV may be formed by the terminal segment of a single vein or by the common stem formed by the union of several veins that empty into the superior petrosal sinus. Tributaries of the SPV are the transverse pontine and pontotrigeminal veins, the veins of the cerebellopontine fissure and the middle cerebellar peduncle, and the common stem of the veins draining the lateral part of the cerebellar hemisphere (Rhoton, 2000a, Rhoton 2000d, Ebner et al. 2009, Koerbel et al. 2009).

Understanding the anatomy of the middle neurovascular complex is crucial for the surgical treatment of vestibular schwannoma (Fig.1) (Rhoton, 2000a, Magnan et al. 2002, Miyazaki et al. 2005). The middle complex includes the anterior inferior cerebellar artery, pons, middle cerebellar peduncle, cerebellopontine fissure, petrosal surface of the cerebellum, and the abducens, facial, and vestibulocochlear nerves (Rhoton, 2000a, Cappabianca et al. 2002, Yuguang et al. 2005).

The anterior inferior cerebellar artery (AICA) arises at the pontine level from the basilar artery, usually as a single trunk. Its origin can be bifurcated or even triplicated. From its origin AICA courses backward around the pons being in contact with the abducens nerve, and proceeds to the cerebellopontine angle where it is related to the facial and vestibulocochlear nerves. After coursing near and sending branches to the facial and vestibulocochlear nerves entering the internal auditory canal and to the choroid plexus protruding from the foramen of Luschka, it passes around the flocculus on the middle cerebellar peduncle to supply the lips of the cerebellopontine fissure and the petrosal surface of the cerebellum. AICA commonly bifurcates near the seventh-eighth nerve complex to form a rostral and a caudal trunk. The rostral trunk sends its branches laterally along the middle cerebellar peduncle to the superior lip of the cerebellopontine fissure and the adjoining part of the petrosal surface, and the caudal trunk supplies the inferior part of the petrosal surface, including a part of the flocculus and the choroid plexus. The AICA gives rise to perforating arteries to the brainstem, choroidal branches to the tela and choroid plexus, and the nerve-related arteries, including the labyrinthine, recurrent perforating, and subarcuate arteries (Rhoton, 2000a, Rhoton 2000b).

The facial nerve arises from the brainstem near the lateral end of the pontomedullary sulcus 1 to 2 mm anterior to the point at which the vestibulocochlear nerve joins the brainstem at the lateral end of the sulcus. The interval between the seventh and eighth nerves is greatest at the level of the pontomedullary sulcus and decreases as these nerves approach the porus of internal auditory canal.

Glossopharyngeal nerve, foramen of Luschka and flocculus can be used as anatomical landmarks to help with identification of the facial nerve at the level of brainstem. The point of origin of the facial nerve from the brainstem is 2 to 3 mm above the most rostral rootlet of the glossopharyngeal nerve. The foramen of Luschka, the sleevelike lateral recess of the fourth ventricle, is situated at the lateral margin of the pontomedullary sulcus, just behind the junction of the glossopharyngeal nerve with the brainstem, and immediately posteroinferior to the junction of the facial and vestibulocochlear nerves with the brainstem. The foramen itself is infrequently well visualized but tuft of the choroid plexus protruding out of the foramen of Luschka over the posterior surface of the glossopharyngeal and vagus nerves, just inferior to the junction of the facial and vestibulocochlear nerves with the brainstem can be well identified (Friedland & Wackym, 1999, Rhoton, 2000a, Koval & Krempaska, 2009). Flocculus, projects from the margin of the lateral recess and foramen of Luschka into the cerebellopontine angle, just posterior to facial and vestibulocochlear nerves.

Proper identification of the foramen of Luschka represent a crucial step in successful placement of the auditory brainstem neuroprosthesis to rehabilitate deafness in the cases of bilateral cochlear nerve loss. Choroid plexus, glossopharyngeal nerve and possibly stump of the eighth nerve represent key anatomical landmarks of the foramen of Luschka (Colleti et al. 2000, Skrivan et al. 2003, Brito Neto et al. 2005).

As stated earlier the facial and vestibulocochlear nerve are in close contact with AICA at the level of the brainstem. In most cases, the AICA passes below the nerves as it encircles the brainstem, but it also may pass above or between the nerves (Rhoton, 2000a, Rhoton, 2000c). Both nerves show relationship with the vein of the pontomedullary sulcus, the veins of the cerebellomedullary fissure, middle cerebellar peduncle, and cerebellopontine fissure veins on the side of the brainstem (Rhoton, 2000a, Rhoton 2000d).

As the seventh-eigth nerve complex runs from the brainstem forward and laterally to the internal auditory canal they usually display contact with the loop of AICA which reaches the porus or protrudes into the canal in almost half of the cases. During the cisternal course the facial nerve is anterior, cochlear portion is inferior and posterior and vestibular portion is superior and posterior. As the nerves approach the porus of the internal auditory canal facial and cochlear portion of the eigth cranial nerve are anterior, and vestibular portion is posterior and lateral. The position of the nerves is most constant in the lateral portion of the internal auditory canal, which is divided into a superior and an inferior portion by the transverse or falciform crest. The facial and the superior vestibular nerves are superior to the transverse crest. The facial nerve is anterior to the superior vestibular nerve and is separated from it at the lateral end of the meatus by the vertical crest or "Bill's bar". The cochlear and inferior vestibular nerves are located below the transverse crest with the cochlear nerve located anteriorly and inferior vestibular nerve posteriorly. Because vestibular schwannoma arise in the posteriorly placed vestibular nerves, they usually displace the facial nerve anteriorly and cochlear nerves inferiorly and anteriorly (Rhoton, 2000a, Magnan et al. 2002, Miyazaki et al. 2005).

The nervus intermedius is usually joined to the ventral surface of the vestibulocochlear nerve a few millimetres adjacent to the brainstem, then has a free segment in the cisternal part as it courses to join the facial motor root.

Labyrinthine artery (or arteries) accompanying the nerves is usually a branch of premeatal segment of AICA, but it can arise from the meatal or postmeatal portion of AICA, basilar artery or posterior inferior cerebellar artery (Rhoton, 2000a, Rhoton 2000c). Injury of the internal auditory artery can hamper hearing preservation during vestibular schwannoma removal.

Looking on the posterior petrosal face we can identify the subarcuate fossa that is enetered by the subarcuate artery. It is located superolateral to the porus of internal auditory canal.

Other important structures are the endolymphatic duct and sac, situated inferolateral to the internal auditory canal. It should be preserved when elevating the dura and opening the canal if there is the possibility of preserving hearing.

The lower neurovascular complex is related to the posterior inferior cerebellar artery, and includes the medulla, inferior cerebellar peduncle, cerebellomedullary fissure, suboccipital surface of the cerebellum, and the glossopharyngeal, vagus, spinal accessory, and hypoglossal nerves (Fig.1) (Rhoton, 2000a, Cappabianca et al. 2002, Yuguang et al. 2005).

The posterior inferior cerebellar artery (PICA) arises from the vertebral artery at the medullary level, encircles the medulla, passing in relationship to the lower cranial and hypoglossal nerves to reach the surface of the inferior cerebellar peduncle, where it dips into the cerebellomedullary fissure and terminates by supplying the suboccipital surface of the cerebellum (Rhoton 2000c).

The glossopharyngeal nerve arises as one or rarely two rootlets from the upper medulla, posterior to the olive in the post-olivary sulcus, just caudal to the origin of the facial nerve. It courses ventral to the choroid plexus protruding from the foramen of Luschka on its way to the jugular foramen. The smaller ventral rootlet has been demonstrated to be motor and the larger dorsal rootlet to be sensory. The glossopharyngeal nerve enters the dural subcompartment of the jugular foramen called the glossopharyngeal meatus (Rhoton, 2000a).

The vagus nerve arises below the glossopharyngeal nerve in the post-olivary sulcus as tightly packed rootlets posterior to the superior third of the olive. The most rostral vagal fibers arise adjacent to the glossopharyngeal rootlets. The vagus nerve is composed of multiple combinations of large and small rootlets that pass ventral to the choroid plexus protruding from the foramen of Luschka on its way to the jugular foramen. The vagal rootlets enter the dural subcompartment of the jugular foramen called the vagal meatus. It is inferior to the glossopharyngeal meatus from which it is separated by a dural septum. The vagus nerve is joined by the accessory nerve as it enters the dura (Rhoton, 2000a).

The accessory nerve arises as a widely separated series of rootlets that originated from the medulla at the level of the lower two-thirds of the olive and from the upper cervical cord.

The cranial rootlets arise as a line of rootlets just caudal to the vagal fibers in the post-olivary sulcus. These are more properly regarded as inferior vagal rootlets, since they arise from vagal nuclei. It may be difficult to separate the lower vagal fibers from the upper accessory rootlets because the vagal and cranial accessory fibers usually enter the vagal meatus as a single bundle. The upper rootlets of the spinal portion of the accessory nerve originate several millimeters caudal to the lowest cranial accessory fibers and either course to join the cranial accessory bundle or enter the lower border of the vagal meatus separate from the cranial accessory rootlets. The spinal accessory fibers pass superolateral from their origin to reach the jugular foramen. Although the cranial and spinal portion of the accessory nerve most frequently enter the vagal meatus together, they may infrequently be separated by a dural septum (Rhoton, 2000a).

The rootlets of the hypoglossal nerve arise from the medulla along the anterior margin of the lower two-thirds of the olive in the preolivary sulcus. The rootlets course anterolateral through the subarachnoid space and pass behind the vertebral artery to reach the hypoglossal canal. Before entering the canal, the rootlets collect into two bundles, and in some cases, the canal is even divided by a bony septum that separates the two bundles (Rhoton, 2000a).

6. Technique of minimally invasive endoscopic and endoscopy-assisted microsurgery of vestibular schwannoma

In its basic aspects the surgery proceeds in a similar fashion as an neurotological procedure. General endotracheal anesthesia is administered, profound and balanced with paralysis avoided. Before durotomy, both controlled hypotension and assisted hyperventilation to obtain a pCO2 of about 25 mm Hg are crucial to lower the intracranial pressure and to help spontaneous cerebellar retraction. Bolus of corticoids at the same moment can be beneficial. Mannitol infusions and lumbar drainage are not needed (Miyazaki et al. 2005, Goksu et al. 2006, Betka et al. 2010). If experience shows that the surgery will take more than 3 hours a Foley catheter is placed. A second generation cephalosporin is used for perioperative prophylaxis.

The patient is placed in supine position with the head rotated away from the ipsilateral ear. Patient positioning is crucial, making sure that the shoulder does not restrict access to the surgical field and proper manipulation with instruments. Fixation of the skull is usually not necessary, fastening of the contralateral forehead with a gel sheet is adequate. Another option is to secure the head in a Mayfield 3-pin head clamp. The table is positioned so that the head is elevated above the level of heart.

For the approach the area to be shaved, only 2 to 3 cm behind the ear is sufficient. The landmarks for skin incison are Frankfurt line joining the outer canthus to the superior part of the external auditory meatus, and a line along the posterior margin on the mastoid. Placement of a minicraniotomy can be marked as a 2 cm circle below and behind from the point where the two lines cross. The incision is outlined as an anterior concave line of 3 to 6 cm in length arching from the tip of the mastoid at a position one finger's width back of the oblique line by passing the backside of the keyhole (Fig.2). Placement of the incision is infiltrated with 1: 200000 Epinephrine. The skin flap is elevated with sharp dissection of the temporalis fascia and the pericranium ending at the level of the external auditory canal. Using the cautery knife and raspatory nuchal muscles are detached from the mastoid and occipital bone backwards and a self retaining retractor is placed in position.

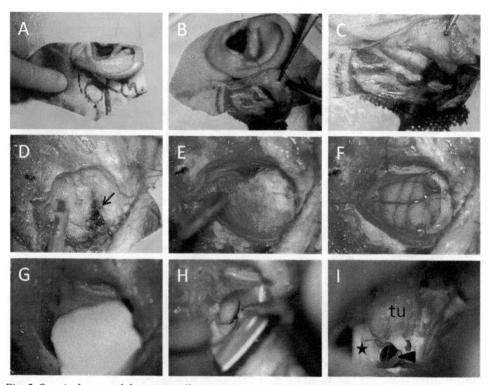

Fig. 2. Surgical steps of the minimally invasive retrosigmoid approach for vestibular schwannoma (*left side*). A: landmarks for skin incison (Frankfurt line and a line along the posterior margin on the mastoid) and place of minicraniotomy (circle) are outlined, B: elevation of the skin flap, C: detachment of the muscles, D: drilling is centered on the emissary vein (arrow), E: minicraniotomy is finished, it is centered on the confluence of sigmoid and transverse sinuses, F: anteriorly based dural flap is elevated and fixated with the suture, G and H: sheet of artificial dura is placed over the cerebellum, the cisterna is opened and cerebrospinal fluid is let to escape and the surgeon waits for the spontaneous cerebellar retraction to occur, H: once adequate cerebellar relaxation has been achieved no brain retractors are needed and dissection of tumor (tu) can proceed (asterisk denotes the seven-eight nerve bundle, arrowhead points on anterior inferior cerebellar artery).

Once adequate exposure of bone is achieved the keyhole craniotomy is performed (Magnan et al. 2002, Miyazaki et al. 2005). Using the cutting burr the drilling starts with the mastoid emissary vein in the centre as the landmark. Asterion represents another anatomic landmark for craniotomy placement as its helps to localize the confluence of sigmoid and transverse sinuses (Rhoton, 2000a, Rhoton, 2000b, Kabil & Shahinian, 2006). All the bone dust is collected to prepare a pate that is solidified with fibrin glue at the end of surgery and used for craniotomy closure. In order to prevent cerebrospinal fluid leakage, all opened mastoid air cells are obliterated with the bone wax. If not used from the beginning it is suggested to use the operating microscope when the dura and posterior margin of sigmoid sinus is approached. It is even safer to use the diamante at this stage of drilling.

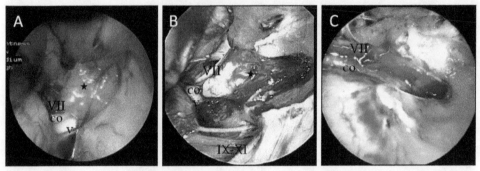

Fig. 3. Minimally invasive endoscopy-assisted removal of small (grade II) vestibular schwannoma (right side). A: anatomic mapping after opening the cisterna (VII: facial nerve, v: vestibular nerves, labyrinthine artery is in between the facial and vestibular nerves), B: internal auditory canal is opened and vestibular nerves sectioned and tumor (asterisk) is exposed, C: control of radicality of resection and integrity of facial and cochlear (co) nerves.

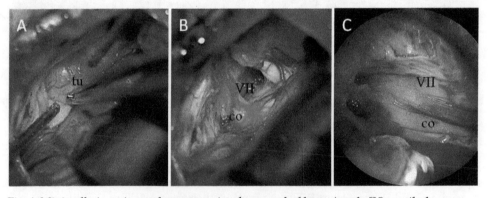

Fig. 4. Minimally invasive endoscopy-assisted removal of large (grade IV) vestibular schwannoma (left side) with preservation of facial and cochlear nerve including preoperatively useful hearing. A: anatomic mapping after opening the cistern, B: cisternal portion of tumor was removed with preservation of cochlear (co) and facial nerve (VII), C: C: control of radicality of resection and integrity of facial and cochlear (co) nerves.

After adequate exposure of the posterior fossa and hemostasis the dura can be incised. An anterior based U-shaped flap is appropriate as its fixation with stay suture helps to retract the sigmoid sinus to gain better access to the cerebellopontine angle. While suctioning of the cerebrospinal fluid, wait for spontaneous cerebellar retraction. Fine neurosurgical cotton 1.5 cm in width and 5 cm in length is placed over the cerebellum to protect it from injury. Cerebellum can be gently pressed by the mid portion of the suction that is gently advanced into the safe corridor between the hemisphere and posterior aspect of the petrous bone until the cerebellopontine cistern is opened at the level of lower cranial nerves. Once adequate cerebellar relaxation has been achieved it is usually not necessary to insert any brain retractor. The endoscopes used are mainly 0° and 30° angled rigid endoscopes of standard 2.7 and 4 mm in diameter and 6, 11 and 14 cm in length according to the situation. If needed 45° and 70° angled rigid endoscopes are used. An irrigation sheath attached to the endoscope clears blood and debris from the lens, eliminating the time consuming and unsafe practice of removing and reinserting the endoscope. A pneumatic holding arm is preferred to secure the endoscope in position, allowing bimanual surgical dissection. Other option is freehand endoscopic technique with an endoscope being moved and held freehand by a second surgeon, with the first surgeon using two other instruments inside the surgical field.

The endoscope and the optical fiber cable used are completely sterilized by autoclaving. By covering the camera cable and the camera adaptor with a sterilized polyethylene cover, endoscopes can be easily exchanged under clean handling conditions. To maintain asepsis, the endoscopic examination is followed on a monitor.

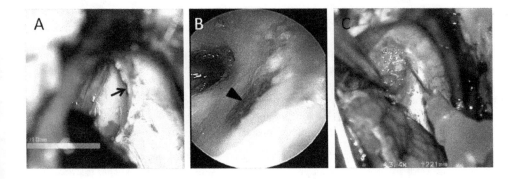

Fig. 5. Endoscopic identification of opened petrous bone air cells. A: with surgical microscope opened air cells might be not visualized with risk for cerebrospinal fluid leakage (position identified by arrow), B: endoscopic view with identification (arrowhead) of opened air cells after drilling of posterior meatal wall, C: sealing of the opened air cells with piece of muscle and tissue glue.

Upon entering the cerebellopontine angle a preliminary survey of the actual neurovascular anatomy including the trigeminal, facial, and lower cranial nerves, as well as the vascular structures is performed (Fig.3 and 4). Neuromonitoring of the facial nerve and hearing is a standard during vestibular schwannoma surgery. Function of the facial nerve stimulator can be checked with stimulation of the accessory nerve rootlets.

Once all the critical structures are identified tumor dissection can take place. The dura overlying the petrous bone posterior to internal auditory canal is cauterized and incised and a diamond bur is used to open the IAC, following the tumor extent laterally within the canal.

No matter whether microsurgical or endoscopic technique is used the basic surgical concept is always to debulk tumor in order to relieve the pressure on the surrounding neurovascular structures. Microdissecting instruments as well as the cavitron ultrasonic aspirator (CUSA) can be used to accomplish this step. Having completed debulking it is easier to appreciate the full anatomical course of the cranial nerves and vessels and to protect them from potential damage. During dissection the most adherent points between the tumor and nerves are recognized and addressed last.

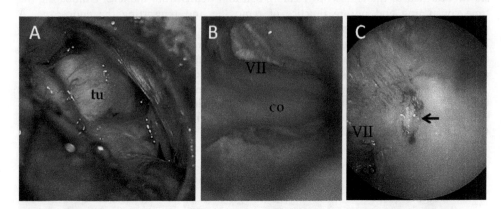

Fig. 6. Minimally invasive endoscopy-assisted removal of large (grade IV) vestibular schwannoma (right side) with preservation of facial and cochlear nerve but "unexplainable" loss of evoked auditory brainstem response during the internal auditory canal opening. A: view of the tumor (tu) after opening the cistern, B:endoscopic control of radicality of resection and integrity of facial (VII) and cochlear (co) nerves, C: loss of hearing was explained with identification of the opened posterior semicircular canal (arrow).

If endoscopic technique is preferred the dissection in the region of the cerebellopontine angle is guided by a 0° endoscope in much the same manner as the microsurgical procedure. Tumor dissection within the internal auditory canal is guided preferentially by the 30° angled endoscope, allowing complete visualization of the lateral extent of the tumor as it is separated from the facial and cochlear nerves. The endoscopes are inserted in the upper part of approach, perpendicular to the sigmoid sinus, or in the angle between the petrous bone and tentorium, while the surgical instruments are inserted below it, along the cerebellar surface. Such position permits both inspection of the relationship between the tumor and critical neurovascular structures, and continuous control of surgical manoeuvres of the instruments, which constantly remain under direct endoscopic view.

Once tumor dissection is completed endoscopic inspection of fundus of the internal auditory canal for residual tumor, integrity of cochlear and facial nerves and meticulous inspection of drilled-out portion of the petrous bone for open air cells that need sealing is performed (Fig.3, 4, 5, 6 and 7). The facial nerve is once again stimulated to confirm its function. Small pieces of fat or muscle together with fibrin glue are used to seal the opened internal auditory canal and petrous bone air cells. Cisterns are repeatedly washed. The dura is reapproximated and sutured to provide a watertight closure.

Bony pate is used to replace the drilled bone at the craniotomy site. Soft tissues of the scalp are closed in anatomical layers without the use of any drains. Following the surgery the patients are typically transferred to intensive care unit for overnight monitoring. Early vestibular rehabilitation is supported postoperatively.

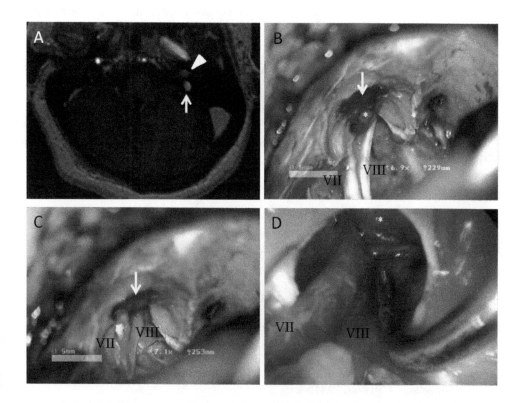

Fig. 7. Minimally invasive endoscopy-assisted removal of intrameatal (grade I) vestibular schwannoma (left side) in case of high jugular bulb. A: MRI showing the high jugular bulb (arrow) being positioned posterior to the internal auditory canal and tumor (arrowhead), B: after drilling the posterior meatal wall high jugular bulb blocks the approach to the medial portion of the tumor, facial (VII) and vestibulocochlear nerve (VIII) can be seen, C: jugular bulb was compressed and major part of the tumor was removed, D: endoscope is used to control tumor removal in the region of fundus of the internal auditory canal.

7. Conclusions

The recent technological advances provided high-quality endoscopes of small diameters and varying lengths and angles, irrigation sheaths for cleaning the lenses inside the operative field, endoscope holders that allow the surgeon to continue using their bimanual microsurgical skills and sophisticated instruments suitable for endoscopic microsurgery. These improvements permit us to use the endoscope, with its wide panoramic, multiangled, and close-up view of the anatomic structures, to ideally express its best properties in deep-seated and narrow space-located lesions of the skull base.

The introduction of endoscopic technique into the repertoire of the surgical methods of treatment of the cerebellopontine angle pathologies has proved to be useful. Although only limited surgical series concerning the employment of the endoscopic techniques for the removal of vestibular schwannomas have been reported recently, it seems clear that the endoscopes offer some advantages over the conventional microsurgical technique either in reducing the invasiveness or in allowing safer and more radical tumor removal, thus helping to lower the complication rate and improving the results. Nevertheless, good equipment and special training are absolutely necessary for attainment of optimal results.

8. Acknowledgements

This work was supported by grants of the Internal Grant Agency of the Ministry of Health of the Czech Republic NS/9909-4, NT/12459-5, NT/11543-6 and Charles University project for support of Specific University Research No. 262510. Authors are grateful to Daniel Kameny M.D. for reading the manuscript.

9. References

Badr-El-Dine M, El-Garem HF, Talaat AM, Magnan J (2002). Endoscopically assisted minimally invasive microvascular decompression of hemifacial spasm. Otol Neurotol 23:122-128.

Betka J, Zverina E, Lisy J, Chovanec M, Kluh J, Kraus J (2008). Vestibular schwannoma. Otorinolaryngol Phoniatr (Prague) 57:221-225.

Betka J, Zverina E, Chovanec M, Kluh J, Lukes P, Kraus J, Lisy J (2009). Minimally invasive endoscopic and endoscopy-assisted microsurgery of vestibular schwannoma. Endoskopie 18:67-71.

Bremond G, Garcin M, Magnan J, Bonnaud G (1974). L'abord a minima de l'espace ponto-cerebelleux. Cah ORL 19:443-460.

Bremond G, Garcin M (1975). Microsurgical approach to the cerebellopontine angle. J Laryngol Otol 89:237-248.

Brito Neto RV, Bento RF, Yasuda A, Ribas GC, Rodrigues AJ Jr (2005). Anatomical references in auditory brainstem implant surgery. Braz J Otorhinolaryngol 71:282-286.

Cakrt O, Chovanec M, Funda T, Kalitova P, Betka J, Zverina E, Kolar P, Jerabek J (2010). Exercise with visual feedback improves postural stability after vestibular schwannoma surgery. Eur Arch Otorhinolaryngol 267:1355-1360.

Cappabianca P, Cavallo LM, Esposito F, de Divitiis E, Tschabitscher M (2002). Endoscopic examination of the cerebellar pontine angle. Clin Neurol Neurosurg 104:387-391.

Chen MJ, Zhang WJ, Yang C, Wu YQ, Zhang ZY, Wang Y (2008). Endoscopic neurovascular perspective in microvascular decompression of trigeminal neuralgia. J Craniomaxillofac Surg 36:456-461.

Cheng WY, Chao SC, Shen CC (2008). Endoscopic microvascular decompression of the hemifacial spasm. Surg Neurol 70 Suppl 1:40-46.

Cheng S, Naidoo Y, da Cruz M, Dexter M (2009). Quality of life in postoperative vestibular schwannoma patients. Laryngoscope 119:2252-2257.

Clemis JD, Ballad WJ, Baggot PJ, Lyon ST (1986). Relative frequency of inferior vestibular schwannoma. Arch Otolaryngol Head Neck Surg 112:190-194.

Colletti V, Fiorino FG, Carner M, Giarbini N, Sacchetto L, Cumer G (2000). Advantages of the retrosigmoid approach in auditory brain stem implantation. Skull Base Surg 10:165-170.

Colletti V, Fiorino F (2005). Is the middle fossa approach the treatment of choice for intracanalicular vestibular schwannoma? Otolaryngol Head Neck Surg 132:459-466.

de Divitiis O, Cavallo LM, Dal Fabbro M, Elefante A, Cappabianca P (2007). Freehand dynamic endoscopic resection of an epidermoid tumor of the cerebellopontine angle: technical case report. Neurosurgery 61:239-240.

Doyen E (1917). In: Surgical therapeutics and operative techniques, vol. 1., 599-602, Balliere, Tindall and Cox, London.

Ebner FH, Roser F, Shiozawa T, Ruetschlin S, Kirschniak A, Koerbel A, Tatagiba M (2009). Petrosal vein occlusion in cerebello-pontine angle tumour surgery: an anatomical study of alternative draining pathways. Eur J Surg Oncol 35:552-556.

Eby JB, Cha ST, Shahinian HK (2001). Fully endoscopic vascular decompression of the facial nerve for hemifacial spasm. Skull Base 11:189-197.

El-Garem HF, Badr-El-Dine M, Talaat AM, Magnan J (2002). Endoscopy as a tool in minimally invasive trigeminal neuralgia surgery. Otol Neurotol 23:132-135.

Friedland DR, Wackym PA (1999). Evaluation of surgical approaches to endoscopic auditory brainstem implantation. Laryngoscope 109:175-180.

Fries G, Perneczky A (1998). Endoscope-assisted brain surgery: Part 2—analysis of 380 procedures. Neurosurgery 42:226-232.

Fukushima T (1978). Endoscopy of Meckel's cave, cisterna magna and cerebellopontine angle. Technical note. J Neurosurg 48:302-306.

Gerganov VM, Giordano M, Herold C, Samii A, Samii M (2010). An electrophysiological study on the safety of the endoscope-assisted microsurgical removal of vestibular schwannomas. Eur J Surg Oncol 36:422-427.

Gerosa M, Mesiano N, Longhi M, De Simone A, Foroni R, Verlicchi A, Zanotti B, Nicolato A (2010). Gamma Knife surgery in vestibular schwannomas: impact on the anterior and posterior labyrinth. J Neurosurg 113 Suppl:128-135.

Goksu N, Bayazit Y, Kemaloglu Y (1999). Endoscopy of the posterior fossa and dissection of acoustic neuroma. J Neurosurg 91:776-780.

Goksu N, Yilmaz M, Bayramoglu I, Aydil U, Bayazit YA (2005). Evaluation of the results of endoscope-assisted acoustic neuroma surgery through posterior fossa approach. ORL J Otorhinolaryngol Relat Spec 67:87-91.

Goksu N, Bayazit YA, Bayramoglu I, Isik B, Yilmaz M, Kurtipek O, Uygur K (2006). Surgical exposure in retrosigmoid approach: do we need cerebellar retractors? Surg Neurol 65:631-634.

Griffith HB (1975). Technique of fontanelle and presutural ventriculoscopy and endoscopic ventricular surgery in infants. Childs Brain 1:359-363.

Guevara N, Deveze A, Buza V, Laffont B, Magnan J (2008). Microvascular decompression of cochlear nerve for tinnitus incapacity: pre-surgical data, surgical analyses and long-term follow-up of 15 patients. Eur Arch Otorhinolaryngol 265:397-401.

Hori T, Okada Y, Maruyama T, Chernov M, Attia W (2006). Endoscope-controlled removal of intrameatal vestibular schwannomas. Minim Invasive Neurosurg 49:25-29.

Jarrahy R, Young J, Berci G, Shahinian HK (1999). Endoscopic skull base surgery II: a new animal model for surgery of the posterior fossa. J Invest Surg 12:335-339.

Jarrahy R, Berci G, Shahinian HK (2000). Endoscope-assisted microvascular decompression of the trigeminal nerve. Otolaryngol Head Neck Surg 123:218-223.

Jarrahy R, Cha ST, Eby JB, Berci G, Shahinian HK (2002a). Fully endoscopic vascular decompression of the glossopharyngeal nerve. J Craniofac Surg. 13:90-95.

Jarrahy R, Eby JB, Cha ST, Shahinian HK (2002b). Fully endoscopic vascular decompression of the trigeminal nerve. Minim Invasive Neurosurg 45:32-35.

Kabil MS, Eby JB, Shahinian HK (2005). Endoscopic vascular decompression versus microvascular decompression of the trigeminal nerve. Minim Invasive Neurosurg 48:207-212.

Kabil MS, Shahinian HK (2006). A series of 112 fully endoscopic resections of vestibular schwannomas. Minim Invasive Neurosurg 49:362-368.

Koval J, Molcan M, Bowdler AD, Sterkers JM (1993). Retrosigmoid transmeatal approach: an anatomic study of an approach used for preservation of hearing in acoustic neuroma surgery and vestibular neurotomy. Skull Base Surg 3:16-21.

Koval J, Krempaska S, Kaliarik L (2009). Minimal retrosigmoidal approach with applied endoscopy. Otorinolaryngol Phoniatr (Prague) 58:8-14.

Koval J, Krempaska S (2009). Anatomic logic of the foramen Luschka in neurootologic surgery. Otolaryngol Pol 63:398-402.

King WA, Wackym PA (1999). Endoscope assisted Surgery for acoustic neuromas Vestibular Schwannomas): early experience using the rigid hopkins telescope. Neurosurgery 44:1095-1102.

Koerbel A, Gharabaghi A, Safavi-Abbasi S, Samii A, Ebner FH, Samii M, Tatagiba M (2009). Venous complications following petrosal vein sectioning in surgery of petrous apex meningiomas. Eur J Surg Oncol 35:773-779.

Linskey ME (2000). Stereotactic radiosurgery versus stereotactic radiotherapy for patients with vestibular schwannoma: a Leksell Gamma Knife Society 2000 debate. J Neurosurg 93 Suppl 3:90-95.

Low WK (1999a). Middle cranial fossa approach to the internal auditory Meatus:A Chinese temporal bone study. ORL J Otorhinolaryngol Relat Spec 61:142-145.

Low WK (1999b). Enhancing hearing preservation in endoscopic-assisted excision of acoustic neuroma via the retrosigmoid approach. J Laryngol Otol 113:973-977.

Magnan J, Chays A, Caces F, Lepetre C, Cohen JM, Belus JF, Bruzzo M (1993). Contribution of endoscopy of the cerebellopontine angle by retrosigmoid approach. Neuroma and neuro-vascular de compression. Ann Otolaryngol Chir Cervicofac 110:259-265.

Magnan J, Chays A, Lepetre C, Pencroffi E, Locatelli P (1994). Endoscopy of the cerebellopontine angle. Am J Otol 15:366-370.

Magnan J, Caces F, Locatelli P, Chays A (1997). Hemifacial spasm: endoscopic vascular decompression. Otolaryngol Head Neck Surg 117:308-314.

Magnan J, Barbieri M, Mora R, Murphy S, Meller R, Bruzzo M, Chays A (2002). Retrosigmoid approach for small and medium-sized acoustic neuromas. Otol Neurotol 23:141-145.

Martin HC, Sethi J, Lang D, Neil-Dwyer G, Lutman ME, Yardley L (2001). Patient-assessed outcomes after excision of acoustic neuroma: postoperative symptoms and quality of life. J Neurosurg 94:211-216.

McKennan K (1993). Endoscopy of the internal auditory canal during hearing conservation acoustic neuroma surgery. Am J Otol 14:259-262.

Mer SB, Derbyshire AJ, Brushenko A, Pontarelli DA (1967). Fiberoptic endotoscopes for examining the middle ear. Arch Otolaryngol 85: 387-393.

Miyazaki H, Deveze A, Magnan J (2005). Neuro-otologic surgery through minimally invasive retrosigmoid approach: endoscope assisted microvascular decompression, vestibular neurotomy, and tumor removal. Laryngoscope 15:1612-1617.

Myrseth E, Møller P, Wentzel-Larsen T, Goplen F, Lund-Johansen M (2006). Untreated vestibular schwannomas: vertigo is a powerful predictor for health-related quality of life. Neurosurgery 59:67-76.

Myrseth E, Pedersen PH, Møller P, Lund-Johansen M (2007). Treatment of vestibular schwannomas. Why, when and how? Acta Neurochir (Wien) 149:647-660.

Myrseth E, Møller P, Pedersen PH, Lund-Johansen M (2009). Vestibular schwannoma: surgery or gamma knife radiosurgery? A prospective, nonrandomized study. Neurosurgery 64:654-661.

O'Donoghue GM, O'Flynn P (1993). Endoscopic anatomy of the cerebellopontine angle. Am J Otol 14:122-125.

Oppel F (1978). Endoscopy of the cerebello-pontine angle: its diagnostic and therapeutic possibilities. In: *Advances and Technical Standards in Neurosurgery, vol. 5*, 269-275, Springer-Verlag, ISBN 0387814418, Berlin.

Oppel F (1981). Indications and operative technique for endoscopy of the cerebellopontine angle. In: *The Cranial Nerves*, Samii M, Jannetta P, 429-437, Springer-Verlag, ISBN 0387106200, Berlin.

Ozluoglu LN, Akbasak A (1996). Video endoscopy-assisted vestibular neurectomy: a new approach to the eighth cranial nerve. Skull Base Surg 6:215-219.

Perneczky A, Fries G (1998). Endoscope-assisted brain surgery: part 1--evolution, basic concept, and current technique. Neurosurgery 42:219-224.

Prott W (1974). Cisternoscopy endoscopy of the cerebello-pontine angle. Acta Neurochir 31:105-113.

Putnam TJ (1942). The surgical treatment of infantile hydrocephalus. Surg Gynecol Obstet 76:171-182.

Rhoton AL Jr (2000a). The cerebellopontine angle and posterior fossa cranial nerves by the retrosigmoid approach. Neurosurgery 47 Suppl 3:93-129.

Rhoton AL Jr (2000b). The temporal bone and transtemporal approaches. Neurosurgery 47 Suppl 3: 211-265.

Rhoton AL Jr (2000c). The cerebellar arteries. Neurosurgery 47 Suppl 3: 29-68.

Rhoton AL Jr (2000d). The posterior fossa veins. Neurosurgery 47 Suppl 3:69-92.

Rosenberg SI, Silverstein H, Willcox TO, Gordon MA (1994). Endoscopy in otology and neurootology. Am J Otol 15:168-172.

Roser F, Tatagiba MS (2010). The first 50s: can we achieve acceptable results in vestibular schwannoma surgery from the beginning? Acta Neurochir (Wien) 152:1359-1365.

Ryzenman JM, Pensak ML, Tew JM Jr (2005). Headache: a quality of life analysis in a cohort of 1,657 patients undergoing acoustic neuroma surgery, results from the acoustic neuroma association. Laryngoscope 115:703-711.

Sakamoto GT, Blevins N, Gibbs IC (2009). Cyberknife radiotherapy for vestibular schwannoma. Otolaryngol Clin North Am 42:665-675.

Saman Y, Bamiou DE, Gleeson M (2009). A contemporary review of balance dysfunction following vestibular schwannoma surgery. Laryngoscope 119:2085-93.

Samii M, Matthies C (1997). Management of 1000 vestibular schwannomas (acoustic neuromas): the facial nerve-preservation and restitution of function. Neurosurgery 40:684-694.

Sandooram D, Grunfeld EA, McKinney C, Gleeson MJ (2004). Quality of life following microsurgery, radiosurgery and conservative management for unilateral vestibular schwannoma. Clin Otolaryngol Allied Sci 29:621-627.

Schroeder HW, Oertel J, Gaab MR (2004). Endoscope-assisted microsurgical resection of epidermoid tumors of the cerebellopontine angle. J Neurosurg 101:227-232.

Schroeder HW, Nehlsen M (2009). Value of high-definition imaging in neuroendoscopy. Neurosurg Rev 32:303-308.

Shahinian HK, Eby JB, Ocon M (2004). Fully endoscopic excision of vestibular schwannomas. Minim Invasive Neurosurg 47:329-332.

Skrivan J, Zverina E, Betka J, Svetlik M, Kluh J, Sollmann WP, Kraus J, Belsan T, Tichy T, Sedlak S, Topol M (2003). Use of the auditory brainstem neuroprosthesis in the Czech Republic. Cas Lek Cesk 142:29-33.

Skrivan J, Zverina E, Betka J, Kluh J, Kraus J (2004). Our surgical experience with large vestibular schwannomas. Otolaryngol Pol 58:69-72.

Springborg JB, Poulsgaard L, Thomsen J (2008). Nonvestibular schwannoma tumors in the cerebellopontine angle: a structured approach and management guidelines. Skull Base 18:217-227.

Stangerup SE, Tos M, Thomsen J, Caye-Thomasen P (2010). True incidence of vestibular schwannoma? Neurosurgery 67:1335-1340.

Sughrue ME, Yang I, Aranda D, Kane AJ, Parsa AT (2010a). Hearing preservation rates after microsurgical resection of vestibular schwannoma. J Clin Neurosci 17:1126-1129.

Sughrue ME, Yang I, Rutkowski MJ, Aranda D, Parsa AT (2010b). Preservation of facial nerve function after resection of vestibular schwannoma. Br J Neurosurg 24):666-671.

Sughrue ME, Kane AJ, Kaur R, Barry JJ, Rutkowski MJ, Pitts LH, Cheung SW, Parsa AT (2011). A prospective study of hearing preservation in untreated vestibular schwannomas. J Neurosurg 114:381-385.

Tallan EM, Harner SG, Beatty CW, Scheithauer BW, Parisi JE (1993). Does the distribution of Schwann cells correlate with the observed occurrence of acoustic neuromas? Am J Otol 14:131-134 .

Tatagiba M, Matthies C, Samii M (1996). Microendoscopy of the internal auditory canal in vestibular schwannoma surgery. Neurosurgery 38:737-740.

Valtonen HJ, Poe DS, Heilman CB, Tarlov EC (1997). Endoscopically assisted prevention of cerebrospinal fluid leak in suboccipital acoustic neuroma surgery. Am J Otol 18:381-85.

Wackym PA, King WA, Barker FG, Poe DS (1998). Endoscope-assisted vestibular neurectomy. Laryngoscope 108:1787-1793.

Wackym PA, King WA, Poe DS, Meyer GA, Ojemann RG, Barker FG, Walsh PR, Staecker H (1999). Adjunctive use of endoscopy during acoustic neuroma surgery. Laryngoscope 109:1193-1201.

Wackym PA, King WA, Meyer GA, Poe DS (2002). Endoscopy in neuro-otologic surgery. Otolaryngol Clin North Am 35:297–323.

Wackym PA (2005). Stereotactic radiosurgery, microsurgery, and expectant management of acoustic neuroma: basis for informed consent. Otolaryngol Clin North Am 38:653-670.

Wackym PA, Hannley MT, Runge-Samuelson CL, Jensen J, Zhu YR (2008). Gamma Knife surgery of vestibular schwannomas: longitudinal changes in vestibular function and measurement of the Dizziness Handicap Inventory. J Neurosurg 109 Suppl:137-143.

Wanibuchi M, Fukushima T, McElveen JT Jr, Friedman AH (2009). Hearing preservation in surgery for large vestibular schwannomas. J Neurosurg 111:845-854.

Yamakami I, Uchino Y, Kobayashi E, Yamaura A (2003). Conservative management, gamma-knife radiosurgery, and microsurgery for acoustic neurinomas: a systematic review of outcome and risk of three therapeutic options. Neurol Res 25:682-690.

Yang I, Sughrue ME, Han SJ, Aranda D, Pitts LH, Cheung SW, Parsa AT (2010). A comprehensive analysis of hearing preservation after radiosurgery for vestibular schwannoma. J Neurosurg 112:851-859.

Yuguang L, Chengyuan W, Meng L, Shugan Z, Wandong S, Gang L, Xingang L (2005). Neuroendoscopic anatomy and surgery of the cerebellopontine angle. J Clin Neurosci 12:256-260.

Zverina E (2010). Acoustic neuroma--vestibular schwannoma--personal experience of up-to-date management. Cas Lek Cesk 149:269-276.

Part 3

Endoscopy in Ophthalmology

Ocular Endoscopy

Durval Moraes de Carvalho[1], Francisco Eduardo Lima[2]
and Durval Moraes de Carvalho Jr[3]
[1,2]Centro Brasileiro de Cirurgia de Olhos
[2]Universidade Federal de Goiás - UFG
[3]Centro Brasileiro da Visão
Brazil

1. Introduction

The ocular endoscopy is available to the ophthalmology since the early 90's, however, until now there has not been consolidated as an essential tool to the world's ophthalmology (Uram, 1992b). The intraocular view is usually possible through adequate light and lens devices, due to the transparency of the part. These tools are practical and they may be also economical; in the cases which the cornea, anterior chamber, crystalline and vitreous are confusing the transparency, the ophthalmology has other resources using ultrasound and x-ray devices which enable the insight of the intraocular problems.

Nowadays the ocular endoscopy is an important resource to ophthalmology practice. Besides the sporadic use of it to the intraocular visualization, there are two other procedures in which it is essential: (a) In glaucoma surgery, Endoscopic cyclophotocoagulation (ECP) (Chen et al., 1997; Lima, 2000; Uram, 1992a; Lima, 1997). (b) In the implantation of intraocular lenses (IOL) in eyes without a capsular support (Scleral fixation) (Carvalho et al., 1996).

2. Glaucoma surgery using endoscopy: The Carvalho-Lima technique

The Glaucoma is an illness of the optical nerve which is irreversible and the intraocular pressure (IOP) is the most frequent cause of it. The primary open-angle glaucoma (POAG) is far the most common type of glaucoma in clinical practice, initially being treated with eye drops. For the cases in which the glaucoma surgery is indicated there are mainly two approaches:

One of them which is classical in all the world is the trying to increase the drainage of aqueous flow, the so called filtering surgeries. The main complications associated with filtering surgeries are due either to scaring process or overfiltration.

The other surgical approach to treat glaucoma is based on diminishing the aqueous production, and have the IOP reduced. Those are the cyclodestructive procedures. These procedures were usually performed by a transscleral route, either by freezing the ciliary body (cyclocryotherapy) or by coagulating the ciliary body with a laser source. Because the surgeon is not able to see the targets being treated, adjacent tissues may be damaged during this process, which may contribute to a relatively high rate of complications, such as pain, visual acuity reduction, inflammation, hypotony and *phthisis bulbi*.

Recently, a new device (Fig. 1) that combines a laser source (Uram, 1992b), endoscopic probe (Fig. 2) and an illumination beam in the same probe has been developed. This instrument has the unique ability of simultaneous visualization and treatment of the ciliary body through a pars plana or anterior segment approach, or even combined with a cataract extraction. Additionally, some authors (Chen et al., 1997; Lima, 2000; Uram, 1992a; Lima, 1997) have demonstrated the safety and efficacy of the endocyclophotocoagulation (ECP) for treatment of refractory glaucoma.

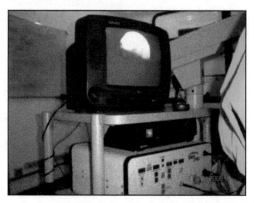

Fig. 1. Ocular endoscopy device; LASER (MicroProbe, ENDOOPTIKS, Little Silver, NJ, USA).

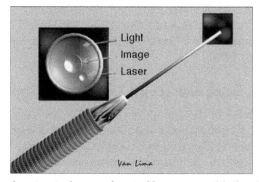

Fig. 2. The ECP probe showing its layers of optic fiber responsible for the light, videoendoscopy and LASER.

The ECP was done with a commercially available device (MicroProbe, ENDOOPTIKS, Little Silver, NJ, USA) with an endoscope with a 110-degree field of view and a focal distance of 2mm, camera and an 810 nm wavelength diode laser source with maximum power of 1.2W. In most of the cases the laser power used is 0.5W, continuous mode for approximately 2 seconds to produce both whitening and shrinkage of the ciliary processes. Laser power and/or duration is decreased if a "pop" is heard.

In phakic eyes the Carvalho-Lima's technique is indicated.

Carvalho-Lima's technique consists of phacoemulsification combined with ECP. ECP is acompplished through the bag and before the intraocular lens implantation (Fig. 3).

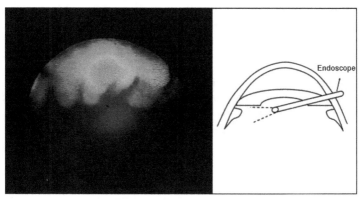

Fig. 3. Photocoagulation of the most bulging part of the ciliary process.

External scleral depression is performed to facilitate the photocoagulation of the entire ciliary process, including the valleys between the the crests of the pars plicata and the anterior third of the pars plana. Additionally, external scleral depression is usefull to guide the surgeon on how much of the ciliary process has been photocoagulated. This technique won a prize in the movies festival of ASCRS in 1999 (Fig. 4).

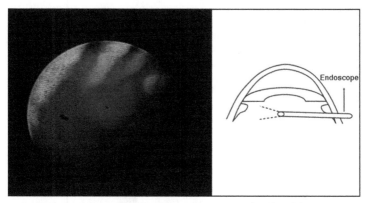

Fig. 4. Photocoagulation of the tail of the ciliary process with scleral depression.

In pseudophakic eyes the procedure is performed by a superior temporal pars plana incision, 3.5mm from the limbus after anterior vitrectomy.

In all eyes ECP is done to 210° of the ciliary body, corresponding to 2 to 9 hours in the right eye and from 3 to 10 hours in the left eye, including the anterior third of the pars plana. Subconjunctival injection of tobramycin and dexamethasone is performed after each procedure. Additionally, 0.1 ml of dexamethasone was injected in the anterior chamber. Topical antibiotics, corticosteroids and atropine were prescribed post-operatively and tapered as the intraocular inflammation decreased.

It is has been observed that when the laser was used in the pars plana just behind the ciliary processes the hypotensive effect was greater. Would pars plana also be a secretor of aqueous? An experimental work done by Dr Durval M. Carvalho JR, MD (Carvalho Jr, 2002) in 2002 was to make it clear most of our doubts. The photocoagulation caused by the ECP causes three different tissue reactions, which varies according to the region of the ciliary body (Fig. 5 and 6), the intensity and time exposed to the laser. The first reaction observed is the whitening of the surface and if the laser exposition continues there is a shrinkage of the ciliary process. If the exposition is excessive, the energy is stored inside the ciliary process and it causes its explosion, emitting a short sound, possible to be heard (pop). The pop indicates overtreatment and is associated with hemorrhage, pigment dispersion and inflammatory reaction. Even though the explosion guarantees the destruction of the ciliary process, it must be avoided so as to cause less side effects.

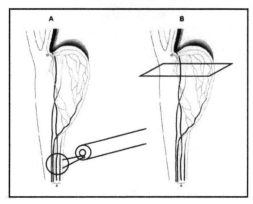

Fig. 5. Photocoagulation of the pars plana.

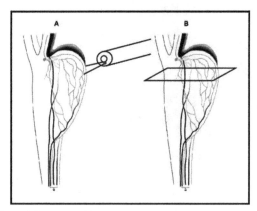

Fig. 6. Photocoagulation of the pars plicata.

In an experimental study (Carvalho Jr, 2002) evaluated the effect of the ECP in the different parts of the ciliary body in rabbit eyes. In the hystopathological analyses (Fig. 7) it was observed an indirect effect of the laser in the microcirculation of the ciliary body and not only the direct lesion to the epithelium. One of the most elucidative founds was the presence of vascular congestion of all the ciliary process when only the pars plana was photocoagulatedm suggesting strong suspect of a coagulative trombosis caused by the laser (Fig. 8).

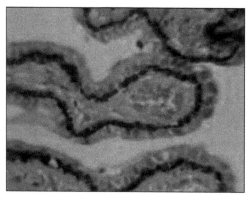

Fig. 7. Hystopathological photograph of a ciliary process of the eye of a rabbit without structure alterations.

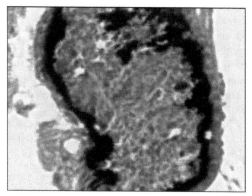

Fig. 8. Ciliary process enlarged with a vascular congestion after recent photocoagulation of the pars plana region.

So these findings may explain in part the variation of results according to the extension to be treated. The applications only in the part of the head (anterior) of the ciliary process can not achieve all the venule arcades, justifying this way an effect bellow the expected, and also explain the eyes treated 360° not to evolute to a bulbar atrophy. On the other hand the treatment only of the pars plana region reaches a higher hypotensor effect, justifying some cases of transcleral cyclophotocoagulation being effective achieving only the pars plana region. The practical application of this found comes to help with the interest of treating a shorter extension of the ciliary body and obtain higher effectivity reducing the IOP, reducing the risk of complications such as the bulbar atrophy. For this the application must be selective and assisted where the endoscopy showed superior itself, although this is an invasive procedure.

Lima and other authors, (Lima et al., 1997; Lima et al., 2004) obtained a clinical evidence in cases of refractory glaucoma treated by ECP, being photocoagulated all the ciliary process including its most posterior portion with the help of a scleral depression in a shorter extension. The reduction of the IOP to acceptable levels and its maintenance as time passes, and also the shorter risk of hypotony and bulbar atrophy has increased the confidence in the technique, that seems to be successesful to other indications and not only as the last option.

Beyond the treatment of glaucoma and cataract combined, the main indications to ECP are:

• Eyes submitted to, at least, a filtration surgery with antimetabolics;
• As a primary procedure in eyes with glaucoma associated to a penetrating keratoplasty;
• As a primary procedure in neovascular glaucoma;
• Eyes submitted to drainage implant surgery;
• Eyes with the conjunctive attached and healed after the cataract surgery, retine surgeries, burn, traumas,etc.;
• Eyes with a congenital glaucoma after goniotomy and or trabeculotoctomy and a trabeculectomy.

Lima and other authors (Lima et al., 2004) have developed a prospective study to compare endoscopic cyclophotocoagulation (ECP) and the Ahmed drainage implant in the treatment of refractory glaucoma.

Sixty-eight eyes of 68 patients with refractory glaucoma were prospectively assigned to either ECP or Ahmed tube shunt implantation. All procedures were performed by a single surgeon. Eyes that were included were pseudophakic with a history of at least one trabeculectomy with antimetabolite, an intraocular pressure (IOP) equal to or above 35 mmHg on maximum tolerated medical therapy, and a visual acuity better than light perception.

Exclusion criteria included eyes that had had previous glaucoma drainage device implantation or a cyclodestructive procedure. Success was defined as an IOP more than 6 mmHg and less than 21 mmHg, with or without topical anti-hypertensive therapy.

The mean follow-up was 19.82 ± 8.35 months and 21.29 ± 6.42 months, for the Ahmed and ECP groups, respectively ($p = 0.4$). The pre-operative IOP, 41.32 ± 3.03 mmHg (Ahmed) and 41.61 ± 3.42 mmHg (ECP) ($p = 0.5$), and the mean post-operative IOP, at 24 months follow-up, 14.73 ± 6.44 mmHg (Ahmed) and 14.07 ± 7.21 mmHg (ECP) ($p = 0.7$), were significantly different from baseline in both groups ($p<0.001$). Kaplan-Meier survival curve analysis showed a probability of success at 24 months of 70.59% and 73.53% for the Ahmed and ECP groups respectively ($p = 0.7$).

Complications included choroidal detachment (Ahmed 17.64%, ECP 2.94%), shallow anterior chamber (Ahmed 17.64%, ECP 0.0%) and hyphema (Ahmed 14.7%, ECP 17.64%).

In conclusion there was no difference in the success rate between the Ahmed Glaucoma Valve and ECP in refractory glaucoma. The eyes that underwent Ahmed tube shunt implantation had more complications than those treated with ECP.

A recent study (Lima et al., 2010) was designed to evaluate the safety and efficacy of phacoemulsification and endoscopic cyclophotocoagulation (ECP) as a primary surgical treatment for glaucoma and cataract.

Three hundred sixty-eight eyes from 243 patients with primary open-angle glaucoma and cataract that underwent an uncomplicated surgery from October 1998 to December 2006 with at least 2 years of follow-up were retrospectively enrolled. The patients were excluded if presented with a previous ocular history of any intraocular surgery or glaucoma laser treatment. Qualified success was defined as 5 mmHg < intraocular pressure (IOP) < 21 mmHg with or without topical antiglaucomatous drugs, and complete success as the same

IOP levels without therapy at all timepoints. Additionally, the needed of any further glaucoma surgery was defined as failure.

The mean follow-up was 35.15 ± 8.14 months. The IOP pre-operatively (23.07 ± 5.52 mmHg) was significantly greater than in the first day post-operatively (13.14 ± 6.09 mmHg), and months 1 (11.03 ± 2.59 mmHg), 6 (12.33 ± 3.01 mmHg), 12 (12.19 ± 2.19 mmHg), 24 (12.14 ± 2.89 mmHg) and in the last appointment (12.29 ± 2.44 mmHg) (p < 0.001 in all timepoints). The number of medications pre-operatively (1.44 ± 0.97) decreased (0.37 ± 0.74) (p < 0,001). Furthermore, there was significantly improvement in the LogMar visual acuity (p = 0.01). 334 (90.76%) eyes achieved qualified success, and 205 (55.7%), complete success.

Complications included immediate post-operative IOP spike 14.4% (53/368), post-operative fibrin exudates in anterior chamber 7.06% (26/368), cystoid macular edema 4.34% (16/368), transitory hypotony 2.17% (8/368), iris *bombé* 1.08% (4/368).

Phacoemulsification associated with Endoscopic Cyclophotocoagulation is safe and effective as a primary procedure for combined glaucoma and cataract.

There is no gold standard for surgical treatment of glaucoma. All the available techiniques are unpredictable as far as the results and complications. Because of the direct approach to the ciliary body, the endoscopic cyclophotocoagulation (ECP) may be a reasonable option in these eyes.

3. Endoscopy in scleral fixation

In the past, cataract surgery just removed the opacified natural lens, living the patient without any substitute lens (aphakia), forced wear glasses with a very high degree. The history began to change in the war of 1945 when fragments of a transparent substance from the airplanes got incrusted in the eye of one of the pilots and it did not caused any reaction; based on this Dr. Nicholas Harold Ridley was able to have a lens of this material which PMMA (polimethilmetracrilate) made and implanted it in the eye of a human; this was the first experience of a lens implantation inside the eye; since then, the technological evolution so as to substitute the glasses by intraocular lens (IOL) has got no limits. There has been a great advance in the industries that make lens of different materials and functions, of equipments that make it easy the surgeries; surgical techniques more and more efficient and surgeons each time more able. Due to these concepts nobody else wants to wear glasses. Even all of this advanced technology, there are complicated cases of cataract surgery that intraocular lens support is lost. Not implant the intraocular lens is a great complication, making necessary use postoperatively glasses with high degrees from 12 to 13 diopters, causing a poor quality of vision. How to implant a intraocular lens in the eye which does not have the capsule to support it anymore? So as to answer these questions we brought togheter our experience with others surgeons experts in different techniques and wrote a book: "Cataract Surgery - Fixation and Secondary Implants" edited by Elsevier in Portuguese (by now). Either in the literature and also in the ophthalmological practice we noticed that we are able to gather the techniques of lens fixation in eyes without a capsular support in the following groups: Anterior Chamber Intraocular Lens; Fixating the lens at the Iris; Fixating the lens at the sclera.

3.1 Anterior chamber intraocular lens

Anterior Chamber Intraocular Lens is a intraocular lens adapted to the anterior segment and implanted at anterior chamber angle , transition between the corneal and iris. The ease of implantation is its advantage and the complications are related to corneal decompensation and iris inflammation.

3.2 Fixation of the lens in the iris

Fixation of the lens in the iris has the advantage of using most of the time the same intraocular lens of a regular cataract surgery. Its complications are most related to deviation of the pupil, iris inflammation, subluxation of the lens to fundus of the eye. This technique depends on good condition of the iris are therefore not for all cases.

3.3 Scleral fixation with endoscopy

We preferred the technique of fixation of the lens at the sclera because it can be applied in most of cases and intraocular lens stay closer to original position of the natural lens. Most of its complications like decentration of lens and cistic macular edema are related to incorrect positioning of the lens. These complications can be avoided by choosing the correct tecnique, its training and application of endoscopic fidings. Part of scleral fixation works behind the iris, exactly where the haptics of the lens are fixated at scleral wall. The haptics are tightened by unabsorbable suture, fixating them in the scleral with buried stitches. The difficulty is that the ideal place for positioning and fixating the lens is just behind the iris, on blind area. Many decentrations of lens had unknown causes, and could not be repaired due to lack of visualization.

With the advent of the endoscope was first presented by Leon and al. in 1991, allowed us expose the blind region. With the technological advance of the ocular endoscopy in the 90's it was supposed to be given a solution to this problem to fixate an intra-ocular lens because with the endoscopy it is possible to have a visualization of the region behind the iris. With endoscopy we find the answer of all decentrations of the lens. However we have this visualization difficulty during the execution of techniques of sclera fixation. We observed that to use the ocular endoscopy in the surgery of sclera fixation it is essential that our technique is used: Finger Crafted Technique (Carvalho et al., 2009). Since we started to work with ocular endoscopy (1996), we perform the surgeries of scleral fixation with total visualization of the ciliary body (behind the iris) at the moment of the line passage and we know exactly where the loop of the lens will be positioned. We have observed that the surgeons have had difficulties on the use of the endoscopy to this procedure recently, not because of the device but due to the surgery technique. Using the Finger Crafted Technique the surgeon handles the needle with the fingers and this permits total security and control to the movement in which the line is passed. In this technique, the other hand gets free enabling the use of the Endoscope easily and with practice. In my conclusion, the scleral fixation is not yet a reproductive technique, standardized and safe, not because of lack of the endoscopy, but because of the non-use of a technique that enable the use of the device with practice similar to what happens when the Finger Crafted Technique is used.

3.4 Surgical technique
3.4.1 Materials

The materials used in this surgical technique include a 30.5-gauge needle that is often used for insulin administration as a guide needle. Suture used in this technique is a 9-0 prolene suture with 2 needles of 0.65 mm. A Blumental type of anterior maintainer is used to keep the anterior chamber from collapsing. A hook with a T tip is used as needed during the surgery. The endoscope provides direct visualization of the ciliary sulcus and aids in good positioning of the sutures and the IOL haptics (MicroProbe; Endooptiks, Little Silver, NJ).

In all the other techniques which the needle is held by a needle holder and not by the fingers, at the moment of transfixation of the sclera, it is almost impossible or at least very hard to visualize with the endoscope and pass the line in the desirable local simultaneously. When the needle is handled with a needle holder, in all the moments, the other hand is needed to replace the needle on the needle holder and it is not possible to handle the endoscope. The details of this technique are complete in the link: Sclera Fixation of Posterior Chamber Lens Implant With Ocular Endoscopy= The Finger-Crafted Technique and Embedded Sclera Suture (Carvalho, D.M. & D.M. Jr., 2007).

3.4.2 Method

Together with our book about sclera fixation, there is a DVD with the videos of each surgical technique. Due to the great diversity of cases that need the sclera fixation, we thought it would be better to gather the cases in 14 situations and so 14 videos. As an example: The eyes that are being operated from the cataract and it was not possible to implant the lens at that moment, and the surgeon decides to wait so as to implant a lens in a second oportunity, in these cases the surgical strategy to make the sclera fixation is completely different for a case that comes with an intraocular lens sprained for the vitreous cavity, as it is different to progam the sclera fixation in the eyes of people that are carriers of a crystalline bad formation syndrome such as the Marfan or Marchesane etc.

We will describe the Finger Crafted Technique when applicated in the surgery of an eye with a good vision potential and a carrier patient of a sprained lens for the vitreous. Let's imagine a patient that has already been operated of cataract for a while,and scratching the eye,the lens were sprained to the macula. Even having restriction in a case like this, there are several strategic possibilities. Let's supose it is a right eye, so we will observe first, what its ocular pressure is. The lens is next to the pupil or it is gathered to the retine? Suposing the ocular pressure over 25mm/hg and the lens next to the pupil we could program:

3.4.3 Preparing the eye to an sclera fixation

With the pupil dilated by eyedrops we make an incision in the conjunctiva in both sides of the eye, next to the EIXO of 3 and 9 hs. The conjunctiva is then folded in 2 equidistant points and the surgeon then performs a 1.5 mm sclerotomy perpendicular to the limbus, starting at 0.5 mm. This sclerotomy should go down almost to the point of reaching the choroid.

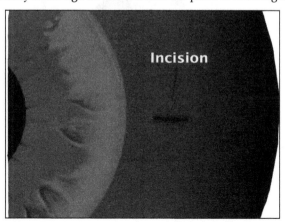

Fig. 9. Scleral Incision.

While preparing the surgery table, the assistent surgeon can hand the surgeon the 9-0 prolene suture material, already cut in half, in the 30.5 gauge guide needle (insulin needle). The surgeon will hold the body of the needle with one hand and Mcpherson forceps are used to pass the threat through the bevel until the other end comes out of the base of the needle. This thread is then pulled until it is the same size as the portion not inserted in the needle.

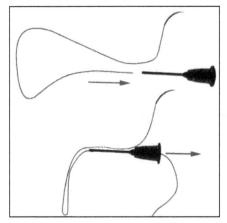

Fig. 10. Preparing the needle and bended needle prepared.

Using his fingers, the surgeon bends the tip of the needle to make it more ergonomic, pushing the eyelids away when the needle is introduced in the eye (fig. 10).
In the temporal limbus, around 7hs we perform a parecentese to the implantation to the chamber maintainer which keeps conected to a balanced salt solution, in a height of 10cm over the eye level so as to keep it with a low pressure. Superior perictomy, opening the conjunctiva in an extension of 6 mm. With the sclera exposed next to the superior limbus an incision is made on the frown (incision as inverted smile) also of 6 mm and it is made a

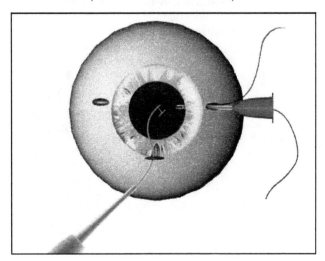

Fig. 11. Needle introduction.

sclera delamination until we get to the cornea. In this phase, the penetration in the anterior chamber must be only of 2 to 2.50 mm in the middle of the incision even though the dilamination is of 6mm; This dilamination typical of the incisions used in the cataract surgeries for extracapsulars.

The surgeon introduces the endoscope through the main incision while, with the other hand, he introduces the previously threaded needle for the sclerotomy, which will be monitored as it penetrates the ciliary sulcus. Using the saline solution, placed about 80 cm above the eye surface, connected by the anterior chamber maintainer.

Once the tip of the needle is inserted, the solution is lowered to 10 cm, the endoscope is removed and the needle is presented until it extends beyond the middle portion of the pupil. It is then retracted to loosen the loop of the thread which is found at the end, forming a loose loop. The other hand captures this loop with a hook, removing it from the eye.

The same maneuver is performed on the other side. Therefore, the main incision should be equidistant from the sclerotomy sites, to facilitate the view with the endoscope.

With the prolenes made apparently by the main incision, the incision is increased to the 6 mm completing the incision of the delamination previously elaborated.

The folded prolene (loops) are positioned on the side of the incision of the sclera delamination so as not to bother the lens to be taken away (fig. 12).

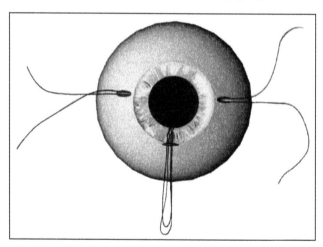

Fig. 12. Position of sutures after its introduction.

3.4.4 Correcting the decentred IOL

It is made one more parecentese of 1.50 mm in 2hs and it is introduced by it a hook with a straight holder so as to reach the haptic of the sprained lens in the vitreous. The lens is hold by the hook and it is moved softly and so as to avoid vitreous tractions in the moment of taking the lens we introduce the vitreofagus by the temporal sclerectomy, it is procedure one vitrectomy so as to totally set free the lens.

The lens is brought and kept in the anterior chamber by the hook and with the introduction of another hook by the main incision the function is passed to this new one which pulls and make it exterior the loop of the lens with the help of a spatula until it is taken from the eye (fig. 13).

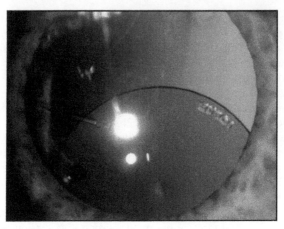

Fig. 13. Intraocular lens decentred.

3.4.5 Implanting the IOL

The chosen foldable, acrylic, monofocal or multifocal IOL in three pieces is placed on a support over the cornea, to prevent contamination.

Using those prolenes that were resting on the side of the main incision the first haptic is tied with three simple knots and so the lens is twisted and the second loop is also tied the same way (fig. 14).

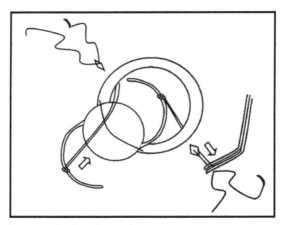

Fig. 14. Introducing lens attached to the prolene.

The anterior chamber is filled with viscoelastic, better if cohesive. In this moment it is closed the entrance of the balanced solution.

Carefully, with the MacPherson forceps the lens is introduced in the eye. In the same moment that it is being introduced, the prolenes that go out from the sclerectomy are pulled and held in the first haptic, so as to direct it to the ciliary sulcus.

The first haptic, positioned, the auxiliar will keep it in the same position holding the prolenes while the surgeon introduces and put in position the second haptic, using a forceps and the holding that keeps it. In this moment sometimes opening the infusion helps in the position of the iol.

After the IOL is positioned, the embedded Sclera Stitch is then put in place with the 2 prolenes from each sclerotomy, which came from the haptics. They are part of the same thread, and one end has been inserted into a needle while the other hasn't . The needle is then used to place a stitch outwards, on one of the borders, and then an inward stitch, on the other border. At the end, then, the embedded bared stitch is then placed in each sclerotomy. By tying the three single knots, the sclerotomy will be closed, thereby embedding the knots and fixating the IOL. After the prolenes are cut close to the sclera, the knots will tend to go deeper into the scleral incision and the tips will remain inside the sulcus (fig. 15).

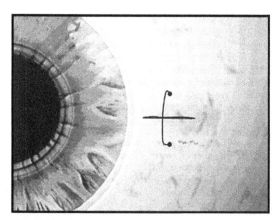

Fig. 15. Final Result of Buried Scleral Suture.

3.4.6 Endocyclophotocoagulation

As in this case the ocular pressure is high and, normally it tends to increase with the surgery, it was planned the endocyclophotocoagulation. When we notice that the lens is well stable in the eye we do not use its visualization by the endoscopy.

When the aim is only the photocoagulation:

The endoscope probe is introduced by the temporal sclerectomy and we perform the photocoagulation as it was already described before, reaching all the possible area of the ciliary body, when we use only an sclera incision. Generally we reach over 220 degrees.

After the endocyclophotocoagulation we take out the probe and introduces the vitreofagus through the same incision trying to take out the vitreous that may be held by the loops and that might get closed in the incisions. During the use of the vitreofagus it is necessary that the vial heigh is higher so as to balance the ocular pressure during the aspiration. At the end so as to avoid that the beams stay in the sclerectomy, we reduce the heigh of the vial before we take the vitreofagus and we also apirate the incision very well.

The sclerectomy is closed, the chamber mainteiner is taken, two or three stitches are made in the main incision so as to avoid the astigmatism, the conjunctiva is closed with absorbable prolenes.

The post operatory period is as simple as the cataract surgery post operatory where we generally use antibiotic eyedrops for 8 days, predinisolone eyedrops for 15 days and non hormonal antinflammatory eyedrops for for 30 days apllyed 4 times a day.

3.4.7 Discussion

The videoendoscopy has a bunch of advantages for the sclera fixation. Before this videoendoscopy the patient and the surgeon used to have some complicationsm such as glaucoma, cystic macular edema, hemorrhage, descentration, IOL inclination without resourses for na immediate clear up.

The ocular endoscopy may help us in the implantation procedures of intraocular lens in eyes without a capsular support in several ways. For example:

3.4.7.1 Diagnosis

a.   Inspect the retroirian region to identify vitreous beams, SINEQUIAS, and if the loop is positioned correctly in the recess.
b.   Inspect the posterior pole about the retinian hemorrhagesm crystalline material, sprained IOL and others.

3.4.7.2 Procedure assistence

a.   Monitoring the entrance of the needle by the sulcus;
b.   Monitoring the vitreofagus point in the retroirian space and posterior pole;
c.   Auxiliating in the repositioning of the sprained IOL;
d.   Auxiliating in the needle penetration, as a support.

3.4.7.3 Treatment

a.   Photocoagulate hemorrhage caused by the needle penetration;
b.   Photocoagulate the ciliary processes for the treatment of associated glaucoma;
c.   Photocoagulate the retine in the presence of associated retinian hemorrhages.

The penetration of the needle through the sclera monitored by the endoscope makes sure the thread fixation in the ciliary sulcus. It is a practical maneuver and it requires the pressurized eye through a maintainer and a protection with viscoelastic in the anterior chamber.As soon as the needle starts to be transfixated in the sclera,the surgeon stops looking through the microscope and follows through the screen the endoscope image. It is observed the showing of the identation through the tip of the needle, allowing its redirection to the ciliary sulcus if it shows in a wrong place.

This technique, besides making sure the correct position of the thread in the ciliary sulcus, it permits the photocoagulation of the hemorrhages that may appear due to the needle penetration, observed more frequently, in hypotensive eyes or with na inflammatory reaction sign.

Another resourse that this technique propotioned is the possibilty of impeding the uveal dislocation, pressing on the sclera the optic fiber itself, working as an opposite point and making it easier the passage of the needle.

With the use of the endoscopy in the sclera fixation it increased the precise to get right the ciliary sulcus during the needle perforation from outside to inside directed by the identation.

After implanting the lens it is possible to perform a review introducing behind the iris the endoscope probe to make sure that the lens is in the correct position. In the presence of descentration or inclination of the IOL in general we find one of the following alterations: Vitreous beam mixed with the haptic and the thread, the inadequate position in the introduction of the IOL, cortical mass lefts promoting kind of a gear over the haptic, fibrosis, rest of capsule gathered in the iris, dislocation of the knot on the holder and others.

When the haptic, of a sprained IOL is on the periferic area, positioned in the vitreous basis, it has its access more difficult and for many times being the cause of the vitreous traction and retine torns , even though specific lens for the vitrectomy surgeries are used. The endoscopy may offer a better angule of vision in the retroirian region, with the advantage of dispersating the sclera depression or the exaggerated twisting of the eye.

The third function of the URAM E2 is the application of laser using the endoscopy, very useful in the last cases of sclera fixation, that frequently are associated to the glaucoma and being worse when the conjunctive is already manipulated.

The association of the videoendoscopy with the photocoagulation brought for us practice for the cases of afacic with glaucoma. It is frequent the surgical reintervention in the eyes which have already being operated due to the cataract and they turn to have glaucoma, mainly the ones that showed a higher ocular pressure. Before the endocyclophotocoagulation we used to avoid the indication for sclera fixation in these cases because we knew that if the glaucoma showed up the consequences would be very hard.

4. References

Althaus, C.; Sundmacher, R. (1993). Intraoperative intraocular endoscopy in transscleral suture fixation of posterior chamber lenses: consequences for suture technique, implantation procedure, and choice of PCL design. *Refract Corneal Surg.* 9(5):333-9.

Busacca, A. (1955)Physiology of the ciliary muscle as studied by gonioscopy. *Ann Ocul.*188(1):1-19. Paris.

Burian, H.M.; Allen, L. (1955). Mechanical changes during accommodation observed by gonioscopy. *AMA Arch Ophthalmol.* 54(1):66-72.

Carvalho, D.M.; Paranhos, F.R.L. (1993). Implante secondário de LIO de câmara posterior: fixação escleral. Rev Bras Oftalmol. 52(1):17-22.

Carvalho, D.; Lima, F.E.; Degani, M.I. (1996). Endoscopia Ocular e Fixaçao de Lente Intra-Ocular. *Revista Brasileira de Oftalmologia 55.* (4):285-7.

Carvalho, D.M. & D.M. Jr. (2007). Fixação escleral: técnica de agulha guia (finger crafted technique) com ponto escleral sepultado. *Cirurgia de catarata: fixação e implantes secundários.* (3):19-47. Elsevier Editora Ltda.

Carvalho Jr, D.M. (2002). Ciclofotocoagulação endoscópica: estudo experimental com aplicação de laser diodo nas diferentes porções do corpo ciliar em olhos de coelhos pigmentados. *Tese de Doutorado.* Universidade de São Paulo. 70p. São Paulo, Brasil.

Chen, J.; Cohn, R.A.; Lin, S.C.; et al. (1997). Endoscopic photocoagulation of the ciliary body for treatment of refractory glaucomas. *Am J Ophthalmol.* 124(6):787-96.

Funk, R.; Rohen, J.W. (1987). SEM studies on the functional morphology of the rabbit ciliary process vasculature. *Exp Eye Res.* 45(4):579-95.

Funk, R.; Rohen, J.W. (1987). Intraocular microendoscopy of the ciliary-process vasculature in albino rabbits: effects of vasoactive agents. *Exp Eye Res.* 45(4):597-606.

Funk, R.; Rohen, J.W. (1988). Experimental studies on the functional morphology of the vascular system of the anterior eye segment in rabbits and primates. *Fortschr Ophthalmol.* 85(2):170-6.

Funk, R.; Rohen, J.W. (1988). Reactions of efferent venous segments in the ciliary process vasculature of albino rabbits. *Exp Eye Res.* 46(1):95-104.

Funk, R.; Rohen, J.W. (1988). SEM studies of the functional morphology of the ciliary process vasculature in the cynomolgus monkey: reactions after application of epinephrine. *Exp Eye Res.* 47(4):653-63.

Funk, R.; Rohen, J.W. (1989). Microendoscopy of the anterior segment vasculature in the rabbit eye. *Ophthalmic Res.* 21(1):8-17.

Leon, C.S.; Leon, J.A. (1991). Microendoscopic ocular surgery: a new intraoperative, diagnostic and therapeutic strategy. Part I: Endoscopic equipment/methodology applied to cataract surgery with intraocular lens implantation. *J Cataract Refract Surg.* 17(5):568-72.

Leon, C.S.; Leon, J.A. (1991). Microendoscopic ocular surgery: a new intraoperative, diagnostic and therapeutic strategy. Part II: Preliminary results from the study of glaucomatous eyes. *J Cataract Refract Surg.* 17(5):573-6.

Leon, J.A.; Leon, C.S.; Aron-Rosa, D.; et al. (2000). Endoscopic technique for suturing posterior chamber intraocular lenses. *J Cataract Refract Surg.* 26(5):644-9.

Lima, F.E.; Carvalho, D.M.; Beniz, J.; Avila, M. (1997). Ciclofotocoagulação endoscópica em glaucomas refratários. *Rev. bras. oftalmol 56.* (6):387-93.

Lima, F.E.; Carvalho, D.M.; Beniz, J.; Ávila, M. (1997). Ciclofotocoagulação Endoscópica em Glaucomas Refratários. *Rev Bras Oft 56.* (6):397-406.

Lima, F.E.; Costa, V. (2000). Management of complex glaucoma: Tube shunt versus cyclodestructive procedure. *Glaucoma Perspectives in Practice – Issue 2.3.*

Lima, F.E.; Magacho, L; Carvalho, D.M.; Susanna, R.; Ávila, M.P. (2004). A Prospective, Comparative Study between Endoscopic Cyclophotocoagulation and the Ahmed Drainage Implant in Refractory Glaucoma. *Journal of Glaucoma 13(3):* 233-237.

Lima, F.E.; Carvalho, D.M.; Ávila, M.P. (2010). Phacoemulsification and endoscopic cyclophotocoagulation as primary surgical procedure in coexisting cataract and glaucoma. *Arquivos Brasileiros de Oftalmologia.* 73(5).

Malbran, E. S. & E. Jr.; Negri, I. (1986). Lens guide suture for transport and fixation in secondary IOL implantation after intracapsular extraction. Int Ophthalmol. *9* (2-3): 151-160.

Mizuno, K.; Asaoka, M. (1976). Cycloscopy and fluorescein cycloscopy. *Invest Ophthalmol.*15(7):561-4.

Mizuno, K.; Asaoka, M.; Muroi, S. (1977). Cycloscopy and fluorescein cycloscopy of the ciliary process. *Am J Ophthalmol.* 84(4):487-95.

Pavlin, C.J.; Rootman, D.; Arshinoff, S.; et al. (1993). Determination of haptic position of transsclerally fixated posterior chamber intraocular lenses by ultrasound biomicroscopy. *J Cataract Refract Surg.* 19(5):573-7.

Pietrabissa, A.; Scarcello, E.; Carobbi, A.; Mosca, F. (1994). Three-dimensional versus two-dimensional video system for the trained endoscopic surgeon and the beginner. *Endosc Surg Allied Technol.* 2(6):315-7.

Scheie, H.G. (1953). Gonioscopy in the diagnosis of tumors of the iris and ciliary body, with emphasis on intraepithelial cysts. *Trans Am Ophthalmol Soc.* 51:313-31.

Uram, M. (1992a). Ophthalmic laser microendoscope ciliary process ablation in the management of neovascular glaucoma. *Ophthalmology 99.* (12):1823-8.

Uram, M. (1992b). Ophthalmic laser microendoscope endophotocoagulation. *Ophthalmology 99.* (12):1829-32.

Zarbin, M.A. et al. (1988). Endolaser treatment of the ciliary body for severe glaucoma. *Ophthalmology 95.* 1639.

Permissions

The contributors of this book come from diverse backgrounds, making this book a truly international effort. This book will bring forth new frontiers with its revolutionizing research information and detailed analysis of the nascent developments around the world.

We would like to thank Cornel Iancu, MD, PhD, for lending his expertise to make the book truly unique. He has played a crucial role in the development of this book. Without his invaluable contribution this book wouldn't have been possible. He has made vital efforts to compile up to date information on the varied aspects of this subject to make this book a valuable addition to the collection of many professionals and students.

This book was conceptualized with the vision of imparting up-to-date information and advanced data in this field. To ensure the same, a matchless editorial board was set up. Every individual on the board went through rigorous rounds of assessment to prove their worth. After which they invested a large part of their time researching and compiling the most relevant data for our readers. Conferences and sessions were held from time to time between the editorial board and the contributing authors to present the data in the most comprehensible form. The editorial team has worked tirelessly to provide valuable and valid information to help people across the globe.

Every chapter published in this book has been scrutinized by our experts. Their significance has been extensively debated. The topics covered herein carry significant findings which will fuel the growth of the discipline. They may even be implemented as practical applications or may be referred to as a beginning point for another development. Chapters in this book were first published by InTech; hereby published with permission under the Creative Commons Attribution License or equivalent.

The editorial board has been involved in producing this book since its inception. They have spent rigorous hours researching and exploring the diverse topics which have resulted in the successful publishing of this book. They have passed on their knowledge of decades through this book. To expedite this challenging task, the publisher supported the team at every step. A small team of assistant editors was also appointed to further simplify the editing procedure and attain best results for the readers.

Our editorial team has been hand-picked from every corner of the world. Their multi-ethnicity adds dynamic inputs to the discussions which result in innovative outcomes. These outcomes are then further discussed with the researchers and contributors who give their valuable feedback and opinion regarding the same. The feedback is then collaborated with the researches and they are edited in a comprehensive manner to aid the understanding of the subject.

Apart from the editorial board, the designing team has also invested a significant amount of their time in understanding the subject and creating the most relevant covers. They scrutinized every image to scout for the most suitable representation of the subject and create an appropriate cover for the book.

The publishing team has been involved in this book since its early stages. They were actively engaged in every process, be it collecting the data, connecting with the contributors or procuring relevant information. The team has been an ardent support to the editorial, designing and production team. Their endless efforts to recruit the best for this project, has resulted in the accomplishment of this book. They are a veteran in the field of academics and their pool of knowledge is as vast as their experience in printing. Their expertise and guidance has proved useful at every step. Their uncompromising quality standards have made this book an exceptional effort. Their encouragement from time to time has been an inspiration for everyone.

The publisher and the editorial board hope that this book will prove to be a valuable piece of knowledge for researchers, students, practitioners and scholars across the globe.

List of Contributors

Jouanneau Emmanuel, Messerer Mahmoud and Berhouma Moncef
Department of Neurosurgery, Skull Base Surgery Unit Pierre Wertheimer, Neurological and Neurosurgical Hospital, Lyon, France

David W.J. Côté and Erin D. Wright
University of Alberta, Canada

W. F. Ezzat
ORL- Head and Neck Surgery, Consultant Pediatric Otolaryngologist, Ain-Shams University, Cairo, Egypt

Miroslav Andrić
University of Belgrade, Faculty of Dentistry, Serbia

Meghan Wilson, Kyle McMullen and Rohan R. Walvekar
Department of Otolaryngology Head & Neck Surgery, Louisiana State, University Health Science Center, New Orleans, Louisiana, USA

Sumeet Anand, Rickul Varshney and Saul Frenkiel
McGill University, Department of Otolaryngology – Head & Neck Surgery, Canada

B.J. Folz and C.G. Konnerth
Department of Otorhinolaryngology, Karl Hansen Medical Center, Bad Lippspringe, Germany

Fabio Pagella, Alessandro Pusateri, Georgios Giourgos and Elina Matti
Foundation IRCCS Policlinico San Matteo and University of Pavia, Italy

P. Grunert and J. Oertel
Johannes Gutenberg University, Germany

Marwan Najjar and Ali Turkmani
American University of Beirut, Lebanon

Betka Jan, Lukes Petr, Skrivan Jiri and Kluh Jan
Charles University in Prague, 1st Faculty of Medicine, Department of Otorhinolaryngology and Head and Neck Surgery, Faculty Hospital Motol, Prague, Czech Republic

Chovanec Martin and Fik Zdenek
Charles University in Prague, 1st Faculty of Medicine, Department of Otorhinolaryngology and Head and Neck Surgery, Faculty Hospital Motol, Prague, Czech Republic
Charles University in Prague, 1st Faculty of Medicine, Institute of Anatomy, Prague, Czech Republic

Zverina Eduard
Charles University in Prague, 1st Faculty of Medicine, Department of Otorhinolaryngology and Head and Neck Surgery, Faculty Hospital Motol, Prague, Czech Republic
Charles University in Prague, 3rd Faculty of Medicine, Department of Neurosurgery, Faculty Hospital Kralovske Vinohrady, Prague, Czech Republic

Profant Oliver
Charles University in Prague, 1st Faculty of Medicine, Department of Otorhinolaryngology and Head and Neck Surgery, Faculty Hospital Motol, Prague, Czech Republic
Department of Auditory Neurosciene, Institute of Experimental Medicine AS CR, Prague, Czech Republic

Durval Moraes de Carvalho
Centro Brasileiro de Cirurgia de Olhos, Brazil

Francisco Eduardo Lima
Centro Brasileiro de Cirurgia de Olhos, Brazil
Universidade Federal de Goiás – UFG, Brazil

Durval Moraes de Carvalho Jr.
Centro Brasileiro da Visão, Brazil

Printed in the USA
CPSIA information can be obtained
at www.ICGtesting.com
JSHW011812301024
72690JS00002B/59

9 781632 411013